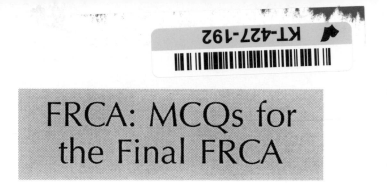

FRCA: MCQs for the Final FRCA

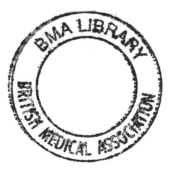

For W.B. Saunders Company Ltd

Publisher Michael Parkinson
Project Editor Jane Shanks
Project Controller Frances Affleck
Design Direction Erik Bigland

FRCA: MCQs for the Final FRCA

Karen Henderson
BSc BM MRCPI FRCA

Consultant Anaesthetist
Royal Sussex County Hospital
Brighton, UK

W.B. Saunders Company Ltd

Edinburgh • London • New York • Oxford • Philadelphia
St Louis • Sydney • Toronto

WB Saunders Company Ltd
An imprint of Elsevier Limited

First published 1998
  Reprinted 2004, 2005

ISBN 0 7020 2347 7

A catalogue record for this book is available from the British Library

ELSEVIER   your source for books,
journals and multimedia
in the health sciences

www.elsevierhealth.com

Working together to grow
libraries in developing countries
www.elsevier.com | www.bookaid.org | www.sabre.org

ELSEVIER   BOOK AID International   Sabre Foundation

Typeset by LaserScript Ltd, Mitcham, Surrey
Transferred to digital printing 2006
B/03

The
publisher's
policy is to use
paper manufactured
from sustainable forests

Contents

With love to Brynjulf in Norway and to Carla in the Sudan.

Foreword

Multiple choice questions are a fundamental part of the Final examination of the Fellowship of the Royal College of Anaesthetists. The questions test knowledge over a wide sphere of areas including physiology, pharmacology, intensive care medicine, medicine, surgery, clinical measurement in addition to questions related to clinical anaesthesia and pain management. Not everyone finds multiple choice papers easy. Mock papers, such as found in this book, enable one to assess the adequacy of knowledge as well as the suitability of technique of answering such questions. Everyone has gaps in their knowledge – Dr Henderson has helpfully given short tutorials on each subject as well as answering the specific questions. Therefore, the reader will be able to answer further questions on the same topic.

The prepared candidate will check on the regulations regarding examinations because they change from time to time. A booklet can be obtained from the Royal College of Anaesthetists, 48/49 Russell Square, London, WC1B 4JY.

Whilst there is no substitute for background hard work, there is no doubt that this book will considerably help in preparation for the FRCA examination.

Good luck!

Acknowledgements

I would like to thank my parents and the many friends and colleagues who gave me encouragement and help with this book. I am particularly grateful to Dr Caroline Thompsett and Dr Sue Milroy for the proofreading. I am also indebted to the postgraduate library of the Royal Sussex County Hospital and Universitetsbiblioteket of Regionsykehuset, Trondheim, Norway.

Introduction

When I was preparing some of the questions for this book, a reviewer suggested that it would be useful to include something at the beginning on how to answer them. I think this may be rather unnecessary as by the time you get to this stage – hopefully the last exam you will ever sit – you will have come across so many MCQs that you will have developed your own particular, and often obscure, method of answering them.

Nevertheless, here are some points worth thinking about:

Negative marking is to be ignored at your peril.

Always read the question and the stems at least twice. However unreasonable, the examiner will occasionally try and confuse you with the wording.

Always read the questions slowly, even if it means following your finger as it traces the question (no one will be looking, honest).

Do *not* spend too much time on one question. Aim to go through the questions once and answer the ones you know (i.e. the easy ones). Repeat the exercise, each time answering ones you know progressively less about, until towards the end of the time available the only questions remaining are the ones you cannot answer.

Do *not* be overwhelmed by a question. To avoid this happening try and organize your approach by attempting to place how much you know about the question and the correct answer to the individual stems into one of three categories:

1. absolute certainty
2. potential certainty
3. haven't got a clue, never heard of it, etc.

The first category is easy to answer. The third category must never be answered unless you can work out the correct answer from first principles. There are no points to be scored if you answer a question you know nothing about. Do not even think about it! The fun is to be had with the questions you have put into the second category. Current thinking is that statistically, if you have some idea about a subject, it is acceptable to guess as you are more likely to get it right than wrong.

Try to avoid answering questions according to a prearranged scheme, i.e. playing the percentages game. Approach each question and answer according to your knowledge.

Finally, love them or hate them, MCQs are part of examination life and I hope these five practice papers will go some way to making your life easier when it comes to the real thing. If by any chance you think any of the answers are incorrect please do not hesitate to let me know. In some of the questions I have included references. This serves two purposes: to let you know where I got my information from and to give you the opportunity to do some further reading on the subject. They are not compulsory reading.

Good luck!

Exam 1

Questions

1.1 **The following are well-recognized causes of amyloidosis:**
  A. tuberculosis (TB).
  B. bronchiectasis.
  C. rheumatic fever.
  D. rheumatoid arthritis.
  E. leprosy.

1.2 **As regards breast cancer:**
  A. hypercalcaemia is a well-recognized complication.
  B. local excision followed by radiotherapy has similar results to mastectomy.
  C. adjuvant therapy with tamoxifen improves symptoms but not length of survival in premenopausal women.
  D. bone metastases are localized earlier with radionuclide scanning compared to plain skeletal X-rays.
  E. endocrine manipulation is useful only in premenopausal women.

1.3 **A 43-year-old dockyard worker sustains an open chest wound. Appropriate management at the site of the accident includes:**
  A. intubation and ventilation.
  B. insertion of a chest drain.
  C. packing the wound and taping it with water-resistant tape.
  D. immediate referral to hospital without disturbing the wound.
  E. telling the patient to cover the wound with his own hand.

1.4 **In an otherwise fit patient, development of postoperative atelectasis can cause:**
  A. an increase in alveolar–arterial oxygen gradient.
  B. hypercarbia.
  C. tachypnoea.
  D. fever.
  E. pleuritic pain.

1.5 **Midazolam:**
  A. inhibits the action of gamma-aminobutyric acid (GABA).
  B. is water-soluble at physiological pH.
  C. acts synergistically with flumazenil.
  D. has an elimination half-life of 2 hours.
  E. is largely excreted unchanged in the urine.

1.6   In the jugular venous pressure (JVP) wave form:
  A. canon waves occur with atrial contraction on a closed tricuspid valve.
  B. the *v* wave is in time with ventricular systole.
  C. the *x* descent follows the *v* waves.
  D. the *a* wave increases in size in atrial fibrillation.
  E. constrictive pericarditis will produce a steep *y* descent.

1.7   Physiological changes in the morbidly obese patient include:
  A. decrease in renal clearance.
  B. decrease in functional residual capacity (FRC).
  C. increase in red cell volume.
  D. increase in volume of distribution.
  E. decrease in systemic vascular resistance (SVR).

1.8   Osteoporosis is a complication of:
  A. Paget's disease.
  B. primary hyperparathyroidism.
  C. chronic renal failure.
  D. osteomalacia.
  E. gastrectomy.

1.9   Immediate treatment of acid aspiration includes:
  A. pulmonary lavage.
  B. intravenous hydrocortisone.
  C. intravenous H_2 blockers such as ranitidine.
  D. immediate intubation and ventilation.
  E. intravenous antibiotics.

1.10   In the surgical management of fractured neck of femur:
  A. regional anaesthesia reduces the incidence of deep vein thrombosis (DVT).
  B. postoperative hypoxaemia may be secondary to air embolism.
  C. general anaesthesia compared to regional anaesthesia decreases perioperative blood loss.
  D. methylmethacrylate cement is a positive inotrope.
  E. there is no difference in 1-year survival between regional or general anaesthesia.

1.11 Caudal analgesia:
- A. is as predictable as a lumbar epidural.
- B. is very unlikely to result in a dural tap.
- C. is recommended for forceps delivery in labour.
- D. may delay micturition.
- E. is ideal for perineal surgery.

1.12 Primary hyperparathyroidism is associated with:
- A. renal calculi.
- B. ectopic calcification.
- C. increased serum phosphate.
- D. an increase in serum alkaline phosphatase.
- E. peptic ulceration.

1.13 The cervical sympathetic chain:
- A. lies superficial to the prevertebral fascia.
- B. terminates near the internal carotid artery.
- C. receives grey rami from the spinal cord.
- D. may be affected by a brachial plexus block.
- E. includes the stellate ganglion close to the 5th cervical vertebra.

1.14 Incidence of nosocomial (hospital-acquired) infection in the intensive care unit (ICU) can be reduced by:
- A. the presence of a hospital infection control team.
- B. regular handwashing.
- C. selective decontamination of the patient's digestive tract.
- D. omeprazole.
- E. use of H_2 antagonists.

1.15 Regarding non-depolarizing neuromuscular blocking agents:
- A. vecuronium has a similar duration of action as rocuronium.
- B. rocuronium has a shorter onset of action than vecuronium.
- C. *cis*-atracurium is associated with histamine release.
- D. doxacurium is longer acting than pancuronium.
- E. vecuronium has no active metabolites.

1.16 The following techniques can be used to reliably assess depth of anaesthesia:
A. bispectral analysis.
B. heart rate.
C. isolated forearm technique.
D. pupillary dilatation.
E. lower oesophageal contractility.

1.17 Placental circulation:
A. is approximately 10% of maternal cardiac output at term.
B. is directly proportional to fetal stroke volume and heart rate.
C. consists normally of two veins and one artery.
D. is independent of perfusion pressure.
E. is significantly impaired by alpha adrenergic stimulation.

1.18 With materno-fetal transfer of drugs given via the epidural route:
A. the placenta is an effective barrier.
B. drugs bound to maternal proteins easily cross to the fetus.
C. persistent fetal bradycardia may occur with LA agents.
D. lignocaine can reduce fetal muscle tone.
E. alfentanil is safe to use in low dose.

1.19 Increased susceptibility to malignant hyperthermia (MH) occurs with:
A. ketamine.
B. propofol.
C. desflurane.
D. lignocaine.
E. prolonged masseter muscle spasm.

1.20 In a young female thyrotoxic patient you would expect to find:
A. atrial fibrillation.
B. pretibial myxoedema.
C. menorrhagia.
D. a large goitre.
E. proximal myopathy.

1.21 The systemic inflammatory response syndrome (SIRS):
- A. can be provoked by acute pancreatitis.
- B. can be initiated by Gram-positive septicaemia.
- C. requires a pyrexia greater than 38°C for diagnosis.
- D. frequently progresses to multiple organ failure.
- E. can be effectively treated with antiendotoxin antibodies.

1.22 The following are safe to use in a patient with poorly controlled epilepsy requiring anaesthesia:
- A. ketamine.
- B. enflurane.
- C. methohexitone.
- D. isoflurane.
- E. spinal anaesthesia.

1.23 Radiographs of the skeleton can help in the diagnosis of:
- A. sickle cell anaemia.
- B. glucose 6 phosphate dehydrogenase (G6PD) deficiency.
- C. extramedullary haematopoiesis.
- D. vitamin C deficiency.
- E. Gaucher's disease.

1.24 Compared to fentanyl, alfentanil:
- A. is more highly protein-bound.
- B. has a smaller volume of distribution.
- C. is more potent.
- D. is more fat-soluble.
- E. has a longer elimination half-life.

1.25 Anatomically:
- A. sensory supply to the umbilicus is supplied by T8.
- B. the median nerve is medial to the palmaris longus.
- C. sensory nerve supply to the thumb is supplied by T1.
- D. the trochlear nerve supplies the inferior rectus.
- E. the subclavian vein is posterior to the subclavian artery.

1.26 Features of small bowel obstruction may include:
- A. bile-stained vomit.
- B. severe abdominal pain worse on movement.
- C. abdominal distension.
- D. constipation.
- E. dullness on percussion in the flanks.

1.27 The following are recognized associations:
   A. thrombocytosis and chronic myeloid leukaemia (CML).
   B. beta thalassaemia major and raised total body iron.
   C. aplastic anaemia and Down's syndrome.
   D. multiple myeloma and gout.
   E. polycythaemia and renal carcinoma.

1.28 Vaporizers for use in the circle breathing system:
   A. are highly efficient.
   B. have a large vaporizing chamber.
   C. have a low resistance.
   D. must be temperature-compensated.
   E. can be placed in the inspiratory or expiratory limb.

1.29 A 36-year-old woman develops a purpuric rash during an undiagnosed septic illness. Possible diagnoses include:
   A. disseminated intravascular coagulation (DIC).
   B. bacterial endocarditis.
   C. acute myeloid leukaemia (AML).
   D. drug toxicity.
   E. systemic lupus erythematosis (SLE).

1.30 Effective pain relief for labour includes:
   A. transcutaneous electrical nerve stimulation (TENS).
   B. intramuscular pethidine.
   C. acupuncture.
   D. patient-controlled analgesia using intravenous morphine.
   E. psychoprophylaxis.

1.31 Regarding nutrition:
   A. a normal adult requires 30–40 g of protein daily.
   B. only L-amino acids are required for protein replacement.
   C. starvation causes loss of lean muscle mass.
   D. a BMI of 22 suggests undernutrition.
   E. kwashiorkor is due to lack of all energy sources.

1.32 Pneumonectomy for a bronchogenic carcinoma is contra-indicated when:
   A. malignant cells are found on sputum cytology.
   B. there is a pleural effusion.
   C. there is a vocal cord palsy.
   D. FEV_1 will be less than 2 l postoperatively.
   E. the patient is aged 70 years or over.

1.33 The following have been successfully used in the treatment of asthma:
  A. ipratropium bromide.
  B. ketamine.
  C. beclomethasone.
  D. halothane.
  E. metoprolol.

1.34 Cigarette-smoking:
  A. triggers release of adrenaline from the adrenal medulla.
  B. delays gastric emptying.
  C. increases variability of fetal heart rate.
  D. requires abstinence for 24 hours prior to surgery to eliminate carbon monoxide.
  E. induces pharmacological dependence.

1.35 Regarding pain measurement:
  A. a visual analogue scale (VAS) measures intensity of pain.
  B. 30% of patients are unable to use a VAS accurately.
  C. self-reporting is superior to observer reporting.
  D. the Magill pain questionnaire (MPQ) is unsuitable for children under 12 years of age.
  E. the Dartmouth pain questionnaire (DPQ) assesses acute pain.

1.36 In DIC:
  A. prothrombin time is normal.
  B. fibrinolysis occurs.
  C. vitamin K is required if severe.
  D. cryoprecipitate is a source of fibrinogen.
  E. heparin may be of value.

1.37 The normal ECG:
  A. has a standard paper speed of 50 mm/s.
  B. has a mean frontal axis between $0°$ and $+110°$.
  C. has a maximal QT interval of 0.42 s.
  D. has a QRS duration of 0.08–0.1 s.
  E. may have an inverted T wave in lead I.

1.38 Parkinson's disease is associated with:
- **A.** bladder dysfunction.
- **B.** intention tremor.
- **C.** peripheral neuropathy.
- **D.** Lewy bodies.
- **E.** depression.

1.39 Tracheo-oesophageal fistula (TOF):
- **A.** is found predominantly in males.
- **B.** can be diagnosed antenatally.
- **C.** is associated with oesophageal atresia in 85% of cases.
- **D.** may present with projectile vomiting.
- **E.** is associated with other major abnormalities.

1.40 Positive end-expiratory pressure (PEEP):
- **A.** reduces mixed venous oxygen content.
- **B.** increases functional residual capacity (FRC).
- **C.** may reduce urine output.
- **D.** increases airway resistance.
- **E.** may reduce cardiac output.

1.41 Carbon dioxide elimination:
- **A.** is exponential.
- **B.** is transported mainly by haem groups.
- **C.** is facilitated by carbonic anhydrase.
- **D.** is normally about 100 ml/min at rest.
- **E.** involves the Bohr effect.

1.42 Unstable blood pressure during a carotid endarterectomy may be due to:
- **A.** chemoreceptor damage.
- **B.** baroreceptor damage.
- **C.** blood loss.
- **D.** vagal stimulation.
- **E.** preoperative hypertension.

1.43 Automated blood pressure monitors:
- **A.** under-read at high pressure.
- **B.** over-read at low pressure.
- **C.** need a cuff width 20% greater than diameter of the arm.
- **D.** extrapolate diastolic pressure.
- **E.** tend to be inaccurate with atrial fibrillation (AF).

1.44 Isoprenaline:
  A. is arrhythmogenic.
  B. causes peripheral vasodilatation.
  C. has an inotropic action.
  D. has a chronotropic action.
  E. can precipitate asthma.

1.45 Recognized complications of chronic renal failure (CRF) include:
  A. peripheral neuropathy.
  B. macrocytic anaemia.
  C. postural hypotension.
  D. diabetes mellitus.
  E. splenomegaly.

1.46 A low arterial oxygen saturation:
  A. is characteristic of pulmonary oedema.
  B. can be due to an alveolar diffusion problem.
  C. is a feature of polycythaemia rubra vera.
  D. tends to cause dilatation of most arteries and arterioles.
  E. stimulates ventilation by an effect on peripheral chemo-receptors.

1.47 The Glasgow Coma Scale (GCS):
  A. ranges from 0 to 15.
  B. reliably assesses brainstem function.
  C. includes scoring up to 6 points for best motor response.
  D. is suitable for use in children under 5 years of age.
  E. suggests elective hyperventilation for a score of 8 is appropriate.

1.48 The following can occur after a stellate ganglion block (SGB):
  A. ipsilateral dilated pupil.
  B. difficulty in swallowing.
  C. supraglottic loss of sensation.
  D. pneumothorax.
  E. hoarse voice.

1.49 Inhaled nitric oxide:
  A. is a bronchodilator.
  B. can be limited by tachyphylaxis.
  C. is responsible for systemic vasodilatation.
  D. is synthesized from aspartate.
  E. can cause methaemaglobinaemia.

1.50 Seminoma:
  A. metastasizes mainly by haematogenous spread.
  B. responds well to radiotherapy.
  C. commonly presents with testicular pain.
  D. has a worse prognosis than teratoma.
  E. can be monitored using human chorionic gonadotrophin (HCG) as a tumour marker.

1.51 Phosphodiesterase inhibitors:
  A. act by blocking the sodium/potassium pump.
  B. increase intracellular cAMP.
  C. cause peripheral vasoconstriction.
  D. represent a homogeneous drug group.
  E. have a positive inotropic action.

1.52 Sickle cell anaemia (Hb SS):
  A. is inherited as a Mendelian dominant.
  B. shifts the oxyhaemoglobin dissociation curve to the left.
  C. is associated with severe haematuria.
  D. can be associated with mild anaemia.
  E. is caused by glutamine replacing lysine in the 6th position of the beta globin chain.

1.53 Syntocinon given quickly often results in:
  A. hypotension.
  B. tachycardia.
  C. a diuresis.
  D. nausea and vomiting.
  E. respiratory arrest.

1.54 The parasympathetic nervous system (PNS):
  A. has long postganglionic fibres.
  B. has myelinated preganglionic fibres.
  C. when stimulated will constrict the sphincter of Oddi.
  D. initiates bladder contraction.
  E. includes fibres carried by fifth (V) cranial nerve.

1.55 Trigeminal ganglion block can cause unilateral anaesthesia of:
  A. interior of ala nasi.
  B. hard palate.
  C. angle of the jaw.
  D. lower lip.
  E. tympanic membrane.

1.56 In near-drowning:
- A. seawater inhalation can cause hypovolaemia.
- B. haemolysis is a recognized complication of freshwater aspiration.
- C. seawater inhalation frequently leads to an increase in serum sodium.
- D. acute renal failure is a common occurrence.
- E. steroids confer neurological protection.

1.57 Prophylactic antibiotics are needed for the following procedures in a patient with a prosthetic heart valve:
- A. insertion of intrauterine contraceptive device.
- B. cystoscopy.
- C. cataract extraction under LA.
- D. dental scaling.
- E. sigmoidoscopy.

1.58 The Système International d'unites (SI) includes:
- A. force: pascal.
- B. mass: gram.
- C. energy: watt.
- D. time: second.
- E. length: metre.

1.59 Gastric acid aspiration at pH 2 may initially cause:
- A. cardiogenic pulmonary oedema.
- B. chemical pneumonitis.
- C. wheezing.
- D. bacterial pneumonitis.
- E. decreased lung compliance.

1.60 Renal cell carcinoma:
- A. initially metastasizes via the lymphatic system.
- B. can be reliably detected by finding malignant cells in the urine.
- C. can present as a pyrexia of unknown origin.
- D. is occasionally found bilaterally.
- E. can present as a chance finding on a chest radiograph.

1.61 A normal plain postero-anterior (PA) chest radiograph of a male adult in full inspiration will show:
  A. anterior ends of the sixth ribs.
  B. cardiac diameter less than 16 cm.
  C. hilar lymph nodes.
  D. right oblique fissure.
  E. right hemidiaphragm higher than the left.

1.62 Type I hypersensitivity:
  A. is invariably mediated by immunoglobulin E (IgE).
  B. can be initiated by direct action of allergen on mast cell membranes.
  C. involves mast cell degranulation.
  D. can result in bronchoconstriction.
  E. is partially mediated by eosinophils.

1.63 Delayed recovery from neuromuscular blockade after vecuronium may be due to:
  A. hyperglycaemia.
  B. hypocalcaemia.
  C. hypokalaemia.
  D. hypoglycaemia.
  E. hypermagnesaemia.

1.64 In paracetamol poisoning:
  A. a raised aspartate transaminase is an early sign.
  B. prolonged prothrombin time is the best guide to liver damage.
  C. renal failure may supervene without liver damage.
  D. loss of consciousness is often delayed.
  E. nausea and vomiting are the only early signs.

1.65 Regarding the heart:
  A. coronary blood flow is regulated by sympathetic innervation.
  B. infarction of the AV node may cause complete heart block.
  C. adenosine constricts coronary arterioles.
  D. the ventricular myocardium responds to an increased workload by hyperplasia.
  E. stroke volume falls with vagal stimulation.

1.66 Sudden onset of complete heart block is associated with:
- **A.** an increase in stroke volume.
- **B.** variable intensity of the first heart sound.
- **C.** variable loudness of the first heart sound.
- **D.** canon waves visible in the neck.
- **E.** syncope.

1.67 The following drug combinations may be disadvantageous:
- **A.** amiodarone and warfarin.
- **B.** trimethoprim and sulphamethoxazole.
- **C.** vecuronium and gentamicin.
- **D.** propranolol and glibenclamide.
- **E.** tranylcypromine and fentanyl.

1.68 A 24-year-old woman in mid-trimester of pregnancy presents with glycosuria but is otherwise well. The following investigations support a diagnosis of gestational diabetes mellitus (GDN):
- **A.** random blood glucose of 9.0 mmol/l.
- **B.** fasting blood glucose of 8.0 mmol/l.
- **C.** a 2-hour post-prandial blood glucose level of 10 mmol/l.
- **D.** 20 g proteinuria in 24 hours.
- **E.** a $P_a\text{CO}_2$ of 3.5 kPa (23 mmHg).

1.69 An intra-aortic balloon pump (IABP) may cause:
- **A.** an increase in heart rate.
- **B.** an increase in left ventricular end-diastolic pressure.
- **C.** an increase in myocardial oxygen demand.
- **D.** an increase in diastolic blood pressure.
- **E.** an improvement in coronary artery perfusion.

1.70 In LA for bronchoscopy:
- **A.** the superior laryngeal nerve (SLN) can be blocked in the piriform fossa.
- **B.** the recurrent laryngeal nerve can be blocked through the thyrohyoid membrane.
- **C.** the external laryngeal nerve must be blocked to achieve vocal cord paralysis.
- **D.** the recurrent laryngeal nerve can be blocked at any level above the vocal cords.
- **E.** the recurrent laryngeal nerve supplies mucosa below the vocal cords.

1.71 Atrial flutter:
  A. is commonly due to ischaemic heart disease.
  B. gives a regular radial pulse.
  C. is identified on the electrocardiogram by 'f' waves.
  D. can be converted to atrial fibrillation by digoxin.
  E. cannot be effectively treated by direct current (DC) cardioversion

1.72 The supraclavicular approach to blocking the brachial plexus differs from the axillary approach by:
  A. having a decreased incidence of pneumothorax.
  B. being a more reliable anaesthetic of the lateral side of the forearm.
  C. requiring a smaller volume of LA.
  D. providing adequate analgesia for surgery to the shoulder.
  E. having a higher failure rate.

1.73 Endotoxins:
  A. are glycoproteins.
  B. are composed of two main components.
  C. are an important trigger of SIRS.
  D. are heat labile.
  E. have O antigen specificity.

1.74 Intrathecal phenol:
  A. is hyperbaric with the addition of glucose.
  B. requires patients to lie still for 30 min after injection.
  C. gives effective pain relief for chronic pancreatitis.
  D. on injection, requires the patient to lie with the bad side down.
  E. is usually used as a 2% solution.

1.75 Techniques for measuring cardiac output include:
  A. measurement of oxygen consumption.
  B. radioactive technetium.
  C. echocardiography.
  D. indocyanine green.
  E. methylene blue.

1.76 As regards cardiopulmonary resuscitation in a 2-year-old child:
- A. the commonest underlying cause is likely to be respiratory failure.
- B. initial dose of adrenaline is 0.1 mg/kg intravenously.
- C. the ratio of ventilation to sternal compressions is 10:1.
- D. the commonest cause of bradycardia is hypoxia.
- E. DC shock, if required, should commence at 10 J/kg.

1.77 The following are normal values:
- A. right atrial pressure   – 8 cm H_2O.
- B. systemic vascular resistance (SVR)   – 1200 dyne s/cm^5.
- C. pulmonary vascular resistance   – 80 dyne s/cm^5.
- D. cardiac index   – 2.0 l/min/m^2.
- E. mean pulmonary artery pressure (PAP) – 10 mmHg.

1.78 Following acute onset of cardiac tamponade:
- A. the pulse may slow.
- B. left and right atrial pressures will be raised.
- C. cyanosis and cool peripheries can occur.
- D. systolic and diastolic blood pressures will be low.
- E. the pulse may disappear on inspiration.

1.79 Koilonychia is:
- A. a common manifestation of pernicious anaemia.
- B. associated with dysphagia.
- C. a consequence of iron deficiency anaemia.
- D. a manifestation of psoriasis.
- E. found in calcium deficiency.

1.80 Ketamine:
- A. is contraindicated in porphyria.
- B. preserves laryngeal reflexes.
- C. is associated with emergence phenomena.
- D. is an antisialogogue.
- E. is water-soluble.

1.81 A pressure-cycled ventilator:
- A. has a linear flow rate.
- B. provides a constant tidal volume.
- C. depends on lung compliance to determine end-inspiratory pressure.
- D. is not suitable for use in children.
- E. is a minute volume divider.

1.82 Recognized causes of stridor in infancy include:
   A. bronchiolitis.
   B. laryngomalacia.
   C. laryngotracheobronchitis.
   D. epiglottitis.
   E. foreign body aspiration.

1.83 Management of a post-partum haemorrhage may include:
   A. uterine packing.
   B. ergometrine.
   C. bimanual uterine compression.
   D. intravenous fluids.
   E. abdominal hysterectomy.

1.84 The following statements are correct:
   A. Avogadro's hypothesis states that at constant temperature and pressure equal volumes of all ideal gases contain the same number of molecules.
   B. Boyle's law states that at constant temperature the volume of a given mass of gas varies inversely with the absolute pressure.
   C. impedance is the resistance to flow of an alternating current in an electrical circuit, and varies with the frequency of the current.
   D. the Beer–Lambert laws describe the basis of oximetry.
   E. critical temperature is the temperature above which a substance cannot be liquefied however much pressure is applied.

1.85 As regards chronic bronchitis:
   A. inspiratory effort is greater than expiratory effort.
   B. *Haemophilus influenzae* is a common pathogen.
   C. it may be associated with a low P_aO_2 and a normal P_aCO_2.
   D. prophylactic antibiotics should be given in the winter months.
   E. steroids may be of value in its management.

1.86 **A 45-year-old woman has the following blood results:**

Sodium	127 mmol/l	Bicarbonate	18 mmol/l
Potassium	6.0 mmol/l	Glucose	3.0 mmol/l

Possible diagnosis includes:
A. acute renal failure.
B. Conn's syndrome.
C. inappropriate ADH secretion.
D. compensated liver failure.
E. fluid overload.

1.87 **The following occur more commonly in ulcerative colitis (UC) than Crohn's disease:**
A. sclerosing cholangitis.
B. rectal sparing.
C. carcinoma of the colon.
D. megaloblastic anaemia.
E. pyoderma gangrenosum.

1.88 **The following can occur after massive transfusion of blood:**
A. metabolic alkalosis.
B. decrease in ionized calcium.
C. decrease in serum potassium.
D. increase in serum magnesium.
E. prolonged TT.

1.89 **Transfusion of mismatched blood is associated with:**
A. wheezing.
B. polyuria.
C. a positive Coombs' test.
D. fever.
E. haemoglobinuria.

1.90 **Regarding the measurement of gas flow:**
A. rotameters are constant flow, fixed orifice devices.
B. rotameters are increasingly inaccurate as flow rate decreases.
C. gas density is important at low flow rates.
D. pneumotachographs are accurate only when gas flow is laminar.
E. pneumotachographs are accurate only when measuring dry gases.

Answers

1.1 **A**.T **B**.T **C**.F **D**.T **E**.T
Amyloidosis is a heterogeneous group of disorders characterized by the deposition of an insoluble fibrillar protein: amyloid.
It may be acquired or hereditary (e.g. familial Mediterranean
fever), localized or systemic. The clinical features are due to
amyloid deposits disrupting normal structure and function of
the affected tissue. As such there are no pathognomonic
features and the patient may present with a wide spectrum of
clinical scenarios including heart failure, nephrotic syndrome,
macroglossia, weakness and peripheral neuropathy. Hepato-
splenomegaly is also seen. The underlying causes of acquired
amyloid are often obscure but include chronic infections (TB,
lepromatous leprosy, bronchiectasis), chronic inflammation
(rheumatoid arthritis) and malignancy (renal, bladder, Hodgkin's disease). Diagnosis requires a high index of suspicion and
is confirmed by Congo red staining of affected tissue or, if
systemic involvement, a rectal biopsy. There is no specific
treatment.

1.2 **A**.T **B**.T **C**.F **D**.F **E**.F
Breast cancer affects 1 in 10 women. The 5-year survival rate is
75%, although a further 17% die in the subsequent 5 years.
Poor prognostic features are: age <35 years or >75 years, obesity
and tumours first diagnosed in pregnancy. Prognosis is
improved if the surgery is performed between days 3 and 12
of the menstrual cycle. Five multicentre trials found little
difference in outcome between conservative treatment and
radiotherapy with mastectomy, particularly if the tumour was
greater than 3 cm in size. Adjuvant chemotherapy with
cyclophosphamide, methotrexate and 5-flurorouracil for 6
months reduces mortality by about 25% in premenopausal
lymph node-positive women. In addition, endocrine manipulation with oophorectomy, radiation ovary ablation, tamoxifen or
progesterone arc useful in premenopausal women if the
tumour is oestrogen receptor-responsive. Adjuvant tamoxifen
(an anti-oestrogen) given for 2–5 years after surgery reduces
mortality by a similar amount in postmenopausal women.
Hypercalcaemia can arise as a result of bone metastases.
Radionuclide scans are highly sensitive but have poor
specificity, and care has to be taken in interpreting any
abnormalities found as they may be the result of trauma,

arthritis or infection for example. Up to 10–40% of metastases are seen on a bone scan in patients with normal skeletal radiographs whilst fewer than 5% of metastatic deposits seen on plain X-rays are missed by radionuclide scan.

1.3   **A.**F   **B.**T   **C.**F   **D.**F   **E.**F

This question assumes that the facilities to carry out the options will be available. However unlikely that may be, the question is really asking what is the immediate management of open lung injuries. All open chest wounds automatically produce a pneumothorax on the same side, as intrapleural pressure increases towards atmospheric pressure and forces the lung to collapse. If the wound is greater than two-thirds of the diameter of the trachea, air preferentially enters through this hole during inspiration. Immediate management is to apply a sterile dressing sealed on three sides. Air can escape via the free edge during expiration but it cannot enter the wound during inspiration as the dressing will be 'sucked' into the wound. A chest drain should be inserted as soon as possible via a freshly created hole to drain the pneumothorax. If the wound acts as a one-way valve, air cannot leave and a tension pneumothorax can arise which can result in fatal cardiovascular collapse unless treated promptly. In this situation, the occluding dressing must be removed to open the wound and allow the air to escape. Long-term management is definitive surgical closure.

1.4   **A.**T   **B.**F   **C.**T   **D.**T   **E.**T

Atelectasis is a common consequence of anaesthesia. It is due to inadequate aeration of alveoli with subsequent resorption of gas. It is more commonly found in dependent areas of the lung, partly as a compression effect from transmitted abdominal pressure as well as a result of mucus plugging of distal bronchi and alveoli. It may persist several days into the postoperative period in patients with pre-existing poor lung function and in fit patients whose chest movement is reduced from pain or upper abdominal surgery. Hypoxaemia occurs even though hypoxic pulmonary vasoconstriction limits the ventilation perfusion mismatch. There is therefore an increase in alveolar–arterial oxygen gradient. Tachypnoea and tachycardia are also seen. Hypocarbia is the norm from increased ventilation. Atelectatic areas of the lung have reduced air entry and if they become infected a pyrexia is possible. Pleuritic chest pain from stretching of parietal pleura is sharp, localized, worse on deep inspiration and coughing, and can occur if atelectasis develops into pneumonia.

1.5   A.F   B.F   C.F   D.T   E.F

Midazolam, like all benzodiazepines, facilitates the effect of GABA, which acts as an inhibitory neurotransmitter within the CNS. Two subgroups of benzodiazepine receptor have also been found: BZ1 receptors are found in the spinal cord and cerebellum, and anxiolytic activity has been attributed to them; BZ2 receptors are located in the cerebral cortex, spinal cord and hippocampus, and may be more related to the sedative effects. It is water-soluble at pH 4 because of its open imidazole ring but becomes lipid-soluble at body pH as the ring closes. This promotes a rapid onset, usually 1–2 min i.v.. The elimination half-life of 2 hours gives a rapid recovery with little hangover effect although this may be prolonged in the elderly: it is almost entirely metabolized in the liver to inactive metabolites (one of which may have slight hypnotic activity). Midazolam has been associated with severe respiratory depression and hypotension. It confers greater anterograde amnesia than diazepam. Serum levels rise markedly with concomitant administration of erythromycin, diltiazem and verapamil. Flumazenil is a competitive reversible benzodiazepine antagonist with a rapid onset and brief duration of action.

1.6   A.T   B.T   C.F   D.F   E.T

The JVP wave form (Fig. 1.1) arises from changes in right atrial pressure. There are three waves, *a*, *c* and *v*, and two descents, *x* and *y*. The *a* wave is due to atrial systole. The *c* wave (rarely seen at the bedside) is possibly transmitted from the carotid pulse. The *v* wave is produced by atrial filling during ventricular systole. The *x* descent is from atrial relaxation and downward displacement of the tricuspid valve in ventricular systole and occurs after the *c* wave. The *y* descent occurs with the fall in pressure when the tricuspid valve opens and occurs after the *v* wave. A canon wave is a giant *a* wave due to atrial contraction on a closed tricuspid valve, most commonly seen with complete heart block. Tricuspid regurgitation produces giant *v* waves. The *a* wave is absent in atrial fibrillation and becomes larger in pulmonary hypertension, right ventricular hypertrophy and tricuspid stenosis. A steep *y* descent due to abrupt fall in diastolic pressure occurs in constrictive pericarditis and tricuspid regurgitation.

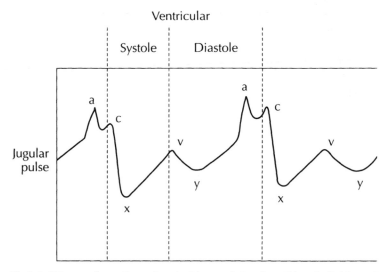

Fig.1.1 JVP wave form. Reproduced with permission from Edwards C, Munro J (1995) *Macleod's Clinical Examination*, 9th edn. Edinburgh, Churchill Livingstone

1.7   A.F   B.T   C.T   D.T   E.T
Normal adults have 15–25% weight as fat. A person is considered obese if fat comprises more than 30% of total body weight. Body mass index (BMI – mass in kg/(height in m)^2) is an easily calculated indicator of obesity; a normal value is 20–24. A BMI of 25–30 indicates moderate obesity, while a BMI >30 (i.e. double expected weight) indicates morbid obesity with serious consequences for health. Renal clearance is increased as a result of increases in both renal blood flow and glomerular filtration rate (GFR). All the other stems are correct. Perioperative problems are considerable and include airway management, increased risk of aspiration, airway difficulty, inadequacy of spontaneous ventilation and the problems of applied ventilation (barotrauma, reduced venous return), adequate monitoring (e.g. finding a large enough blood pressure (BP) cuff), safe positioning and increased blood loss, to name but a few. Postoperative problems include increased incidence of wound infections, dehiscence, deep vein thrombosis (DVT) and respiratory failure (hypoventilation, atelectasis). Mortality is increased, 6.6% as opposed to 2.7% for patients of normal weight. Regional anaesthesia may be preferrable but has little proven benefit on outcome. (See: Shenkman Z, Shir Y,

Brodsky JB (1993). Perioperative management of the obese patient. *British Journal of Anaesthesia* **70**, 349–359.)

1.8   A.F   B.F   C.T   D.F   E.F

Osteoporosis is a reduction in bone mass as a result of the loss of all components of bone, not just calcium as in primary hyperparathyroidism. Although found in both sexes it is more common in postmenopausal women as a result of oestrogen deficiency, and can also be secondary to endocrine disease (e.g. Cushing's syndrome, thyrotoxicosis). Biochemical screening is normal. Radiographs show fractures (femur, wrist, vertebrae) and osteopenia but the condition is best detected with bone densitometry. Regular exercise is the best preventative treatment. Oestrogen is possibly useful if postmenopausal, and biphosphonates can be used in late-stage disease to inhibit bone resorption. Osteomalacia mimics osteoporosis but is due to defective mineralization of bone ('adult' rickets). Paget's disease arises from excessive osteoclastic bone resorption with disordered osteoblastic new bone formation. Although the new bone is abundant it is structurally abnormal and weak. The bone disease of chronic renal failure (renal osteodystrophy) is complex and results from a combination of osteomalacia, osteitis fibrosa and osteoporosis, the latter being thought to be due to mild malnutrition. If anything, gastrectomy may cause malabsorption resulting in osteomalacia.

1.9   A.F   B.F   C.F   D.F   E.F

Immediate management of acid aspiration is supportive. The patient must be turned on his/her side and tilted head-down to prevent further aspiration or at least to localize the aspiration to one lung. Suction and supplementary oxygen should be applied and the patient monitored by pulse oximetry and arterial blood gases to assess gas exchange. Bronchoscopy is of value for particulate matter. Pulmonary lavage is ineffective as aspirated fluid disperses too quickly. The threshold for intubation and ventilation should be low but no immediate intervention is necessary unless consciousness is reduced or severe respiratory distress is present. Bronchodilators, e.g. salbutamol, are helpful and aminophylline may also be considered although additional bronchodilator effect is minimal and side-effects are significant Physiotherapy may be useful. Shock requires fluid and inotropes for cardiovascular support. The initial use of antibiotics is controversial as gastric acid is usually sterile but, as secondary colonization of chemically damaged tissue may lead to pneumonia, they are often given, particularly if aspirate is infected (e.g. faecal material in bowel obstruction) or particulate matter is present. Steroids may slow pulmonary healing and increase the risk of infection. Sodium bicarbonate is not useful. Ranitidine increases pH and decreases production of gastric acid but has no effect on acid already in the lung. It is used prophylactically for the 'at risk' patient. (See: Kallar SK, Everett LL (1993) Potential risks and preventive measures for pulmonary aspiration. *Anesthesia and Analgesia* **77**, 171–182.)

1.10 A.T **B.**T **C.**F **D.**F **E.**T

It has been long debated whether regional or general anaesthesia is better. There is no doubt that regional techniques reduce the incidence of DVT (in one study from 76% to 40%) but little else has been shown to differ, including perioperative blood loss and mortality, either in the immediate postoperative period or at one year (20–30%). Survival is probably improved as a result of two manoeuvres. One is early repair as immobilization even for a short time exponentially increases the incidence and severity of pulmonary complications, and the other is involvement of an experienced surgeon and anaesthetist. Methylmethacrylate cement is an acrylic polymer which produces an expanding exothermic interface between bone and prosthesis. It has been associated with hypotension, hypoxaemia and pulmonary and cardiovascular dysfunction, the proposed mechanisms for which include fat, air and bone marrow embolism, toxic effects of the cement and neurovascular effects from increase in intramedullary pressure. (See: Sorenson RM, Pace NL (1993) Anesthetic techniques during surgical repair of femoral neck fractures. *Anesthesiology* **77**, 1094–1104.)

1.11 A.F **B.**T **C.**F **D.**T **E.**T

Caudal analgesia is achieved by injection of local anaesthetics (LAs) and/or other agents (ketamine, buprenorphine, clonidine and opiates) into the sacral canal to produce block of sacral and lumbar nerve roots. It is ideal for perineal analgesia in circumcision, haemorrhoidectomy and anal dilatation. It is particularly good for providing postoperative analgesia for inguinal herniotomy and orchidopexy in children as there is less extradural fat, allowing greater spread of analgesic solution and thus higher blocks. In adults, higher blocks require greater volumes and, in combination with a variable sacral anatomy, are less predictable and have a higher failure rate compared to lumbar extradurals. The dura ends at S2 (S4 at birth), at the level of the posterior iliac spines, and dural puncture is rare. Other complications are as for lumbar epidural anaesthesia but are much less common. Difficulty in micturition after a caudal may occur but is uncommon. Insertion of the needle into the presenting part of a fetus in labour has been reported and its use for forceps delivery is not recommended. Catheter insertion into the caudal space has been performed for continuous caudal block as well as being the site of entry for an epidural catheter that is 'fed' up to the desired position. Difficulty in maintaining strict asepsis limits both uses.

1.12 A.T **B.**T **C.**F **D.**T **E.**T
Primary hyperparathyroidism arises from either a single adenoma (>90%), hyperplasia or, rarely, malignancy. The elevated parathyroid hormone (PTH) stimulates calcium release from bones and in 50% of cases asymptomatic hypercalcaemia is the only indication of the disease. Serum phosphate is usually low and alkaline phosphatase – an index of osteoblastic activity – may be elevated. Non-specific features include nausea, vomiting, constipation, tiredness and depression. Osteitis fibrosa results from calcium being replaced by fibrous tissue in the bones and causes tenderness, swelling, deformities and fractures. Renal calculi are common and calcium can be deposited in renal parenchyma (nephrocalcinosis) leading to loss of renal function. Ectopic calcification can also be found in the cornea and arterial wall. Peptic ulceration, hypertension, myopathy and pruritis are also possible. Definitive treatment is parathyroidectomy.

1.13 A.T **B.**F **C.**F **D.**T **E.**F
Peripheral sympathetic supply arises from T1–L2. White rami communicantes are the only connection from the spinal cord to the peripheral sympathetic system. They carry myelinated preganglionic fibres to the sympathetic ganglia. The cervical sympathetic chain is organized into three groups of ganglia: superior, medial and inferior. All fibres to the medial and superior (the largest) must pass through the inferior (stellate) ganglion first. This lies above the pleura, with the subclavian and vertebral arteries in front and the neck of the first rib and

the prevertebral fascia and transverse process of the seventh cervical vertebra behind. Postganglionic sympathetic fibres are unmyelinated grey rami communicantes which pass to spinal nerves to be distributed to somatic areas. Brachial plexus block can lead to unintentional block of the stellate ganglion, owing to its relative proximity.

1.14 A.T B.T C.T D.F E.F
Of all patients in hospital, 5–10% develop a nosocomial infection, with ICUs responsible for 25% of all hospital-acquired bloodstream and pulmonary infections. The main infecting organisms are Gram-negative and antibiotic-resistant Gram-positive cocci. The commonest is infection of the urinary tract followed by surgical wounds and pneumonia. Prevention of nosocomial infections is critical as morbidity, mortality and hospital stay are otherwise prolonged, with obvious implications for cost. The presence of an infection control team reduces the incidence of all types of nosocomial infections compared with hospitals without one. Improving handwashing technique has been shown to reduce infections by 20–25%. A significant proportion of chest infections in ICU patients are thought to arise from the use of H_2 antagonists which, by reducing gastric acid production, encourage bacterial overgrowth. Selective decontamination of the digestive tract using oral non-absorbable antibiotics (polymixin, gentamicin, etc.) was devised to break the colonization–infection cycle of bacterial overgrowth thought to be an important cause of nosocomial pneumonia. Results suggest that this does reduce the incidence of infection but a reduction in length of ICU stay and mortality remains unproven. Sucralfate may be a suitable replacement for H_2 antagonists as it exerts an equally protective effect on the gut mucosa with little effect on normal gastric pH. Unfortunately trials have been inconclusive. The same is true of cisapride. Omeprazole is a proton pump inhibitor which reduces gastric acidity and volume and, for the same reason as H_2 blockers, is unlikely to be of value. (See: Baxby D, Van Saene HK *et al.* (1996) Selective decontamination of the digestive tract. What it is and what it is not. *Intensive Care Medicine* **22** (**7**), 699–706.)

1.15 A.T B.T C.F D.T E.F
Vecuronium is a monoquaternary ammonium homologue of the bisquaternary aminosteroid pancuronium. It has active

metabolites, one of which has 60% of the potency of the parent drug whilst the others are only weakly active. They do not cross the blood–brain barrier. It undergoes hepatobiliary elimination, and both liver and renal failure prolongs its action. Rocuronium is similar to vecuronium but its molecular structure differs by four positions. It is 5–10 times less potent than vecuronium and has a shorter onset (60–90 s, but suxamethonium is still faster at 20–40 s) but same length of action as vecuronium. An analogue of vecuronium, ORG 9487, is thought to improve speed of onset further and maintain the hope that suxamethonium can ultimately be replaced. *Cis*-atracurium is a more potent non-histamine releasing isomer of atracurium. Other relatively new neuromuscular blocking agents include pipecuronium and doxacurium. Both are cardiostable with no histamine releasing action at clinical doses, a slow onset (2–3 min) and prolonged action (1–2 hours). The former is a more potent analogue of pancuronium excreted renally, whilst the latter is metabolized by plasma esterases without Hoffmann degradation. (See: Durcan T, Philpott G (1995) The metabolic fate of newer anaesthetic drugs. *Anaesthesia Review,* vol. 12, ch. 10, pp. 165–180. London, Churchill Livingstone.)

1.16 A.T B.F C.T D.F E.F
Much time and effort has gone into finding a consistently reliable method to measure depth of anaesthesia and so combat the problems of awareness and overdose. The large range available suggests that none has been entirely successful. Autonomic changes in BP, heart rate, sweating and lacrimation are useful but may also be associated with other events. Pupil diameter was originally described to be of value with ether (dilates with increasing dose) but the polypharmacy of contemporary anaesthesia renders it unreliable. Lower oesophageal contractility, like heart rate and BP, is under autonomic control and it exhibits regular spontaneous contractions in awake patients. During anaesthesia it is possible to measure reduction in frequency and amplitude of contractions but as it is not under control of conscious thought it is unreliable in predicting awareness. The isolated forearm technique involves the use of a tourniquet on an arm prior to neuromuscular blockade. The arm is free to move during surgery and purposeful movements in response to instruction indicate light anaesthesia. The EEG records the responses of

many thousands of neurones in the cerebral cortex and is useful in assessing depth. The results are difficult to interpret, vary according to the anaesthetic given and are subject to considerable interference. The cerebral function monitor and bispectral analysis simplify the EEG data and appear to be the monitors with greatest success. Auditory, visual and somatosensory evoked potentials are depressed by anaesthesia and also appear to be a promising guide to depth of anaesthesia. (See: Newton DEF (1993) Editorial: depth of anaesthesia. *Anaesthesia* **48**, 367–368. Also: Cormack RS (1993) Editorial II: conscious levels during anaesthesia. *British Journal of Anaesthesia* **71**, 469–471.)

1.17 A.T **B.**F **C.**F **D.**F **E.**T
Placental blood flow near term is approximately 600 ml/min. There is usually one umbilical vein carrying oxygenated blood to the fetus and two arteries carrying deoxygenated blood to the placenta. At term, the placental circulation is maximally dilated and therefore depends mostly on maternal blood pressure and is not related to fetal stroke volume or heart rate. The uteroplacental arteries have mostly alpha adrenergic receptors. Any event that lowers systemic BP (aortocaval compression, hypovolaemia) may induce release of catecholamines to cause uterine artery constriction thereby decreasing blood flow to the placenta. This can occur independently from maternal blood pressure.

1.18 A.F **B.**F **C.**F **D.**F **E.**T
The placenta is a simple lipid membrane. Drugs, particularly if lipid-soluble and non-ionized, cross primarily by simple diffusion down a concentration gradient. Maternal protein binding of drugs limits transfer, e.g. 80% of bupivacaine is protein-bound and 30% traverses whilst lignocaine is 70% bound but 57% crosses. Fetal hypoxia and acidosis can create a greater pH differential (normally only 0.1) between maternal and fetal circulation which can lead to weakly basic drugs becoming more ionized and trapped in the fetal circulation after transfer. Lignocaine is not associated with any adverse fetal neurobehavioural effects but is rarely used owing to tachyphylaxis. Bupivacaine has been associated with reduced variability of fetal heart rate. Fetal complications are more likely to arise from LA-induced hypotension reducing uteroplacental circulation. Fentanyl is a lipophilic, highly protein-bound (69%) opiate. By the epidural route, it improves quality

and length of analgesia with minimal fetal side-effects. Significant neonatal depression occurs if given intravenously. Alfentanil is less lipid-soluble and has been associated with neonatal hypotonia at a dose of 30 μg/kg, but it is now considered safe to use at a lower dose.

1.19 A.F B.F C.T D.F E.T

MH can be induced by all the currently available volatile inhalational agents, including desflurane and sevoflurane, as well as suxamethonium and other depolarizing muscle relaxants. Other possible trigger agents include phenothiazines and haloperidol. The amide LAs are no longer considered to initiate MH at clinical doses (the original work used doses far exceeding the therapeutic range), nor are nitrous oxide, ketamine and propofol. Other safe agents include intravenous induction agents, ester LAs, non-depolarizing neuromuscular blocking agents, opioids, droperidol and benzodiazepines. Masseter muscle spasm is commonly seen in children after suxamethonium. When prolonged, it can be one of the earliest signs of an MH episode.

1.20 A.F B.T C.F D.T E.T

In the young age group, hyperthyroidism is most commonly due to Graves' disease, i.e. circulating IgG antibodies activating thyroid-stimulating hormone (TSH) receptors on the thyroid gland to produce thyroid hormones. This is classically associated with eye signs (proptosis, limitation of eye movements, lid lag), pretibial myxoedema (purple plaques on shins) and thyroid acropachy (clubbing, swollen fingers, periosteal new bone formation.) Goitres are more common in young women. Other features of hyperthyroidism include oligomenorrhoea, heat intolerance, weight loss, tremor, diarrhoea, irritability and a marked proximal myopathy. The elderly tend to develop toxic multinodular goitres and atrial fibrillation. Treatment includes drugs (carbimazole, beta blockers), radioactive iodine and surgery. Prior to surgery, patients must be euthyroid and conventional practice is to stop antithyroid drugs 10 or so days prior to operation and to give potassium iodide to reduce vascularity of the gland. A thyroid crisis is a rare but life-threatening acute exacerbation of hyperthyroidism with hyperpyrexia, tachycardia and restlessness. It is most commonly precipitated by infection, stress, surgery or after radioactive iodine is given in hyperthyroid patients. Treatment is with propranolol, potassium iodide, antithyroid drugs and corticosteroids.

1.21 A.T **B.**T **C.**F **D.**T **E.**F

SIRS is seen with a wide variety of severe clinical insults including trauma, pancreatitis, extensive tissue injury, ischaemia and haemorrhagic shock. Diagnosis requires at least two or more of the following:

1. Temperature >38°C or <36°C.
2. Heart rate >90 beats per min.
3. Respiratory rate >20 breaths per min or $P_a co_2$ <4.3 kPa.
4. White cell count >12 000 cells/mm^3 or <4000 cells/mm^3.

Sepsis is a term reserved for patients with SIRS who have a documented infection.
Severe sepsis is sepsis with organ dysfunction, hypoperfusion or hypotension.
Septic shock is severe sepsis with hypotension unresponsive to fluid resuscitation.
Refractory shock is shock unresponsive to therapy (fluids, inotropes) within 1 hour of onset.

SIRS frequently leads to multiple organ failure and once three or more organs have failed mortality is in excess of 80%. Management is supportive. Adjunctive therapy including steroids, prostaglandins, opiate antagonists, antiendotoxin antibodies, anticytokines and nitric oxide synthetase inhibitors has been largely disappointing. (See: American College of Chest Physicians *et al.* (1992) Definitions for sepsis and organ failure and guidelines for the use of innovative therapies in sepsis. *Critical Care Medicine* **20**, 864–874.)

1.22 A.T **B.**F **C.**F **D.**T **E.**T

Enflurane produces abnormal EEG activity which may resemble grand mal epilepsy in children and focal seizures in adults. The effect is potentiated by hypocarbia and EEG charges may last for several weeks. *Methohexitone* can precipitate convulsive activity in patients with an abnormal EEG or a history of focal epilepsy. *Ketamine* can cause involuntary movements and tremor severe enough to suggest seizure activity but no associated EEG evidence of cortical seizure activity has been found. *Thiopentone, halothane* and *isoflurane* have anticonvulsant activity and are the agents of choice. *Regional anaesthesia* is not contraindicated but is sometimes avoided for fear of a convulsion during the procedure. *Propofol* has been implicated in a number of case reports of causing seizures and epilepti-form EEG changes. Nevertheless, it has been used as an anticonvulsant and a number of studies have shown that it does not induce ictal activity, even in patients with intractable epilepsy. (See: Cheng MA *et al.* (1996) Large dose propofol alone in adult epileptic patients: electrocorticographic results. *Anesthesia and Analgesia* **83**, 169–174. Also: Ebrahim ZY *et al.* (1994) The effect of propofol on the EEG of patients with epilepsy. *Anesthesia and Analgesia* **78**, 275–279.)

1.23 A.F **B.**F **C.**F **D.**F **E.**F

This is a difficult question to answer as **A**, **C**, **D** and **E** will show radiological changes with their disease. However, radiographs would not normally be the first line in investigation, nor are the changes specific for each disease. Nevertheless, sickle cell anaemia can cause aseptic necrosis of femoral and humeral heads and bone infarcts. Extramedullary haematopoiesis is a feature of myelosclerosis. This causes progressive fibrosis of the bone marrow, resulting in patchy osteosclerosis. Gaucher's syndrome is a lysosomal storage disease in which Gaucher's cells invade bone marrow, leading to decreased bone growth, poor mineralization, pathological fractures, avascular necrosis of the femoral heads and a flask-like expansion of the lower end of the femur. Subperiosteal haemorrhages and widening of the provisional zone of calcification (white line of Frankel) with rarefaction are found with vitamin C deficiency. G6PD deficiency is an inherited condition which may result in haemolytic anaemia, either spontaneously or with infections, drugs or broad beans (favism).

1.24 A.T **B.**T **C.**F **D.**F **E.**F

	Morphine	Fentanyl	Alfentanil
Equivalent i.v. dose	10 mg	0.1 mg	0.5 mg
Onset of action	>15 min	4–10 min	1–2 min
Duration of action	3 h	25 min	12 min
% Protein-bound	35%	84%	92%
Vol. distribution	100–300 l	240–400 l	50 l
Half-life	1–4 h	2–7 h	1–3 h

Fentanyl and alfentanil are both phenylpiperidine derivatives of pethidine. Although alfentanil is less fat-soluble than fentanyl, solubility is still sufficient to allow for rapid penetration of membranes, including the CNS. This gives it a short onset time but less is redistributed to fat and muscle, giving a smaller volume of distribution. Despite a lower clearance, this gives alfentanil a shorter elimination half-life and duration of action compared with fentanyl. Both have minimal cardiovascular effects although bradycardia and hypotension may occur. Both are hepatically cleared. Excretion is delayed in the elderly and in those with pre-existing liver disease. High doses of both are associated with muscle rigidity, possibly from an interaction with central dopamine receptors; this can be reversed by naloxone or the new longer-acting opioid antagonist, nalmephene (which can also be given orally). Both are used perioperatively and by infusion for sedation in ICUs.

1.25 A.F B.F C.F D.F E.F
The umbilicus is supplied by the ventral rami of T10. The sensory supply to the thumb is supplied by the median nerve (C6, 7, 8), which lies both behind and lateral to the palmaris longus. The ulnar nerve contains T1 which supplies the medial part of the hand, including the medial half of the ring finger and all of the little finger. The trochlear (IVth cranial) nerve supplies the superior oblique muscle of the eye. An isolated lesion is rare and causes diplopia when looking down and away from the affected side. The inferior rectus is supplied by the oculomotor (IIIrd cranial) nerve along with the superior and medial recti, the inferior oblique and the levator palpebrae superioris muscles. The abducens (VIth cranial) nerve supplies the lateral rectus muscle. The subclavian vein is the continuation of the axillary vein. It extends from the outer border of the first rib to the medial border of the scalenus anterior where it unites with the internal jugular vein to form the brachiocephalic vein. The clavicle lies in front and the subclavian artery lies behind and above but separated by the scalenus anterior.

1.26 A.T B.F C.T D.T E.T
Small bowel obstruction produces copious amounts of bile-stained vomit. Abdominal distension is due to gas-filled loops of bowel proximal to the obstruction – the more distal the obstruction, the greater the distension. It can also give rise to

abdominal pain but is rarely severe unless strangulation has occurred. Constipation is absolute: neither faeces nor flatus are passed rectally as bowel gas is absorbed distal to the obstruction and propulsion of bowel contents is arrested. On percussion, the centre of the abdomen tends to be resonant and the flanks dull because bowel gas rises to the most elevated point. This can be confused with ascites. Bowel sounds are traditionally described as being loud, high-pitched and frequent. They can also be echoing or sound like gentle lapping of water owing to fluid sloshing about in the gas-filled bowel. Visible peristalsis may be observed in thin patients with subacute obstruction of long duration.

1.27 A.T B.T C.F D.T E.T
Of all the leukaemias, CML is the only one where the platelet count may be raised. Beta thalassaemia is a failure to synthesize β haemoglobin and survival is not possible without frequent blood transfusions. This results in iron overload – transfusion haemosiderosis – the complications of which, despite chelating agents, are often the cause of death. Down's syndrome is associated with leukaemia. Aplastic anaemia can be primarily congenital (e.g. Fanconi's) or be acquired as a result of agents such as drugs, insecticides, ionizing radiation or infections. All lymphoproliferative diseases, including multiple myeloma, lymphomas and leukaemias, can cause gout due to excessive purine synthesis. A raised haemoglobin with renal malignancy is the result of an inappropriate increase in erythropoietin production.

1.28 A.F B.F C.T D.F E.T
The use of in-circle vaporizers such as the Goldman vaporizer is becoming rare. In-circle vaporizers are simple and must have a low resistance and a small vaporizing chamber. They are neither efficient nor temperature-compensated and can be placed in the inspiratory or expiratory limb. Anaesthetic depth with spontaneous ventilation is self-regulating as respiration will be depressed as uptake of volatile agent increases. This safety factor relies on the production of an excessive depth of anaesthesia and it is no longer considered a safe method of controlling anaesthetic administration. In addition, controlled ventilation will rapidly produce a high and potentially dangerous concentration of anaesthetic owing to the loss of this negative feedback mechanism. Thus, the use of an in-circle

vaporizer for spontaneous or applied ventilation nowadays requires monitoring of the inspired concentration of the volatile agent.

1.29 **A**.T **B**.F **C**.T **D**.T **E**.T
Purpura is the result of bleeding into the skin. Causes are many but can be classified as arising from a disorder of platelets, vessels or coagulation. *DIC* can complicate a severe septic illness and the coagulopathy can result in florid purpura. *AML* not infrequently presents with an intercurrent illness from impairment of immune function and thrombocytopaenia resulting in spontaneous haemorrhages. If the septic illness was treated with *sulphonamide antibiotics*, purpura can occur secondary to a vasculitis. *SLE* is a multisystem connective tissue disorder associated with antinuclear antibodies. Although mainly found in women, it can also occur in men. Clinical presentation is variable but results from the consequences of a vasculitis and therefore purpura is possible. In addition, an acute exacerbation commonly presents with a non-infective pyrexia which can be easily misinterpreted as a septic episode. *Bacterial endocarditis* is associated with a pyrexia. Cutaneous manifestations include petechial haemorrhages, Janeway lesions, splinter haemorrhages, Roth spots and Osler's nodes but not purpura.

1.30 **A**.F **B**.F **C**.F **D**.F **E**.F
Labour is extremely painful and there is no evidence to suggest that it is beneficial to the mother or the fetus. Deleterious effects for example include increased oxygen debt from hyperventilation and sympathetic catecholamine release; these can lead to a decrease in uteroplacental blood flow and reduced oxygen transfer to the fetus. Regional techniques are superior to any other method in providing effective pain relief. TENS is of limited value helping only for backache at the onset of labour. Acupuncture provides inconsistent, incomplete and unpredictable analgesia. Intramuscular pethidine is used routinely with little justification as efficacy and patient satisfaction are low. Side-effects include nausea and vomiting in the mother and respiratory depression in the neonate. Intravenous morphine, longer acting than pethidine, has long been abandoned because of respiratory depression in neonates. Psychoprophylaxis involves reconditioning mothers to believe that labour can be a pain-free event by relaxation and breathing exercises. Good education does allay anxiety and

reduce analgesic requirements but only in combination with other procedures.

1.31 A.F B.T C.T D.F E.F
Protein intake should be approximately 1 g/kg per day and must supply the eight essential amino acids. The others can be made *in vivo* by amination of carbohydrate and fat residues. All naturally occurring amino acids are in the L form. In complete starvation there is an initial protein sparing effect at the expense of fat (protein: 4 kcal/g, fat: 9 kcal/g) but ultimately protein catabolism of muscle, liver and spleen occurs, with preferential sparing of heart and brain. Optimal BMI (weight divided by height squared) is 20–25 kg/m^2. Malnutrition in childhood ranges from kwashiorkor, where there is relatively adequate energy intake but protein deficiency, to marasmus, where all energy sources are inadequate.

1.32 A.F B.F C.T D.F E.F
Lung cancer is the commonest cause of death from malignancy and surgical resection is the best chance of cure. Even then, the 5-year survival rate is only 25%. Operability depends on the nature of the tumour, its spread and patient fitness. Surgery is feasible if local spread is limited to the ipsilateral hilum or peribronchial nodes with no known distant metastases. A pleural effusion may be caused by a tumour but is not a contraindication as it may also arise from infection due to bronchial obstruction by a tumour. Preoperative pulmonary function tests provide a reasonable guide to whether a patient has sufficient lung capacity to cope with a pneumonectomy. This is possible if the FEV_1 >1.5–2 l, maximal voluntary ventilation >50% of predicted, and residual volume to total lung capacity ratio <50%. Even if these criteria are not met surgery may still be possible if the diseased lung makes little contribution to ventilation – something that can be demonstrated by perfusion scanning. A predicted postoperative FEV_1 of 0.8–1.0 l is also needed. Positive sputum cytology is useful for diagnosis but it is not a contraindication to surgery. Patients over 70 years do not tolerate pneumonectomy well, particularly if in poor general condition, but it is not a contraindication. Surgery should not be performed with intrathoracic spread involving sympathetic trunk, recurrent laryngeal and phrenic nerves, trachea, oesophagus, pleura and pericardium. Nor should it be contemplated in the presence

of a widened fixed carina and if the tumour is within 1.5 cm of the origin of the main contralateral bronchus. (See: Dunn WF, Scanlon MD (1993) Preoperative pulmonary function testing for patients with lung cancer. *Mayo Clinic Proceedings* **68**, 371–377.)

1.33 A.T B.T C.T D.T E.F
Asthma is defined as 'reversible airways obstruction resulting from bronchoconstriction'. It can be reversed with β_2 adrenoceptor agonists such as salbutamol and terbutaline. Parasympathetic stimulation of the lungs also causes bronchoconstriction; therefore the anticholinergic ipratropium bromide is useful, particularly with coexisting chronic obstructive pulmonary disease (COPD). Ketamine is a bronchodilator. Inhaled beclomethasone is a steroid which dampens the inflammatory responses of the triggering agents. This can otherwise result in an exudate containing eosinophils, lymphocytes, kinins and other inflammatory mediators into the lumen of the airways contributing to oedema, mucus plugging, decreased mucociliary clearance and further narrowing. Halothane has a well-recognized bronchodilator action. Metoprolol is a selective β_1 adrenoreceptor antagonist and as such has less effect on the lungs compared with non-specific beta blockers, e.g. propranolol. Nevertheless, it is not recommended.

1.34 A.T B.F C.F D.T E.T
Upwards of 30% of the population smoke. It often begins in adolescence for psychosocial reasons but the pharmacological properties of nicotine confer dependence. Carbon monoxide has a greater affinity for haemoglobin than oxygen and carboxyhaemoglobin levels of up to 15% (2% in non-smokers) are sufficient to shift the oxyhaemoglobin dissociation curve to the left, thus promoting tissue hypoxia. Abstinence of 12–24 hours is sufficient to reduce levels to normal thus improving oxygenation. Other pulmonary effects include impaired ciliary activity, reduced immunological defences and increased bronchial reactivity which all require 6–8 weeks of non-smoking before returning to normal. Smokers are more likely to suffer increased sputum production and retention, bronchospasm, coughing, atelectasis and chest infections postoperatively. Nicotine activates the sympathoadrenergic system which increases oxygen demand, coronary vascular resistance and

the risk of arterial thromboembolism and coronary vasospasm, all of which may lead to cardiovascular compromise. Smoking during pregnancy leads to placental impairment from nicotine-induced vasoconstriction. Fetal nicotine levels often exceed maternal levels and at term fetal heart rate is increased with decreased variability in smokers. Some earlier studies suggested gastric emptying was delayed in smokers but these findings have not been sustained in more recent work. (See: Nel MR, Morgan M (1996) Editorial: smoking and anaesthesia revisited. *Anaesthesia* **51**, 309–311. Also: Egan TD, Wong KC (1992) Perioperative smoking cessation and anesthesia: a review. *Journal of Clinical Anesthesia* **4**, 63–72.)

1.35 A.T   B.F   C.T   D.T   E.F
Pain is defined as 'an unpleasant sensory and emotional experience associated with actual or potential tissue damage, or described in terms of such damage'. As the perception of pain is influenced by behavioural, emotional, economic and socio-cultural factors, self-reporting is more reliable than observer opinion. The VAS and NRS (numerical rating scale) measure one modality of pain, such as pain intensity. Although quick and easy to use, e.g. for postoperative pain relief, they have a failure rate of about 10%. The MPQ assesses different modalities of pain (affective, evaluative, sensory and miscellaneous) by selection of the appropriate words in these categories to describe the pain; each word is ranked to give a score known as the patient rating index (PRI). It is more suited to chronic pain and is unsuitable for children under 12 years of age. The DPQ is used in conjunction with the MPQ and focuses more on pain intensity, its time course and effect on behaviour.

1.36 A.F   B.T   C.F   D.T   E.T
DIC arises when the normal balance between intravascular coagulation and fibrinolysis is disturbed. The initial event is activation of the coagulation cascade resulting in thrombin converting fibrinogen to fibrin to produce widespread thrombus formation. Platelets and coagulation factors are consumed and secondary activation of fibrinolysis occurs, leading to production of fibrin degradation products, which may themselves contribute to the coagulation defect by inhibiting fibrin polymerization. Causes are many and include sepsis, obstetric complications (amniotic fluid embolism, abruption), burns, trauma and malignancy. Clinical presentation varies from

chronic (with little bleeding) to acute (with complete haemo-static failure and widespread haemorrhage). When severe, all the common tests of coagulation (prothrombin time (PT), partial thromboplastin time (PTT), thrombin time (TT)) are prolonged, fibrinogen levels are low, fibrin degradation products (FDP) high and thrombocytopenia from consumption is the norm. Management aims to eliminate the cause and replace blood and coagulation factors with fresh-frozen plasma, platelet concentrates and cryoprecipitate rich in fibrinogen and factor VIII. The aim of therapeutic anticoagulation with heparin is to halt the coagulation process and remove the trigger for fibrinolysis. Its use is controversial and it would be a brave person who gave it in established DIC. However, it may be of value early in the development of DIC, particularly if chronic or where the vasculature (sepsis, neoplasia) is intact. Antith-rombin III may cause less bleeding and be superior to heparin. Vitamin K is used in coagulopathies associated with liver disease and in the newborn.

1.37 A.F B.F C.T D.T E.F
Normal values include:

> Standard speed: 25 mm/s.
> One small square represents 0.04 s, one large square 0.2 s.
> Two large squares vertically = 1 mV.
> PR interval: 0.12–0.2 s (3–5 small squares).
> P wave: maximum height 2.5 mm; maximum duration 0.11 s.
> Mean frontal QRS axis: −30° to +110°; maximum duration 0.1 s.
> Maximum QT interval: less than 0.42 s.
> Normal QRS duration of 0.08–0.1 s.

Lead I is between the right and left arms. The T wave should be positive but may be inverted in left ventricular strain, infarction, conduction defects and dextrocardia.

1.38 A.T B.F C.F D.T E.T
Parkinson's disease is a disease of the elderly with an incidence of 1 in 200 if over 70 years of age. It is due to progressive cell degeneration in the pars compacta of the substantia nigra with the appearance of eosinophilic inclusion bodies (Lewy). Biochemically, there is depletion of dopamine resulting in the unopposed action of acetylcholine. The principal symptoms are

tremor at rest, rigidity ('cogwheel' or 'leadpipe'), and poverty and slowing of movement. The sufferer develops a stoop, a shuffling festinant gait and an expressionless face. Muscle strength, sensation and reflexes remain normal until advanced akinesia makes assessment difficult. Balance is often impaired and falls are common. As the disease advances dysphagia, depression and mild dementia also occur. Bladder dysfunction is a recognized feature of both the disease and the anticholinergic agents used in the treatment of the tremor and rigidity (e.g. benzhexol). Other drugs of value are L-dopa in combination with a peripheral decarboxylase inhibitor to limit peripheral breakdown and reduce side-effects, selegiline to inhibit dopamine catabolism in the brain, and amantadine to increase synthesis and release of dopamine. Remissions are unknown and cure is not possible. The rate of progression varies but survival after diagnosis is usually 10–15 years with death most commonly as a result of bronchopneumonia.

1.39 A.F B.F C.T D.F E.T

TOF is due to imperfect embryological division of the foregut into the trachea anteriorly and the oesophagus posteriorly. Its incidence is 1 in 4000 live births, with an equal sex incidence. Definitive antenatal diagnosis is not possible but it may be suspected in cases of maternal polyhydramnios and premature labour. 85–90% of cases have a proximal oesophageal atresia with a TOF fistula between the posterior aspect of the trachea and the distal portion of the oesophagus. Other congenital abnormalities are present in about 50% of cases and are collectively termed the VACTERL association (**v**ertebral defects, **a**nal atresia, **c**ardiac lesions, **t**racheo-**o**esophageal fistula, **r**adial or **r**enal anomalies, and **l**imb defects). Neonates presenting with excessive salivation, choking, cyanosis on feeding and respiratory distress should be investigated for a TOF. Diagnosis can be confirmed by radiographic evidence of failure to pass a catheter (Replogle tube) into the stomach. It is seen curled up in the proximal oesophagus. Projectile vomiting is anatomically impossible. Preoperatively, the patient should be cared for in a head-up position. Surgical intervention must be prompt to prevent pneumonitis. A right thoracotomy allows extrapleural ligation of the fistula and usually primary anastomosis of the oesophagus. Survival is near 100% in otherwise healthy full-term infants.

1.40 A.F **B.**T **C.**T **D.**F **E.**T

PEEP aims to expand and recruit underventilated alveoli to minimize airway collapse. This has the benefit of reducing airway resistance and the work of breathing as well as increasing compliance and FRC. It also helps to redistribute lung water from the alveoli to the interstitium. If hypoxaemia is due to shunting from alveolar collapse, this will result in a decrease in ventilation perfusion mismatch. This reduces venous admixture thereby improving oxygenation and thus mixed venous oxygen content. Recruitment of atelectatic areas also leads to less ventilator-induced lung injury from shear forces. PEEP is indicated when an F_iO_2 of >0.5 is unable to maintain an S_aO_2 of > 90% in ventilated patients. Levels used are normally in the order of 5–20 cm H_2O. PEEP increases intrathoracic pressure (and therefore central venous pressure (CVP)) which, in turn, may reduce venous return and increase pulmonary vascular resistance resulting in a fall in cardiac output. This can ultimately reduce oxygen delivery to the tissues and care has to be taken to provide 'best' PEEP, i.e. minimal side-effects for maximal gain. Nevertheless patients with low compliance, as in adult respiratory distress syndrome (ARDS), may be protected to some extent from these deleterious effects as stiff lungs limit transmission of raised airway pressures to the central veins. High levels of PEEP are associated with ventilator-induced lung injury (barotrauma) and an increase in dead space. In addition, intracranial pressure is increased and urine output can be reduced as a result of an increase in antidiuretic hormone (ADH) release from the posterior pituitary. PEEP is not a panacea for all patients with hypoxia; in COPD and asthma for example, where air-trapping is a problem, it may significantly compromise lung function at more than moderate levels (>10 cm H_2O).

1.41 A.F **B.**F **C.**T **D.**F **E.**F

Carbon dioxide is the end-product of aerobic metabolism. It is transported to the lungs for removal in three forms, the majority as bicarbonate (70%) and the rest either in solution (10%) or combined with terminal amino groups – mainly reduced haemoglobin (20%). When CO_2 is released from cells it passes into the bloodstream and into red blood cells. Under the influence of carbonic anhydrase it undergoes conversion with water to carbonic acid and from there to bicarbonate and hydrogen ions:

$$CO_2 + H_2O \rightleftharpoons H_2CO_3 \rightleftharpoons H^+ + HCO_3^-$$
$$\uparrow$$
carbonic anhydrase

Once generated, the bicarbonate ions diffuse quickly from the red blood cells into the plasma where they rapidly pass to the lungs. To maintain electrochemical neutrality, chloride ions enter the red blood cells to compensate for the loss of HCO_3^- ions (chloride shift). The remaining H^+ ions – in turn – are buffered by the reduced haemoglobin (as it is more basic than oxyhaemoglobin). This is the basis for the Bohr effect. That is, the more acidic the environment, the lower affinity there is for haemoglobin and oxygen, thus promoting oxygen delivery to the tissues (right shift of the oxyhaemoglobin dissociation curve). The Haldane effect promotes CO_2 elimination as reduced haemoglobin can be reversibly bound with CO_2 as carbaminohaemoglobin and its greater buffering action (compared with oxyhaemoglobin) allows more bicarbonate ions to be formed. The reverse occurs in the lungs whereby haemoglobin becomes saturated with O_2. The H^+ ions are released and then combine with HCO_3^-, which is converted back to CO_2 and eliminated from the lungs (down a concentration gradient).

1.42 A.F   B.T   C.T   D.T   E.T

Carotid endarterectomies reduce the risk of stroke in patients with symptomatic carotid stenosis. Hypotension and hypertension, both intraoperatively and in the immediate postoperative period, are common (30–35%), and strict control of blood pressure is required throughout to reduce the incidence of neurological deficit (1–7% regardless of whether local or general anaesthesia is used). Preoperative hypertension, pain, agitation, confusion and a new neurological deficit are all valid explanations for unstable BP in the early postoperative period. Intraoperatively, the likeliest hypothesis for unstable blood pressure centres on carotid manipulation from either cross-clamping of the artery or dissection around the carotid sinus. The former can disrupt the carotid baroreceptor reflex, while the latter results in transmission of impulses to the vasomotor centre which stimulates vagal efferent activity, causing vasodilatation and bradycardia. Another possible explanation could be vasoconstriction in the contralateral artery with inhibition of vagal activity via the brainstem. Some attempt may be made to attenuate the BP response by infiltrating the carotid sinus with local anaesthetic. Blood loss resulting in hypovolaemia can also cause hypotension. Chemoreceptor damage affects ventilatory responses, not blood pressure. (See: Garrioch MA, Fitch W (1993) Anaesthesia for carotid artery surgery. *British Journal of Anaesthesia* **71**, 569–579. Also: White JS *et al.* (1981) Morbidity and mortality of carotid endarterectomy. *Archives of Surgery* **116**, 409–413.)

1.43 A.F **B.**F **C.**T **D.**T **E.**T
Non-invasive blood pressure (NIBP) machines inflate a cuff above systolic pressure and, during incremental deflation, pressure fluctuations within the cuff are sensed by an electronic transducer. Systolic and mean blood pressures are taken to be the beginning of the point of maximum amplitude and the lowest pressure where maximum amplitude is maintained, respectively. Diastolic pressure is derived from these figures. Such monitors do tend to over-read at high pressures and under-read at low pressures. A short cuff over-reads, as does a narrow cuff (too wide a cuff may give low readings). Recommendations for an adult suggest the cuff should be 14 cm wide, cover two-thirds of the upper arm or be 20% greater than arm diameter, and 36 cm long. Machines rely heavily on a regular cardiac cycle to compare systolic pulsations and it may be difficult to obtain consistent values with AF or any other cardiac arrhythmia.

1.44 A.T **B.**T **C.**T **D.**T **E.**F
Isoprenaline is a synthetic catecholamine with non-selective β adrenoceptor action. It is predominantly a chronotrope but also has some inotropic action. As the tachycardia is achieved at the expense of increased myocardial oxygen consumption, its use is now reserved for short-term management of bradyarrhythmias, particularly those associated with atrioventricular (AV) block. It is also an effective bronchodilator. However, its use in asthmatics was associated with an increase in sudden death thought to be due, in part, to its arrhythmogenic potential. As such, it has long been abandoned in favour of safer and equally effective drugs. Hypotension may also result from isoprenaline-induced peripheral vasodilatation. One question in the final FRCA has been whether the effect of isoprenaline is decreased by the concomitant administration of propranolol, nifedipine, guanethidine, methyldopa or trimetaphan. I shall leave you to find the correct answers!

1.45 **A**.T **B**.F **C**.T **D**.T **E**.F

Complications from CRF affect every system in the body. Polyuria and nocturia result from inability to concentrate urine. Hypochromic anaemia arises from bone marrow depression, low erythropoietin production, shortened red cell survival and increased blood loss (gut or haemodialysis). A uraemic autonomic neuropathy responsible for postural hypotension occurs late in the course of the disease, as˙does a mixed peripheral neuropathy; both can improve with dialysis. Other problems include peptic ulceration, metabolic acidosis, myopathy, endocrine dysfunction (particularly thyroid), atherosclerosis, hypertension, and impairment of cellular and humoral immunity. Splenomegaly would be coincidental. Poor diabetic control causes renal failure.

1.46 **A**.T **B**.T **C**.F **D**.F **E**.T

The main causes of a low arterial oxygen saturation (P_aO_2) (hypoxaemia) include:

1. a low inspired oxygen concentration, e.g. high altitude
2. alveolar hypoventilation, e.g. excess opiates, neuromuscular diseases, e.g. myasthenia gravis
3. increased ventilation/perfusion mismatch, e.g. pneumonia
4. increased shunting, e.g. pulmonary oedema
5. diffusion abnormality with limitation of transfer of oxygen through the alveolar capillary membrane, e.g. fibrosing alveolitis

All but hypoventilation are associated with a normal P_aCO_2 level. All but increased shunting will respond to oxygen therapy. Hypoxaemia below 9 kPa stimulates the peripheral chemoreceptors to increase ventilation although overall changes in carbon dioxide and hydrogen ion concentration have a greater influence. Peripheral vasodilatation is due to hypercapnia. A low oxygen saturation causes hypoxic pulmonary vasoconstriction. Polycythaemia rubra vera is a myeloproliferative disorder resulting in an increased red cell mass and therefore greater oxygen-carrying capacity.

1.47 **A**.F **B**.F **C**.T **D**.F **E**.T

The GCS is a scoring system initially devised for assessing patients 6 hours or more after a head injury but its use has been extended to include other causes of coma. Changes in scores over time are more useful than single values. Brainstem function (pupillary reactions, corneal reflexes, oculovestibular response, etc.) is best assessed using brainstem death criteria. A GCS score of 8 or less indicates a severe head injury requiring intubation and moderate hyperventilation. Children under 5 years of age cannot score normally for verbal and motor responses and, despite modifications to the GCS, doubts remain as to its accuracy and reproducibility. The range is from 3 to 15, with points distributed as follows:

Eye opening	spontaneous	4
	to speech	3
	to pain	2
Best verbal response	orientated	5
	confused	4
	inappropriate	3
	incomprehensible	2
	nil	1
	intubated	T
Best motor response	obeys commands	6
	localizes to pain	5
	withdraws to pain	4
	abnormal flexion	3
	extensor response	2
	nil	1

(See: Teasdale G, Jennett B (1977) Assessment of coma and impaired consciousness. *Lancet* **ii**, 81–84. Also: Reilly PL *et al.* (1988) Assessing the conscious level in infants and young children: a paediatric version of the Glasgow Coma Scale. *Childs Nervous System* **4**, 30–33.)

1.48 A.F B.T C.F D.T E.T
SGB aims to block the outflow from the upper four to six thoracic and lower cervical sympathetic ganglia. It is of diagnostic and therapeutic value in Raynaud's syndrome, hyperhidrosis, reflex sympathetic dystrophy (RSD) and phantom limb pain, amongst others. The presence of ipsilateral Horner's syndrome (ptosis, miosis, enophthalmos, anhidrosis) and venous engorgement of the hand suggest a successful block. Complications include subarachnoid and intravascular injection, pneumothorax and paralysis of recurrent laryngeal nerve leading to hoarseness, subglottic loss of sensation and difficulty in swallowing.

1.49 A.T   B.F   C.F   D.F   E.T

Nitric oxide (NO) is produced by nitric oxide synthetase in vascular endothelium using the amino acid L-arginine as substrate. It acts on guanylate cyclase to convert cGMP from GTP to effect smooth muscle relaxation and vasodilatation. Endogenous NO has been implicated in the pathogenesis of many diseases including hypertension, coronary artery disease and SIRS. However, its therapeutic value is based on inhaled NO acting as a specific pulmonary vasodilator, decreasing pulmonary vascular resistance and pulmonary artery pressure. Given in this way systemic effects are minimal as NO combines readily with haemoglobin to give a short half-life of 5 s. It has been used with some success in pulmonary hypertension of varying aetiology including acute lung injury (where hypoxic pulmonary vasoconstriction causes pulmonary hypertension) and persistent pulmonary hypertension of the newborn. It also has some bronchodilator action and, although not as potent as salbutamol, it may be useful in treating asthma and bronchospasm. It has been difficult to determine its overall value as its use has been associated with a marked and often unpredictable variation in its effect, both among different patients and within the same patient at different times of the underlying illness. Doses range from 5–80 ppm. Tachyphlaxis has not been observed even if NO is continued for several weeks. NO is toxic (common constituent of cigarette smoke) as are its by-products nitrogen dioxide and peroxynitrite ($OONO^-$). Levels of NO and N_2O must be measured regularly. NO should be less than 25 ppm and N_2O should be <5 ppm. Methaemaglobinaemia is also a potential problem requiring daily measurement. (See: Kam PCA, Govender G (1994) Nitric Oxide: basic science and clinical applications. *Anaesthesia* **49**, 515–521.)

1.50 A.F   B.T   C.F   D.F   E.F

About 99% of testicular tumours are malignant, and seminomas account for 40%. They are rare before puberty and tend to occur in the 35- to 45-year-old age group. They tend to be locally invasive with metastases predominantly from lymphatic spread. Following orchidectomy radiotherapy is standard, the amount and distribution being dependent on disease staging. The commonest presentation is accidental discovery of a hard mass which is rarely painful. The 5-year survival rate for seminomas is 95% without metastases, 75% with. The cure rate for teratomas is improving but is not as good, standing at 85%

and 60%, respectively. Non-seminomatous tumours secrete HCG and this is a useful guide to disease progression.

1.51 A.F **B.**T **C.**F **D.**F **E.**T

Enoximone and milrinone belong to a heterogeneous group of drugs which act by selective inhibition of type III phosphodiesterase isoenzyme found specifically in the myocardium, smooth muscle and platelets. They exert a positive inotropic action by enhancing cAMP activity leading to an increase in intracellular calcium levels. This in theory improves cardiac output by increasing stroke volume but without significant tachycardia or much increase in myocardial oxygen demand. They also reduce systemic vascular resistance by vasodilatation. Sustained haemodynamic benefits have been seen in some patients with acute heart failure after myocardial infarction. Unfortunately their action in chronic heart failure refractory to other therapies (e.g. angiotensin converting enzyme (ACE) inhibitors) has been disappointing, with little evidence of an overall reduction in mortality. The vasodilatory action may precipitate or worsen systemic hypotension so these drugs are relatively contraindicated in hypotensive patients. Their use has been further compromised by other side-effects including tachyarrhythmias, nausea and vomiting, oliguria and limb pain. (See: Skoyles JR, Sherry KM (1992) Pharmacology, mechanisms of action and uses of selective phosphodiesterase inhibitors. *British Journal of Anaesthesia* **68**, 293–302.)

1.52 A.F **B.**F **C.**T **D.**T **E.**F

Sickle cell disease is an autosomal recessive condition arising from the substitution of valine for glutamine in the 6th position of the beta globin chain. Hb SS is the homozygote form which usually manifests itself when Hb F decreases to adult levels at about 6 months of age. Symptoms vary from a mild to a severe haemolytic anaemia in combination with a variable number of recurrent severe painful crises arising from occlusion of small vessels by sickled cells. This can typically result in bone pain, pleurisy, haematuria from renal papillary necrosis, convulsion from cerebral involvement, and splenic and liver infarcts. Infection, dehydration, cold, acidosis and hypoxia are the main precipitating factors. Long-term problems include susceptibility to infections, particularly *Streptococcus pneumoniae* (meningitis or pneumonia), as well as leg ulcers, gallstones, aseptic bone necrosis (commonly of the femoral heads), blindness due to retinal detachment and proliferative retinopathy, and chronic renal failure. Hb S releases oxygen to the tissues more easily than normal Hb (i.e. oxyhaemoglobin dissociation curve moves to the *right*). The heterogeneity of the disease means anaemia may be minimal although it is usually in the order of 6–8 g/dl with a high reticulocyte count at 10–20%. Haemoglobin electrophoresis confirms the diagnosis by absence of Hb A, presence of 80–95% Hb SS and 2–20% Hb F. Management includes avoiding precipitating factors and supportive treatment during a crisis with intravenous fluids, oxygen, antibiotics and adequate analgesia. Prior to surgery, reducing Hb S to about 20% by transfusion reduces the potential for adverse sequelae.

1.53 A.T B.T C.F D.F E.F
Syntocinon is a synthetic preparation of oxytocin, a posterior pituitary hormone causing uterine contraction. It is a nonapeptide differing from vasopressin (ADH) in only two of its nine amino acids. Syntocinon is used clinically in obstetrics as an infusion to increase force and frequency of uterine contractions, either for induction (following spontaneous or deliberate rupture of the membranes) or augmentation of labour. It has a direct but transient action on vascular smooth muscle resulting in flushing, hypotension and reflex tachycardia, which may, rarely, lead to myocardial ischaemia. The main concerns with its use include the potential for fetal hypoxia and uterine rupture. It is therefore mandatory to monitor both fetal activity and heart rate. If uterine resting tone increases, or contractions are too frequent or forceful, or there is evidence of fetal distress, the infusion must be discontinued immediately. Particular care is needed with its use in women of high parity or with a history of Caesarean section. Not surprisingly, it has an antidiuretic action which may lead to water intoxication when given in excess. Nausea and vomiting are unlikely, as is respiratory arrest, although they have been documented and were thought to be due to an anaphylactoid response. Half-life is 12–17 min.

1.54 A.F B.T C.F D.T E.T
The PNS consists of long myelinated preganglionic fibres which pass directly to ganglia on their target organ, which in turn synapse with short postganglionic fibres. This limits their action to a small area (the reverse is true for sympathetic

fibres). Acetylcholine is the neurotransmitter at nicotinic (ganglia) and muscarinic (postganglionic) synapses. Parasympathetic outflow is associated with cranial nerves (III, VII, IX, X) and via S2–S4 spinal routes. Actions mediated by PNS include miosis, ciliary contraction, lacrimal secretion, bradycardia, vasodilatation, bronchoconstriction, increased gastrointestinal motility, relaxation of sphincters, bladder contraction, detrusor relaxation, penile erection and increased sweating. Three types of muscarinic receptor exist: M1 occurs in the brain and gastric parietal cells; M2 in the heart; and M3 in smooth muscle and glands. Clinically useful muscarinic agonists and antagonists show little selectivity for the different subtypes.

1.55 A.T B.T C.F D.T E.F
The trigeminal (Vth cranial) nerve arises from the Gasserian ganglion in the middle cranial fossa. The sensory root divides into three. The *ophthalmic* passes through the superior orbital fissure to supply the forehead, nose and upper jaw. The *maxillary* passes through the foramen rotundum to supply lower eyelids, cheek and upper jaw. The largest, the *mandibular* nerve, supplies lower jaw, chin, mandibular and temporal regions. There is only one small motor root which joins the mandibular nerve to supply the muscles of mastication. The angle of the jaw is supplied by the second cervical nerve (C2) of the cervical plexus. The tympanic membrane is supplied by branches from the mandibular, vagus and glossopharyngeal nerves.

1.56 A.T B.T C.F D.F E.F
Near-drowning is a common problem and 1500 deaths are estimated to occur in the UK each year (150 000 worldwide). Over 50% of cases are aged under 20 years. Hypoxaemia and metabolic acidosis are the commonest sequelae but whereas hypertonic seawater draws fluid from plasma to the alveoli (which can lead to hypovolaemia), hypotonic freshwater rapidly enters the circulation and inactivates surfactant to cause alveolar collapse. In either situation an ARDS-type picture can develop. Electrolyte abnormalities do occur but are rare as large amounts of fresh- or seawater have to be aspirated before they occur (unless the victim is unlucky enough to be in the Dead Sea) – similarly for haemolysis with freshwater aspiration. Renal function is rarely impaired

although acute tubular necrosis has been noted. A wide range of arrhythmias have been observed which are largely related to the degree of hypothermia. Bradycardia is the most frequent but ventricular fibrillation (hyperkalaemia from haemolysis) from freshwater aspiration is also a possibility. The correct immediate management is vital to survival and involves basic resuscitation – establishing a clear airway and giving mouth-to-mouth resuscitation and external cardiac massage as required. Hospital care centres on providing continuing respiratory and cardiovascular support. Neither steroids nor prophylactic antibiotics are recommended. Despite aggressive measures to treat neurological damage, one-third of the children who arrive at hospital comatose die, one-third survive with permanent brain damage and one-third have no long-lasting sequelae. (See: Golden F St. C, Tiplon MJ, Scott RC (1997) Immersion, near drowning and drowning. *British Journal of Anaesthesia* **79**, 214–225.)

1.57 A.T   **B.**T   **C.**F   **D.**T   **E.**T
Patients with a heart valve lesion, septal defect or a patent ductus should be given prophylactic antibiotics for dental (extractions, scaling and surgery involving gingival tissues), upper respiratory tract and genitourinary procedures. Patients with a prosthetic valve or a history of endocarditis are 'special risk' and should also have antibiotics for all of the above, as well as for obstetric, gynaecological and gastrointestinal procedures and when foreign material is implanted, e.g. joint replacements. Normal practice is either an oral, intravenous or intramuscular dose of amoxycillin 1 hour prior to induction, followed by a second oral dose 6 hours later. Gentamicin is usually added at induction if at 'special risk'. If the patient is allergic to penicillin or has received more than a single dose of penicillin in the previous month, vancomycin with gentamicin, clindamycin or teicoplanin can be used. Cataract extraction does not require prophylactic antibiotics. (See: Recommendations of the Working Party of the British Society for Antimicrobial Chemotherapy (1982) *Lancet* **ii**, 1323–1326. Also: (1993) *Journal of Antimicrobial Chemotherapy* **31**, 437–438; or any current copy of the *British National Formulary* (*BNF*) under 'prophylactic antibiotics'.)

1.58 A.F B.F C.F D.T E.T

SI units of measurement were introduced in 1960. The seven base units include:

length	– metre (m)
mass	– kilogram (kg)
time	– second (s)
current	– ampere (A)
temperature	– Kelvin (K)
luminous intensity	– candela (cd)
amount of substance	– mole (mol)

Some of the derived units are:

temperature	– degrees Celsius (°C)
force	– Newton (N)
pressure	– pascal (Pa)
energy	– joule (J)
power	– watt (W)
frequency	– hertz (Hz)

A few unofficial units are still in common use, e.g. energy (calorie = 4.18 J) and pressure (mmHg and bar), with 7.5 mmHg = 1 kilopascal, 1 bar = 100 kilopascals or 750 mmHg.

1.59 A.F B.T C.T D.F E.T

Lung damage from acid aspiration is proportional to the volume and pH of the aspirate. There is a danger of severe chemical pneumonia if the aspirate exceeds 0.4 ml/kg and/or the pH is <2.5. There is a 100% mortality with an aspirate of pH <1.8. Bacterial pneumonitis is unlikely in the initial stages as aspirate is normally sterile due to the low pH. With time, secondary airway colonization of the damaged lung tends to occur. When aspiration is severe, vagally mediated broncho-spasm resulting in wheezing occurs immediately, followed within minutes by damage to the alveolar epithelium, and ultimately atelectasis from surfactant inactivation. Fluid and protein leak into alveoli and bronchi to produce non-cardiogenic pulmonary oedema and a decrease in lung compliance. Alveolar consolidation and hyaline membrane formation occur within the following 48 hours. Clinically, there is dyspnoea, wheezing and hypoxaemia often accompanied by hypovolaemia and hypotension. Chest radiographs show diffuse bilateral pulmonary infiltrates frequently indistinguish-able from ARDS (aspiration is responsible for up to 25% of all cases of ARDS). Sepsis, multiple organ failure and mortality are high (25–100%).

1.60 A.F B.F C.T D.T E.T

Renal cell carcinomas arise from proximal tubular epithelium and are the commonest renal tumour in adults. The average age of presentation is 55 years, and is rare under 40 years. Tumours are either solitary or multiple, and only infrequently bilateral. Local spread invades renal veins and lymph nodes which often leads to solitary metastases in liver, bone and lungs. The latter are occasionally picked up on a chest radiograph as the first presenting feature. Presenting features are often non-specific and include malaise, anorexia, weight loss and, in about 20%, pyrexia. More specific findings include haematuria, loin pain, mass in the flank and polycythaemia. Diagnosis can be confirmed by a combination of excretion urography, ultrasound and computerized tomography (CT), although magnetic resonance imaging (MRI) is proving to be better than CT for tumour staging. Urine cytology is of no value. Surgery is the treatment of choice, even in the presence of metastases, as their regression has been noted with removal of the primary tumour. Medroxyprogesterone acetate is of some value in controlling metastatic disease and interferon-α produces a 20% response rate in the short term. Prognosis depends on the degree of differentiation and presence of metastases (about 25% at diagnosis). The 5-year survival rate is 60–70% if the tumour is confined to the renal parenchyma, 15–35% with lymph node involvement, and only 5% if distant metastases are present.

1.61 A.T B.T C.F D.F E.T

A normal chest radiograph should be centred with medial ends of clavicles equidistant from the vertebral spinous processes at the T4–5 level. The vertebral bodies and disc spaces should be just visible through the cardiac shadow. On full inspiration the anterior ends of the 6th ribs and posterior ends of the tenth are above the diaphragm. Two-thirds of the cardiac shadow lies to the left of the midline, one-third to the right, and cardiothoracic ratio should not exceed 50% or 16 cm (15 cm for women). Hilar lymph nodes are not visible unless pathological. The right frontal fissure is visible on a PA film but oblique fissures are seen only in lateral view. The right hemidiaphragm is higher because the heart depresses the left – not because the liver pushes up the right.

1.62 A.T **B**.T **C**.T **D**.T **E**.T

Type I is immediate (anaphylactic) hypersensitivity. It occurs clinically when an allergen such as a drug (or any foreign protein or carbohydrate) combines covalently with normal plasma and tissue proteins to form an antigenic complex. This stimulates production of IgE which then binds to and sensitizes mast cells and, to a lesser extent, eosinophils, basophils and macrophages. Subsequent exposure can result in cross-linking of IgE antibodies or binding of allergen to sensitized cells to cause degranulation and release of inflammatory mediators including histamine, prostaglandins, leukotrienes, kinins, etc. It covers a wide range of severity from minor hay fever and urticaria to asthma and systemic anaphylaxis. *Type II* cytotoxic hypersensitivity has IgG and IgM antibodies forming a complex with antigens in the tissues or on cell surfaces to effect lysis (e.g. incompatible blood transfusion and autoimmune diseases). *Type III* are immune complex reactions when IgG and IgM combine with soluble antigen and resultant complexes are deposited in blood vessel walls, joints and the glomerulus. These are the basis of some systemic diseases including glomerulonephritis and rheumatoid arthritis. *Type IV* are cell-mediated delayed hypersensitivity reactions when antigens combine with specific T lymphocytes which then recruit other cell types, including macrophages, to the site of reaction. Type IV reactions are responsible for contact hypersensitivity, granulomatous disease and some immune-mediated food intolerance such as intolerance to cow's milk.

1.63 A.F **B**.T **C**.T **D**.F **E**.T

Hypokalaemia alters the intracellular:extracellular potassium gradient (which maintains the resting membrane potential at around -90 mV). This hyperpolarizes the cell membrane, making it more resistant to depolarization by acetylcholine and thus more sensitive to the effect of non-depolarizing muscle relaxants. Magnesium produces a dose-dependent presynaptic inhibition of neurotransmitter release in peripheral nerves due to competition with calcium for membrane channels on the presynaptic terminal. In this way, both hypermagnesaemia and hypocalcaemia can cause significant neuromuscular blockade (NMB), to potentiate and prolong the duration of non-depolarizing NMBs. Although tetracyclines, aminoglycosides and clindamycin can produce NMB in their own right, this is unusual unless there is an underlying neuromuscular disease.

They are more likely to cause an increased sensitivity to muscle relaxants. The mechanism of action is complex and not fully elucidated but may be related to a reduction in release of acetylcholine or a decrease in sensitivity of the nicotinic receptor. Plasma glucose level has no effect on recovery from NMB.

1.64 A.F B.T C.T D.T E.T
Paracetamol poisoning is responsible for approximately 7% of all deaths and 15% of all admissions for drug overdose. On average, 10–15 g are needed but poisoning can occur with 5 g. Normally, paracetamol metabolites are inactivated by conjugation with glutathione. In most cases of overdose, patients recover fully but occasionally toxic paracetamol metabolites overwhelm hepatic glutathione reserves and bind to sulphydryl groups in liver macromolecules to produce centrilobular liver necrosis 3–4 days after ingestion. Renal tubular necrosis can also occur even in the absence of liver failure. The only early symptoms are nausea and vomiting. Loss of consciousness comes with development of hepatic encephalopathy. Treatment depends on the time interval between ingestion and presentation. Between 4 and 16 hours after ingestion the paracetamol level can be referred to a graph of log concentration against time to determine whether hepatic toxicity is likely (anything above 200 mg/l at 4 hours to 50 mg/l at 12 hours). Gastric lavage should be considered within 4 hours of ingestion but the best treatment is to increase glutathione availability by giving an acetylcysteine infusion (oral methionine is unreliable if vomiting occurs). This should be given as soon as possible, even before blood levels are known and certainly within 8 hours of ingestion for maximum benefit. If this is not possible, some benefit may be seen up to and over 24 hours after overdose, particularly if there is any evidence of encephalopathy. Pregnant women should be treated the same way as neither acetylcysteine nor methionine are fetotoxic. Some patients (e.g. chronic alcoholics and those taking enzyme-inducing drugs such as phenytoin) are at greater risk of liver damage and should be treated at concentrations of paracetamol half as great as those indicated on the nomogram. Outcome is poor if international normalized ratio (INR) >3, serum creatinine raised, blood pH <7.3 at 36 hours after ingestion. Liver transplantation may be necessary.

1.65 A.F **B**.T **C**.F **D**.F **E**.T

Blood to the coronary arteries flows mainly in diastole. In systole the left ventricle is at a higher pressure than the aorta and little flow can occur. The autonomic nervous system plays little part in coronary blood flow and any increase principally relies upon a build-up of locally produced metabolites (lactate, bradykinin, prostaglandins, adenosine, etc.) to produce vaso-dilatation. Myocardial cells hypertrophy (increase in size, not number) with increasing load. An increase in stroke volume is dependent on increasing ventricular contractility during systole. This in turn depends on an increase in end diastolic volume (Starling's law of the heart whereby increasing volume of the blood in the ventricle results in a more forceful contraction) and increased sympathetic activity. As vagal stimulation decreases ventricular contractility, stroke volume will fall. When conduction from the atria to the ventricles is completely interrupted, as with infarction of the AV node, the atria continue to beat independently at the normal sinus rate but the ventricular rate is usually 25–50 beats per minute and complete or third-degree heart block is said to be present.

1.66 A.T **B**.T **C**.T **D**.T **E**.T

Complete heart block occurs when normal AV conduction fails so the atria and ventricles beat independently. It is most commonly found in the elderly as a result of idiopathic fibrosis of the bundles of His. Other underlying causes include congenital heart disease (e.g. transposition of the great arteries) after an inferior myocardial infarction and rheumatic fever. Ventricular contractions of 25–50 beats per minute are maintained by a spontaneous escape rhythm initiated by a ventricular myocardial cell below the level of the block. The ECG will show regular P waves and QRS complexes occurring independently of each other. The duration of the QRS complexes depends on the site of the block and the position of the ventricular pacemaker. If the block is high enough the idioventricular impulse can follow the normal pathway to allow the QRS complex to be of normal duration (< 0.12 s). If not, the QRS complex will be prolonged. The pulse is regular and does not vary with exercise, resulting in a decreased exercise tolerance as well as periods of dizziness and syncopal (Stokes–Adams) attacks. To compensate, stroke volume usually in-creases and a large volume pulse and systolic flow murmurs are present. Canon waves may be visible in the neck and the intensity of the first heart sound varies owing to the loss of AV synchrony.

1.67 A.T **B.**F **C.**T **D.**T **E.**F

The dose of amiodarone needs to be decreased when used in combination with warfarin (inhibits its metabolism) and digoxin (reduces renal clearance to increase half-life) but increased with phenytoin. Trimethoprim and sulphamethoxazole comprise co-trimoxazole (ratio 1:5). They act synergistically by blocking sequential steps in the production of tetrahydrofolate, essential for bacterial replication. It is now reserved for *Pneumocystis carnii* pneumonia owing to adverse drug reactions from the sulphonamide component. Aminoglycosides produce neuromuscular blockade by competing with calcium ions thereby inhibiting release of acetylcholine at preganglionic terminals. This action can be antagonized by calcium salts. Tetracyclines and polymixins also prolong blockade. Propranolol, as a non-selective β_2 adrenoceptor antagonist, will block sympathetically mediated tachycardia, a sign of impending hypoglycaemia in diabetics. Monoamine oxidase inhibitors (MAOIs), e.g. tranylcypromine, irreversibly inhibit the action of monoamine oxidase, important for the breakdown of catecholamines and 5-hydroxytryptamine (5-HT). When combined with pethidine excessive central activity of 5-HT can occur, which may result in hyperpyrexia, neurological and cardiovascular collapse. Fentanyl and phenoperidine are structurally related to pethidine but are considered safe, although morphine has been suggested as the opioid of choice.

1.68 A.T **B.**T **C.**T **D.**F **E.**T

Fasting glucose in pregnancy is below that of a non-pregnant individual (as the fetus utilizes maternal glucose) so a random glucose level of >6.0 mmol/l or >9.0 mmol/l 2 hours after a 75 g glucose load suggests GDM. Care should be taken with timing of the screening as glucose tolerance varies with gestation and may improve in the first half of pregnancy. Microalbuminuria can be detected by radioimmunoassay above 30 mg/day but significant proteinuria in diabetes occurs at >50 g/day. Diabetic ketoacidosis with hyperventilation could explain the low $P_a\text{co}_2$. The incidence of GDM in Europe is 1–2%; risk factors include obesity and a positive family history. It is seldom symptomatic, so screening is essential. Normoglycaemia should be attempted in the first instance by diet, although insulin is often required.

The condition resolves on delivery but 50% present within 5 years with overt diabetes. (See: Mazze RS, Krogh MD (1992) Gestational diabetes mellitus: now is the time for detection and treatment. *Mayo Clinic Proceedings* **67**, 995–1002.)

1.69 A.F B.F C.F D.T E.T
An IABP was first used in 1968. It is a sausage-shaped balloon which is inserted either via the femoral artery or via the ascending aorta to lie just distal to the left subclavian artery. Early in diastole the balloon is rapidly inflated so that the pressure in the aortic root rises and coronary blood flow increases. Not surprisingly, this leads to an increase in diastolic pressure which can be as much as 90%. Rapid deflation, triggered by the R wave to occur at the onset of systole, creates an instant pressure drop in the proximal aorta facilitating left ventricular emptying. This reduction in afterload leads to a decrease in left ventricular end-diastolic pressure, stroke work and myocardial oxygen requirement. This results in an increase in cardiac output between 20% and 50%. An IABP is used preoperatively to support patients with cardiogenic shock who have a surgically correctable condition, e.g. postmyocardial infarction, ventricular septal defect (VSD) or acute mitral regurgitation, and postoperatively it can be helpful in weaning patients from cardiopulmonary bypass.

1.70 A.F B.F C.T D.F E.T
The vagus nerve supplies the larynx, trachea and bronchi via its superior and recurrent laryngeal branches. The SLN divides into an external laryngeal nerve which provides motor function to the cricothyroid muscle and an internal branch which provides sensation to the epiglottis, aryepiglottic folds and larynx down to the vocal cords. The recurrent laryngeal nerve supplies motor function to all the muscles of the larynx except the cricothyroid, as well as sensation below the cords and into the trachea and bronchi. The SLN can be blocked percutaneously at the inferior border of the hyoid bone. The internal branch of the SLN can be blocked by applying LA to the piriform fossa. The trachea can be anaesthetized by injecting LA through the cricothyroid membrane. The recurrent laryngeal nerve can be blocked at any level below the cricoid cartilage. As the cricothyroid muscle tenses the vocal cords, it does need to be blocked to achieve paralysis.

1.71 A.T **B.**T **C.**T **D.**T **E.**F

Atrial flutter normally has a fast atrial discharge at about 300 per min compensated by a 4:1 or 2:1 AV block to give a ventricular rate of 75–150 per min. The pulse is normally regular. The ECG shows a saw-tooth pattern ('f' waves) instead of a straight isoelectric line between QRS complexes. The commonest cause is ischaemic heart disease but other causes include mitral valve disease, hyperthyroidism, cardiomyopathy and acute hypovolaemia. For effective management all must be excluded and/or treated. Most patients will return to sinus rhythm after low-energy DC (i.e. current delivery synchronized to occur with the R wave as delivery during ventricular repolarization may produce ventricular tachycardia (VT)) cardioversion. If this fails, rapid atrial pacing of about 20–30% over the atrial rate may work. Drug therapy is aimed at reducing AV node conduction. Digoxin is the drug of choice in the hope that it may induce atrial fibrillation. Sinus rhythm may then be restored on digoxin withdrawal. If atrial flutter persists with digoxin, chronic prophylaxis with verapamil and disopyramide can be considered, although amiodarone may be more effective for otherwise refractory cases.

1.72 A.F **B.**T **C.**T **D.**F **E.**F

The brachial plexus arises from C5–T1 spinal nerve roots. There are four main approaches for blocking: interscalene, supraclavicular, infraclavicular (least used) and axillary. Each has its own advantages and disadvantages. The supraclavicular route is the most reliable in providing anaestheia for all branches of the plexus as the LA is injected where the plexus is most compactly arranged. For the same reason, the volume of LA needed is less and the onset time is faster compared with the other approaches. The axillary approach is best reserved for hand surgery because the musculocutaneous nerve and (less frequently) the radial nerve can be missed as they leave the perivascular bundle high up in the axilla. Thus, axillary block may fail to anaesthetize the lateral aspect of the forearm. The complication rate is proportional to the inexperience of the operator. The axillary approach is the safest with potential complications minimal with the exception of the suggested transarterial approach. Complications of supraclavicular block include pneumothorax (most commonly), accidental intravascular, epidural or subdural injection, phrenic nerve palsy and Horner's syndrome from sympathetic blockade. The interscalene block is more useful for operations to the shoulder, which can be missed by the supraclavicular approach. (See: Brockway MS, Wildsmith JAW (1990) Axillary brachial plexus block: method of choice? *British Journal of Anaesthesia* **64**, 224–231.)

1.73 A.F B.F C.T D.F E.T
Endotoxins are heat-stable lipopolysaccharides derived from the outer membrane of Gram-negative bacteria. They consist of a lipid moiety (lipid A), a core polysaccharide and an oligosaccharide side chain, which differs considerably between strains and confers O antigen specificity to the molecule. They are released when bacteria die and activate lymphocytes, macrophages and endothelium to produce cytokines such as tumour necrosis factor and interleukin-1. Cytokines, in turn, influence thermoregulation, endocrine function, metabolic responses and immune function and are pivotal in the host response to infection including development of SIRS. Gram-negative bacteria are normally located in the gut, which explains the rationale for trying to preserve splanchnic blood flow in critically ill patients and thus reduce bacteria translocation. *Exotoxins* are heat-labile antigenic proteins produced by microorganisms (bacteria, fungi) which can also be harmful to the host.

1.74 A.F B.F C.F D.T E.F
Phenol is a neurolytic chemical used to interrupt nerve pathways in the treatment of chronic pain conditions particularly when associated with malignant disease. A weak acid, it is used in concentrations of 5–10% in aqueous solution, and dissolved in glycerine for intrathecal use. The hyperbaricity (sp. gr. 1025) means that the patient must lie with the bad side down. The neurolytic effect is more pronounced in the small-diameter, pain-conducting Aδ and C fibres, thus preserving motor function transmitted by relatively larger diameter Aα fibres. An initial LA effect lasts 15–30 min, followed by nerve destruction in nerve roots between the spinal cord and dural cuff. The cord remains undamaged but progressive destruction of the posterior columns has been noted with repeated injections. Less than 0.5% phenol remains after 15 min, and it is then safe to change positions. Alcohol, glycerol and chlorocresol are also used for neurolysis. Treatment of chronic pancreatitis can be: *dietary* (small meals); *pharmacological*, e.g.

omeprazole and H_2 antagonists to reduce acid load to the duodenum pancreatic supplements, antidepressants and non-narcotic analgesics; and *alternative*, e.g. hypnosis, acupuncture and TENS. If pain persists coeliac, but more commonly splanchnic, nerve blocks with a combination of LAs and steroids or neurolytic agents can be performed repeatedly for severe persistent pain including that from carcinoma of the pancreas.

Note: nerve fibres are divided into A, B, C. A fibres are 1–20 μm in diameter and are divided into α, somatic motor and propriosensation; β, touch and pressure sensation; γ, motor to muscle spindles; and δ, pain, cold touch. B fibres are preganglionic autonomic fibres (1–3 μm diameter) and C are unmyelinated postganglionic fibres for pain and temperature sensation (<1 μm diameter).

1.75 A.T B.T C.T D.T E.F

The Fick principle utilizes oxygen consumption. Radionuclide technetium binds to red cells and a gamma camera over the precordium measures the difference in radioactive content during systole and diastole, allowing calculation of ejection fraction and stroke volume; it is rarely used. End-diastolic and end-systolic ventricular diameters can be estimated using echocardiography and converted into stroke volume. Dilution techniques use temperature differences with cold crystalloid or dye such as indocyanine green (safe, short half-life). Methylene blue interferes with saturation monitors. Other possibilities include Doppler ultrasonography, thoracic electrical bioimpedance and cardiac catheterization with angiography.

1.76 A.T B.F C.F D.T E.F

Respiratory failure, typically from bronchiolitis, pneumonia or asthma, is the commonest underlying cause of cardiac arrest in children, circulatory failure from fluid and blood loss or sepsis is the next commonest. A primary cardiac event is rare. Bradycardia leading to asystole is the commonest arrhythmia and hypoxia is the main cause. Thus, following the 'ABC' rule, ventilation and oxygen therapy are essential. The sternal compression to ventilation ratio should be 5 : 1, with a depth of compression of about 3 cm at a rate of 100 per min. Adrenaline is the only drug of proven benefit in cardiac arrest. Initial dose is 0.01 mg/kg (0.1 ml/kg of a 1 : 10 000 solution). Subsequent doses are 0.1 mg/kg. Ventricular fibrillation is an unusual arrhythmia in a child but defibrillation commencing at 2 J/kg, increasing to 4 J/kg after two attempts is the correct management. (See: Zideman D *et al.* (1994) Guidelines for paediatric life support. *Resuscitation* **27**, 91–105.)

1.77 A.T B.T C.T D.F E.T
Normal values are:

right atrial pressure	– 1–6 mmHg.
SVR	– 800–1500 dyne s/cm^5.
pulmonary vascular resistance	– 20–120 dyne s/cm^5.
cardiac index	– 2.5–4.2 l/min/m^2.
mean PAP	– systolic/diastolic 12–30/0.8 mmHg, mean 10–15 mmHg.

Right atrial pressure can be measured in either mmHg or cm H_2O. The conversion factor is 1 mmHg = 1.36 cm H_2O. SVR is the resistance against which the heart pumps and can be calculated using the principle of Ohm's law. Pulmonary vascular resistance is analogous to SVR and can be calculated in the same way although is rarely of use clinically. The cardiac index is the cardiac output corrected for body surface area. PAP is usually about 20% of systemic pressure. Absolute values do vary according to the source used!

1.78 A.F B.T C.T D.F E.T
Cardiac tamponade arises from an increase in intrapericardial pressure from a collection of fluid or blood, which reduces ventricular volume and increases diastolic pressure. This is associated with an increase in right and left atrial pressures. Reduced ventricular filling leads to a reduction in stroke volume, cardiac output and systolic blood pressure. There is a compensatory tachycardia and the combination of a fixed low cardiac output and peripheral vasoconstriction leads to cyanosis and cool peripheries. Other signs include elevation of the venous pressure with a paradoxical rise during inspiration (Kussmaul's sign), soft heart sounds and pulsus paradoxus where there is a large fall in blood pressure during inspiration and when the pulse may also be impalpable. Tamponade occurs with trauma, myocardial rupture, malignancy, connective tissue diseases or can complicate any form of pericarditis.

1.79 A.F B.T C.T D.F E.F
Koilonychia is a spoon-shaped deformity of the nails and is classically associated with iron deficiency anaemia. Dysphagia,

post-cricoid web and iron deficiency anaemia are the principal features of Paterson Kelly syndrome, which in turn can herald an oesophageal malignancy. Repetitive trauma such as vibration is also a cause, e.g. 'rickshaw boys' (toe) nails'. Psoriasis can be associated with onycholysis, pitting and thickening of the nails but not koilonychia.

1.80 A.F **B.**F **C.**T **D.**F **E.**T

Ketamine is a water-soluble, acidic, phencyclidine derivative producing 'dissociative' anaesthesia with amnesia and excellent analgesia. Its analgesic action is thought to be due to its effect on afferent pain pathways in the spinoreticular tracts and the antagonizing action of the excitatory neurotransmitter glutamate on NMDA (*N*-methyl-D-aspartate) receptors. Onset of action is slow (90 s or so). Ketamine causes a tachycardia and hypertension due to CNS action but arrhythmias are uncommon. Respiration is unchanged, and ketamine is the only anaesthetic agent not to affect pulmonary function significantly, i.e. no change in FRC, incidence of atelectasis, etc. Coughing and laryngospasm are rare and as a bronchodilator it is safe to use in asthmatics. Muscle relaxation is poor and involuntary movements commonly occur. Neurologically, ketamine increases intracranial pressure (ICP) and cerebral blood flow (CBF) and so is not recommended in head injuries. Preservation of laryngeal reflexes is not guaranteed and so ketamine cannot be used in patients in danger of aspirating. Its use is limited by emergence phenomena mainly presenting as hallucinations and vivid dreams, which can last more than 24 hours. These are more common in young women but are rare in children and the elderly. Such effects can be modified by concomitant administration of opiates or benzodiazepines and recovery in a quiet area. As it is a potent sialogogue, patients often require concomitant atropine. Severe adverse drug reactions are rare but ketamine can cause skin rashes, nausea and vomiting, and an increase in uterine tone. It undergoes hepatic metabolism to weakly active metabolites and is renally excreted. It is safe with porphyria and, contrary to popular belief, does not increase intraocular pressure. Useful in developing countries, war surgery and in children, notably for burns dressings and radiotherapy. Dose: 2 mg/kg i.v. 5–10 mg/kg i.m. Increasing the dose does not intensify the effect but merely prolongs the duration of action.

1.81 A.F B.F C.F D.F E.F

Classification of ventilators is somewhat arbitrary since they all depend on the same variables of time, pressure, volume and flow. Nevertheless, a pressure-cycled ventilator delivers inspiratory gas until a preset pressure is achieved in the airway resulting in cycling from the inspiratory to the expiratory phase. The flow rate is non-linear because at the start of inspiration airway pressure is low and flow is rapid, but as the pressure within the lungs increases the flow diminishes. As the pressure generated is low, the tidal volume achieved depends on the resistance of the ventilator tubing *and* the patient's respiratory dynamics, such as compliance and airway resistance. Thus, decreased compliance or increased resistance means a given airway pressure will be reached sooner resulting in a smaller tidal volume being delivered before the ventilator cycles to expiration. This makes the ventilator unsuitable for patients with underlying airway narrowing, as seen in asthma or COPD. However, it is ideal for infants or small children as it compensates for the leak around an uncuffed endotracheal tube and limits the risk of barotrauma. A minute volume divider is a volume-controlled ventilator.

1.82 A.F B.T C.T D.T E.T

Stridor is caused by upper airway obstruction and is commonly congenital or infective. Most cases are supraglottic in origin but some originate in the trachea and major bronchi. *Congenital* stridor can be due to craniofacial dysmorphology (Pierre Robin, Treacher Collins, Beckwiths, etc.) or malformation of the larynx (subglottic stenosis, laryngeal web, vocal cord paralysis, etc.). In laryngomalacia stridor is due to weak posterior cricoarytenoid muscles allowing the larynx to be sucked together on inspiration. The stridor appears at or soon after birth, and is often croaking and inspiratory in nature. It is exacerbated by exertion, often settles with rest, and frequently disappears by 2–5 years of age. The main underlying cause of croup laryngotracheobronchitis is parainfluenza virus type 1. Although it is normally self-limiting, stridor at rest indicates severe obstruction requiring hospitalization, nebulized adrenaline and rarely intubation and ventilation. Other infective causes include epiglottitis and diptheria. Inhalation of foreign bodies, postintubation laryngeal trauma (e.g. mechanical, thermal, chemical) and neoplasms are other potential causes. Bronchiolitis, due to respiratory syncytial virus (RSV), does not cause stridor as it involves the lower respiratory tract to produce a cough, tachypnoea, wheezing and occasionally severe respiratory distress.

1.83 A.T **B.**T **C.**T **D.**T **E.**T

Blood loss of >500 ml after vaginal delivery of a baby is considered pathological and requires immediate treatment. Main causes are retained placenta or placental fragments, uterine atony, cervical tears and acute inversion of the uterus. Ergometrine and abdominal massage to stimulate uterine contraction are the first line of management. At the same time, fluid resuscitation and blood cross-matching should be commenced. Initial cardiovascular compensation of blood loss is temporary and when clinical shock develops it is rapid and profound. If initial measures fail, manual removal of the placenta or evacuation of retained products of conception should be performed as soon as possible. This usually requires anaesthesia. If bleeding continues and the uterus remains lax, bimanual compression is indicated with one hand on the abdomen and the other inside the uterus. If this is effective, the pressure is maintained by packing the uterus for at least 24 hours and providing cover with broad-spectrum antibiotics. As a last resort, a hysterectomy may be life-saving. The level of intervention increases sequentially for management of this life-threatening condition (mortality 1.3 in 100 000 deliveries) and must be continued until haemostasis is secured.

1.84 A.T **B.**T **C.**T **D.**T **E.**T

Avogadro's number is the number of particles found in 12 g of carbon and is equal to 6.02×10^{23}, or one mole. One mole of any ideal gas will occupy 22.4 l. *Beer's law* states that the intensity of transmitted light decreases exponentially as concentration of the substance increases. *Lambert's law* states intensity of transmitted light decreases exponentially as distance travelled through the substance increases. 'Other laws' worth remembering include: *Charles's law*, which states that at constant pressure the volume of a given mass of gas varies directly with the absolute temperature. *The third perfect gas law* states that at constant volume the absolute pressure of a given mass of gas varies directly with the absolute temperature. *Henry's law* states that at constant temperature the amount of gas dissolved in a liquid is proportional to the partial pressure of the gas above the liquid.

1.85 A.F **B**.T **C**.T **D**.F **E**.T

Chronic bronchitis is defined as 'sputum production on most days for three consecutive months for more than one year'. It is due to a combination of airway narrowing from hypertrophy of the mucous glands and poor mucous clearance producing airflow obstruction requiring greater expiratory rather than inspiratory effort. *H. influenzae* and *Streptococcus pneumoniae* are commonly isolated from sputum, particularly when it is purulent. Arterial blood gases will initially show hypoxaemia. As the disease progresses a permanent rise in $P_a\text{CO}_2$ and a fall in $P_a\text{O}_2$, reflecting alveolar hypoventilation, occurs. Antibiotics should be given when sputum is purulent. Prophylactic antibiotics are not recommended because of the danger of developing drug resistance. A trial of steroids is often indicated as some patients have an element of reversibility of airway narrowing. They should be continued only if there is >15% improvement in FEV_1 after 2 weeks of treatment with oral prednisolone.

1.86 A.F **B**.F **C**.F **D**.F **E**.F

It is important to have a 'system' for answering this type of question and one of the easiest ways is to do so by exclusion; that is, find a value that does not fit with the suggested possibilities. For example, inappropriate ADH (vasopressin) increases intravascular volume causing a dilutional hyponatraemia *and* hypokalaemia. Fluid overload does the same. Knowing one value does not fit means the answer must be false and it doesn't matter whether there is an acidosis (low bicarbonate) or hypoglycaemia in those conditions. Acute renal failure is slightly more difficult as it can cause hyponatraemia, hyperkalaemia and an acidosis but an association with hypoglycaemia is not well recognized. Chronic liver failure has relatively few electrolyte abnormalities unless decompensation has occurred. Conn's syndrome is an adrenal adenoma resulting in primary hyperaldosteronism. It is a rare syndrome where high aldosterone levels exist independently of the renin–angiotensin syndrome. Conn's syndrome clinically presents with hypertension (<1% of all cases) and predominantly asymptomatic hypokalaemia. The data actually fit Addison's disease or primary hypoadrenalism which results in loss of glucocorticoids, mineralocorticoids and sex steroids.

1.87 A.T B.F C.T D.F E.T

UC and Crohn's disease overlap and a diagnosis of one or the other is not possible in about 10% of cases. Histologically, UC tends to produce superficial inflammation throughout the bowel whilst Crohn's disease is characterized by deep ulcers and fissures. Rectal involvement is almost pathognomonic of UC whilst in Crohn's disease it is rare (although, paradoxically, oral disease is common). UC tends to be associated with sclerosing cholangitis (a progressive narrowing of the bile ducts leading to obstructive jaundice) and carcinoma of the colon. Risk of malignancy is still present even when symptom-free. Anaemia in both UC and Crohn's is usually the normocytic, normochromic of chronic disease but can also be iron deficiency due to bloody diarrhoea. Megaloblastic anaemia is rare even in Crohn's disease with terminal ileum involvement. Pyoderma gangrenosum occurs three times more commonly in UC. It consists of intradermal bullae which coalesce and burst leaving large denuded areas. Other manifestations more typical of UC include pericholangitis and cirrhosis of the liver. Seronegative arthritis, kidney and gall-bladder stones and erythema nodosum are more common in Crohn's disease.

1.88 A.T B.T C.T D.F E.F

A massive transfusion of blood (e.g. whole blood volume in 24 hours) results in increased bleeding as stored blood has few platelets and there is also reduced activity of clotting factors V and VIII. PT and the activated PTT are prolonged but TT (sensitive to fibrinogen deficiency) is normal. Ionized hypocalcaemia and a low serum magnesium arise from the inability to metabolize citrate (preservative in stored blood) rapidly. Hypokalaemia occurs more commonly than hyperkalaemia because the transfused red cells absorb potassium from the plasma. Transfused blood can cause a metabolic alkalosis owing to citrate metabolism generating bicarbonate. Excess lactate, ammonia and hydrogen ion found in transfused blood are usually rapidly buffered, but a metabolic acidosis will result if the patient is not fully resuscitated or is hypotensive, hypothermic or has inadequate liver perfusion. Warmed blood is less likely to give rise to metabolic abnormalities.

1.89 A.T B.F C.T D.T E.T

Symptoms arise from complement activation and intravascular haemolysis of donor cells to produce both haemoglobinaemia and haemoglobinuria. The earliest symptom is fever, which unfortunately cannot be distinguished from an uncomplicated febrile reaction. Urticaria, flushing, headache and rigors are also common. Acute respiratory and/or cardiovascular collapse with or without renal failure (from formation of antigen–antibody complexes rather than free haemoglobin) and DIC may supervene. The clinical picture includes wheezing, hypotension, pulmonary oedema, tachycardia, oliguria and oozing from wounds. The Coombs' test becomes positive because of coating of transfused cells with antibodies. Mortality is related to the volume of mismatched blood given but averages around 20%. Apart from halting the transfusion, treatment includes measures to combat shock, maintain renal function and correction of any coagulopathy.

1.90 A.F B.T C.F D.T E.F
Rotameter is the trade name given to constant flow variable orifice flow meters. They give a continuous indication of gas flow. Each rotameter is calibrated for a specific gas. At the bottom of the rotameter the distance between the bobbin and the glass tube is big enough for the flow to be laminar, obey Poiseuille's law, and viscosity to be important. Density becomes important at higher flow rates. Rotameters are depressed by applied back pressure such as from a ventilator or a nebulizer. They become increasingly inaccurate at low flow rates. A pneumotachograph is a variable pressure drop, fixed orifice flow meter used to record respiratory volume and flow rate. For accuracy flow has to be laminar and gases are heated to prevent condensation from moist gases.

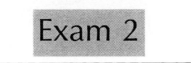

Exam 2

Questions

2.1 **Stroma-free haemoglobins:**
   A. have a half-life greater than 24 hours.
   B. strongly activate complement.
   C. are scavenged by the reticuloendothelial system.
   D. have vasopressor action.
   E. can cause intravascular coagulation.

2.2 **A 2-year-old child presents with fever and limitation of movement and pain in the right hip joint. Possible diagnoses include:**
   A. haemophilia A.
   B. scurvy.
   C. juvenile rheumatoid arthritis.
   D. osteomyelitis.
   E. brucellosis.

2.3 **A fit patient develops a blood pressure of 240/110 during surgery. Appropriate management includes:**
   A. phenoxybenzamine.
   B. labetolol.
   C. increasing inhalational agents.
   D. measurement of vanillylmandelic acid (VMA) levels post-operatively.
   E. abandoning the procedure.

2.4 **Which of the following are true:**
   A. a cystic hygroma may be transilluminated.
   B. the commonest bladder malignancy is a transitional cell tumour.
   C. maldescended testes can be found in the perineum.
   D. the appendix is rarely retrocaecal.
   E. the commonest bone to be fractured in the wrist is the scaphoid.

2.5   **A confused 60-year-old man has the following arterial blood gases (ABGs):**

P_aO_2 7.5 kPa,
P_aCO_2 7.5 kPa,
Hb   16.9 g/dl.

These values are compatible with:
A.   type 1 respiratory failure.
B.   the presence of central cyanosis.
C.   pulmonary embolus.
D.   central depression of respiration.
E.   oxygen therapy.

2.6   **Cytokines:**
A.   are glycoproteins.
B.   include tumour necrosis factor (TNF).
C.   are released from macrophages.
D.   have autocrine function.
E.   mediate development of systemic inflammatory response syndrome (SIRS).

2.7   **Transdermal absorption is possible with:**
A.   atropine.
B.   hyoscine.
C.   morphine.
D.   fentanyl.
E.   paracetamol.

2.8   **The Goldman cardiac risk index gives a score for:**
A.   atrial fibrillation.
B.   hypertension.
C.   hypokalaemia.
D.   previous cardiac surgery.
E.   recent myocardial infarction (MI).

2.9   **The trachea in the adult:**
A.   is 1.5–2.0 cm wide.
B.   begins at the level of the 4th cervical vertebra.
C.   bifurcates at the 6th thoracic vertebra.
D.   is lined with transitional epithelium.
E.   receives most of its blood supply from the bronchial arteries.

2.10 Intestinal carcinoid is associated with:
  A. aortic valve lesions.
  B. severe flushing.
  C. urine turning pink on standing.
  D. constipation.
  E. hyperpyrexia.

2.11 Which of the following anaesthetic breathing systems requires a fresh gas flow (FGF) in excess of minute ventilation to prevent rebreathing during spontaneous ventilation:
  A. Mapleson A.
  B. Mapleson C.
  C. Mapleson D.
  D. Mapleson F.
  E. Humphrey ADE.

2.12 A prolapsed intravertebral disc causing right-sided sciatica:
  A. can result in loss of tendon reflex in the right knee.
  B. can cause loss of sensation over the medial side of the calf.
  C. requires urgent surgical intervention if there is rapid onset of urinary retention.
  D. is best treated by bedrest.
  E. can cause a foot drop.

2.13 A low fixed cardiac output is a feature of:
  A. constrictive pericarditis.
  B. cor pulmonale.
  C. aortic stenosis.
  D. cardiac tamponade.
  E. aortic regurgitation.

2.14 Ondansetron:
  A. can be given orally.
  B. causes diarrhoea with chronic use.
  C. stimulates the chemoreceptor trigger zone.
  D. can cause cardiac arrhythmias.
  E. has active metabolites.

2.15 Pregnanolone:
   A. is insoluble in water.
   B. is a steroid.
   C. causes pain on injection.
   D. is less potent than propofol.
   E. is associated with significant hypotension.

2.16 Insulin-dependent diabetes mellitus (IDDM) may be associated with:
   A. decreased insulin requirement in pregnancy.
   B. retinal haemorrhages.
   C. postural hypotension.
   D. renal papillary necrosis.
   E. proximal myopathy.

2.17 Is it true that:
   A. urinary tract infection is the commonest cause of abdominal pain in children?
   B. acute pancreatitis is rare under the age of 40 years?
   C. carcinoma of the breast is more often found in the upper outer quadrant?
   D. torsion of the spermatic cord is more likely in a maldescended testis?
   E. following thyroidectomy, pre-existing exophthalmos may worsen?

2.18 The following values are appropriate for cerebrospinal fluid (CSF):
   A. protein: 400 mg/l.
   B. glucose: 6 mmol/l.
   C. chloride: 80 mmol/l.
   D. pressure: 8 cm H_2O.
   E. cells: less than 5 lymphocytes per mm^3.

2.19 Characteristic features of salicylate overdose include:
   A. coma.
   B. tinnitus.
   C. hypoventilation.
   D. hyperpyrexia.
   E. epigastric pain.

2.20 In sarcoidosis:
   A. a Kveim test is the diagnostic procedure of choice.
   B. there is depression of delayed hypersensitivity reaction.
   C. spontaneous remission occurs in less than 10% of cases.
   D. pulmonary fibrosis is a not uncommon outcome.
   E. the granulomata are caseating.

2.21 For effective cricoid pressure the following are essential:
   A. extension of the neck.
   B. one hand supporting the back of the neck.
   C. a complete ring of cricoid cartilage.
   D. preoxygenation for a minimum of 3 min.
   E. absence of a nasogastric (NG) tube.

2.22 Tetanus:
   A. commonly has an incubation period of more than 20 days.
   B. can be complicated by severe autonomic dysfunction.
   C. can be reliably diagnosed by culture of *Clostridium tetani* from the wound.
   D. has a worse prognosis if severe spasms are present.
   E. should be treated with intrathecal antitoxin.

2.23 The following features would lead you to doubt a diagnosis of appendicitis in a 5-year-old boy:
   A. pain in the right iliac fossa (RIF) when pressing on the left iliac fossa.
   B. diarrhoea the evening prior to admission.
   C. microscopic examination of the urine revealing 5 white blood cells/mm^3.
   D. heart rate of 90 beats per minute.
   E. pyrexia of 39.6°C.

2.24 Perioperative aspiration is more likely with:
   A. sliding hiatus hernia.
   B. achalasia of the oesophagus.
   C. obesity.
   D. lithotomy position.
   E. polyhydramnios.

2.25 Phantom limb pain (PLP):
   A. is often effectively treated by cordotomy.
   B. is more likely if the limb is painful prior to amputation.
   C. can be precipitated by spinal anaesthesia.
   D. is equally common in children and adults.
   E. can be controlled by non-steroidal anti-inflammatory drugs (NSAIDs).

2.26 Synchronized direct current (DC) cardioversion is indicated in:
   A. pulseless ventricular tachycardia (VT).
   B. atrial fibrillation.
   C. atrial flutter.
   D. ventricular fibrillation (VF).
   E. supraventricular tachycardia.

2.27 Acute intermittent porphyria (AIP) is associated with:
   A. psychiatric disturbance.
   B. abdominal pain.
   C. raised porphobilinogen and δ-aminolaevulinic acid levels.
   D. autosomal dominant inheritance.
   E. raised faecal porphyrins.

2.28 Postoperative nausea and vomiting (PONV):
   A. has the same incidence in men and women.
   B. is more common in children.
   C. is increased with longer operations.
   D. is increased by the use of dopamine antagonists.
   E. rarely occurs with spinal or epidural anaesthesia.

2.29 In an acute severe asthma attack:
   A. pulsus paradoxus is a reliable indicator of severity.
   B. a high $P_a\text{co}_2$ is an indication for immediate ventilation.
   C. sodium chromoglycate is of no immediate benefit.
   D. oxygen therapy should be at 28% until arterial blood gases are available.
   E. corticosteroid therapy should be given promptly.

2.30 In tetralogy of Fallot:
   A. there is right axis deviation.
   B. there is an overriding aorta.
   C. palliative surgery is all that is available.
   D. cyanotic spells are worsened by squatting.
   E. pulmonary plethora is present radiographically.

2.31 Postoperative shivering:
   A. can usually be avoided by active warming of the patient.
   B. is associated with hypoxaemia.
   C. causes a respiratory acidosis.
   D. occurs rarely with spinal anaesthesia.
   E. responds to the administration of opiates.

2.32 The Severinghaus CO_2 electrode:
   A. has CO_2-sensitive glass.
   B. uses sodium bicarbonate as a buffer.
   C. is an indirect method of measuring carbon dioxide tension.
   D. is accurate to within 130 Pa (1 mmHg).
   E. is temperature-dependent.

2.33 Pulmonary artery occlusion pressure (PAOP) is a good indicator of left ventricular (LV) diastolic pressure:
   A. in aortic regurgitation.
   B. after a pneumonectomy.
   C. with constrictive pericarditis.
   D. following a myocardial infarction.
   E. in pulmonary hypertension.

2.34 Features of cor pulmonale include:
   A. third heart sound.
   B. pleural effusion.
   C. barely palpable liver.
   D. hypertrophic pulmonary osteoarthropathy (HPOA).
   E. pulmonary valve incompetence.

2.35 As regards magnetic resonance imaging (MRI):
   A. the magnetic field strength is measured in gauss.
   B. patient screening with a metal detector is useful.
   C. cardiac pacemakers are likely to malfunction.
   D. it is contraindicated in patients with a prosthetic heart valve.
   E. ferromagnetic gas cylinders are safe within the 5 gauss line.

2.36 Complications of central venous line insertion include:
   A. cardiac tamponade.
   B. pneumothorax.
   C. Horner's syndrome.
   D. phrenic nerve palsy.
   E. thrombosis.

2.37 Cerebral damage after hypotensive anaesthesia is worsened by:
  A. anaemia.
  B. isoflurane.
  C. extreme head-up positioning.
  D. hyperventilation.
  E. open-heart surgery.

2.38 Cataract is a recognized complication of:
  A. thyrotoxicosis.
  B. Down's syndrome.
  C. non-insulin-dependent DM.
  D. primary hypoparathyroidism.
  E. Marfan's syndrome.

2.39 Effective neuroprotection following a severe head injury includes:
  A. steroids.
  B. hypothermia.
  C. hyperventilation below a $P_a\text{co}_2$ of 3.5 kPa.
  D. thiopentone.
  E. calcium channel blockers.

2.40 When investigating a patient with a haemorrhagic disease:
  A. an increased prothrombin time (PT) is found with haemophilia A.
  B. an increased PT occurs with factor V deficiency.
  C. a decreased PT indicates increased plasma fibrinogen.
  D. an increased bleeding time indicates factor VIII deficiency.
  E. a low platelet count occurs in von Willebrand's disease.

2.41 The following indicate a poor prognosis after a myocardial infarction (MI):
  A. age over 70 years.
  B. pulmonary oedema.
  C. primary VF.
  D. complete heart block with an anterior myocardial infarction.
  E. pre-existing non-insulin dependent DM.

2.42 Sevoflurane is similar to desflurane as regards:
  A. minimum alveolar concentration (MAC).
  B. irritation to upper airway.
  C. proportion metabolized.
  D. fluoride ion production.
  E. analgesic properties.

2.43 Responses to starvation include:
  A. a decrease in insulin secretion.
  B. hyperglycaemia.
  C. an increase in growth hormone secretion.
  D. increased production of ketone bodies.
  E. increase in gluconeogenesis.

2.44 Inappropriate antidiuretic hormone secretion may be caused by:
  A. diuretic therapy.
  B. pneumonia.
  C. cerebral abscess.
  D. acute intermittent porphyria.
  E. severe burns.

2.45 A drug with a pK_a of 9.4:
  A. is extensively bound to albumin.
  B. is 50% ionized at pII 7.4.
  C. has increased excretion with acidic urine.
  D. is likely to be a gastric irritant.
  E. has a rapid onset of action.

2.46 Prognostic indicators for a parotid tumour include:
  A. preservation of the facial nerve.
  B. rapid growth.
  C. presence of enlarged lymph nodes.
  D. palpable swelling on opening of the mouth.
  E. local pain.

2.47 Typical features of Cushing's disease include:
  A. generalized obesity.
  B. menorrhagia.
  C. peripheral neuropathy.
  D. increased susceptibility to infections.
  E. hypotension.

2.48 As regards double lumen tubes:
  A. a right-sided tube is preferred to a left-sided tube.
  B. a right-sided tube is easier to insert than a left-sided tube.
  C. a Robertshaw tube has a carinal hook.
  D. they cannot be used in children under 8 years of age.
  E. rupture of the bronchus is a well-recognized problem.

2.49 A rise in intracranial pressure (ICP) can be evidenced by:
  A. hypotension.
  B. tachycardia.
  C. pupillary constriction.
  D. reduced conscious level.
  E. rhinorrhoea.

2.50 Acute pulmonary contusion is closely associated with:
  A. interstitial lung damage.
  B. crackles on auscultation within 6 hours of the accident.
  C. opacities on chest radiograph within 6 hours of blunt trauma to the chest.
  D. pulmonary laceration.
  E. progressive pulmonary fibrosis.

2.51 Regarding explosions:
  A. a stoichiometric mixture of gases is less likely to explode.
  B. oxygen is highly explosive.
  C. nitrous oxide is a useful diluent in an explosive mixture.
  D. the current inhalational agents are non-flammable.
  E. the risk of explosions is increased at high humidity.

2.52 Epistaxis:
  A. usually arises from the lateral wall of the nose.
  B. can be commonly caused by Vincent's angina.
  C. may be associated with sinusitis.
  D. may require ligation of the external carotid artery.
  E. is more common in hypertensive patients.

2.53 Streptokinase therapy:
  A. reduces mortality following myocardial infarction.
  B. is contraindicated in diabetic patients.
  C. can give rise to massive haemorrhage.
  D. is inhibited by concurrent aspirin therapy.
  E. can be effective up to 12 hours after a myocardial infarction.

2.54 Radiological change of the pituitary sella is associated with:
- A. raised ICP.
- B. craniopharyngioma.
- C. Cushing's disease.
- D. glioma of the optic chiasma.
- E. primary hyperaldosteronism.

2.55 Etomidate:
- A. belongs to the imidazole group.
- B. is metabolized by esters.
- C. alters function of the adrenal medulla.
- D. is insoluble in water.
- E. is associated with epileptiform discharges on EEG.

2.56 Gas chromatography employs:
- A. a carrier gas.
- B. electron deflection.
- C. the Venturi principle.
- D. haemodilution.
- E. transillumination.

2.57 Myoglobin:
- A. binds reversibly with carbon dioxide.
- B. has a larger molecular weight than haemoglobin.
- C. provides a reservoir of oxygen in muscles.
- D. does not show the Bohr effect.
- E. has an oxygen dissociation curve to the right of the oxyhaemoglobin dissociation curve.

2.58 Disequilibrium syndrome with haemodialysis:
- A. is more commonly found than with peritoneal dialysis.
- B. is a result of autonomic nervous system dysfunction.
- C. can be overcome by using bicarbonate dialysate.
- D. causes hypertension
- E. may cause convulsions.

2.59 Suction for anaesthetic use:
- A. can be achieved using the Venturi principle.
- B. requires a low volume displacement.
- C. requires a high negative pressure.
- D. requires a minimum flow of 25 l/min.
- E. may share the same vacuum system as that for scavenging waste anaesthetic gases.

2.60 Weight loss in a patient with a normal or increased appetite could be due to:
A. gastric ulcer.
B. untreated DM.
C. Addison's disease.
D. thyrotoxicosis.
E. tuberculosis.

2.61 The femoral nerve:
A. lies lateral to the femoral artery below the inguinal ligament.
B. block provides adequate analgesia for a femoral shaft fracture.
C. provides cutaneous sensation over the lateral side of the calf.
D. arises from the anterior spinal roots of L2, L3, L4.
E. block can be used as the sole technique for arthroscopy.

2.62 The following can be used in the measurement of cardiac output by the Fick principle:
A. arterial oxygen content.
B. venous oxygen content.
C. oxygen consumption.
D. respiratory quotient.
E. arterial carbon dioxide content.

2.63 Appropriate treatment of raised temperature and dehydration caused by severe exercise can include:
A. aspirin.
B. external cooling.
C. dantrolene.
D. crystalloid infusion.
E. prophylactic antibiotics.

2.64 Effects of H_1 blockers include:
A. excitation of the CNS.
B. cholinergic effects.
C. adrenergic effects.
D. an antiemetic action.
E. haemolytic anaemia.

2.65 Diseases more commonly seen in males include:
- A. SLE.
- B. primary adrenocortical deficiency (Addison's disease).
- C. primary biliary cirrhosis.
- D. congenital hypertrophic pyloric stenosis.
- E. Parkinson's disease.

2.66 Consistently reliable methods to detect oesophageal intubation include:
- A. pulse oximetry.
- B. capnography.
- C. condensation seen in a clear tracheal tube.
- D. light wand.
- E. chest auscultation.

2.67 Intravenous patient-controlled analgesia (PCA) with opiates:
- A. cannot be used with other analgesic regimens.
- B. is not possible with fentanyl.
- C. avoids the risk of respiratory depression.
- D. can be successfully used by a 5-year-old child.
- E. has a reduced incidence of nausea and vomiting compared with intramuscular opiates.

2.68 As regards colloids:
- A. hydroxyethyl starch can interfere with blood coagulation.
- B. Haemaccel has a half-life of 6–8 hours.
- C. dextran 70 infusion can increase bleeding time.
- D. all forms of dextran are antigenic.
- E. gelatin solutions can interfere with blood cross-matching.

2.69 The following are true of the T wave of the ECG:
- A. it represents ventricular depolarization.
- B. it is normally more than 2 mV in the standard leads.
- C. the amplitude is increased in hyperkalaemia.
- D. the amplitude is increased in digoxin toxicity.
- E. it is normal in atrial fibrillation.

2.70 Digoxin:
  A. increases intracellular sodium levels.
  B. can be used in the management of Wolff–Parkinson–White syndrome (WPW).
  C. can cause bradycardia and prolonged PR interval.
  D. can produce abnormal red-green colour perception.
  E. toxicity increases with hyperkalaemia.

2.71 Non-parametric tests include:
  A. Student's *t*-test.
  B. Wilcoxon rank sum test.
  C. Mann–Whitney rank sum test.
  D. chi-squared test.
  E. McNemar test.

2.72 Physiological changes in the third trimester of pregnancy include:
  A. increase in stroke volume.
  B. increase in red cell mass.
  C. decrease in glomerular filtration rate (GFR).
  D. decrease in fibrinogen level.
  E. decrease in gastric emptying.

2.73 Features of a hydatidiform mole may include:
  A. pre-eclampsia.
  B. a coagulopathy.
  C. an increase in human chorionic gonadotrophin hormone (HCG).
  D. increased incidence of nausea and vomiting.
  E. liver metastases.

2.74 Immediate management of acute anaphylaxis includes:
  A. chlorpheniramine.
  B. hydrocortisone.
  C. adrenaline.
  D. isoprenaline.
  E. 0.9% normal saline.

2.75 Volatile anaesthetics can be measured by:
  A. mass spectrometry.
  B. Raman spectrometry.
  C. acoustic difference.
  D. piezoelectric effect.
  E. ultraviolet absorption.

2.76 Trigeminal neuralgia:
  A. may remit spontaneously.
  B. is characterized by loss of the corneal reflex.
  C. is associated with ipsilateral loss of sensation.
  D. is effectively treated with chlorpromazine.
  E. can resolve after radiofrequency thermocoagulation.

2.77 A 'three in one' nerve block acts on:
  A. the femoral nerve.
  B. the ilio-inguinal nerve.
  C. the obturator nerve.
  D. the genitofemoral nerve.
  E. the lateral cutaneous nerve of the thigh.

2.78 A urinary specific gravity of 1.030 is compatible with:
  A. diabetes insipidus.
  B. pre-renal failure.
  C. dehydration.
  D. normal renal function.
  E. chronic renal failure.

2.79 Mixed venous oxygen saturation is increased in:
  A. anaemia.
  B. cyanide toxicity.
  C. hypothermia.
  D. sepsis with peripheral shunting.
  E. strenuous exercise.

2.80 Reliable indicators of nutritional status in the critically ill include:
  A. lymphocyte count.
  B. urinary nitrogen excretion.
  C. weight loss.
  D. triceps skinfold thickness.
  E. serum albumin.

2.81 In one-lung ventilation, hypoxic pulmonary vasoconstriction in the non-dependent lung is inhibited by:
  A. clonidine.
  B. inhalational agents.
  C. intravenous induction agents.
  D. hypocapnia.
  E. positive end-expiratory pressure (PEEP) to the dependent lung.

2.82 Chronic administration of phenytoin can cause:
  A. ataxia.
  B. megaloblastic anaemia.
  C. hepatic damage.
  D. skin rashes.
  E. neural tube defects in children of mothers taking phenytoin.

2.83 Predisposing factors for postoperative deep vein thrombosis (DVT) include:
  A. sickle cell anaemia.
  B. congestive cardiac failure.
  C. hypotensive anaesthesia.
  D. presence of varicose veins.
  E. antithrombin III deficiency.

2.84 Signs of a lower motor neurone lesion include:
  A. fasciculation.
  B. reduced reflexes.
  C. muscle wasting.
  D. reduced joint position sense.
  E. reduced temperature sensation.

2.85 Adults breathing 100% oxygen at sea level may develop:
  A. convulsions.
  B. reversible loss of vision.
  C. dizziness.
  D. fall in residual volume.
  E. retrosternal pain.

2.86 The following statements are true:
  A. Morton first used ether in 1846.
  B. Simpson was the first to use chloroform in 1847.
  C. Quincke first demonstrated a lumbar puncture in 1891.
  D. tracheal intubation was first introduced in 1910.
  E. Ralph Waters was the first professor of anaesthesia.

2.87 Haematuria is more likely to be glomerular in origin if:
  A. red cell casts are present in the urine.
  B. heavy proteinuria coexists.
  C. red cells are of normal morphology.
  D. hyaline casts are present in the urine.
  E. epithelial casts are present in the urine.

2.88 As regards anticholinergic agents:
   A. glycopyrrolate is a more potent antisialogogue than atropine.
   B. atropine increases physiological dead space.
   C. hyoscine undergoes extensive metabolism in the liver.
   D. hyoscine is excreted unchanged in the urine.
   E. glycopyrrolate is longer-acting than atropine.

2.89 Blood platelets are important in haemostasis as they:
   A. adhere to collagen.
   B. help to initiate the coagulation cascade.
   C. stimulate local vasoconstriction.
   D. encourage fibrinolysis.
   E. play a part in clot retraction.

2.90 A mid-thigh amputation requires the following nerves to be blocked:
   A. genitofemoral nerve.
   B. obturator nerve.
   C. femoral nerve.
   D. sciatic nerve.
   E. lateral femoral cutaneous nerve.

Answers

2.1 **A**.F **B**.F **C**.T **D**.T **E**.F

Much research has been concentrated on the development of stroma-free haemoglobin solutions for oxygen carriage. Initial problems, such as the left shift of the oxyhaemoglobin dissociation curve, very short half-life and osmotic diuresis, have been largely overcome. Other side-effects include a transient rise in blood urea and precipitation of trace amounts of the product in the kidneys. Because of this, it is probably safer to avoid stroma-free haemoglobins where renal function is already compromised, even though no long-term damage has been reported in healthy subjects. Immune reactions have occurred (but not complement activation) but their importance has yet to be fully determined. They have no precoagulant or anticoagulant function but do have intrinsic vasopressor activity. Their intravascular retention time is about 6–8 hours. Overall results from clinical trials look promising. Advantages include better laminar flow characteristics (molecules are 10^4 times smaller than red blood cells) and thus potentially better oxygen delivery to poorly perfused tissues. They may also have a use in cardioplegia, organ preservation for transplantation and major surgery in Jehovah's witnesses. Anticipated problems include lack of coagulation factors, short half-life, and breakdown products which are taken up by the reticuloendothelial system and may affect immunity. (See: Mallick A, Bodenham AR (1996) Modified haemoglobins as oxygen transporting blood substitutes. *British Journal of Hospital Medicine* **55**, 443–447. Also: Dietz NM *et al.* (1996) Blood substitutes: fluids, drugs or miracle solutions. *Anesthesia and Analgesia* **82**, 390–405.)

2.2 **A**.T **B**.T **C**.T **D**.T **E**.T

In *haemophilia A*, reduced factor VIII results in bleeding into a joint which can cause fever, pain and limitation of movement. Such bleeding can be caused by mild trauma in patients whose factor VIII levels are below 10% of normal: when the levels are below 2% bleeding can occur spontaneously. *Scurvy*, or ascorbic acid deficiency, reduces factor VIII levels and platelet adhesiveness. *Juvenile rheumatoid arthritis* has the same symptoms as in an adult and a worse prognosis. Although it is not a likely diagnosis at this age, initial presenting features include fever and joint pain, which in approximately 15% affect only one joint. *Osteomyelitis* can be due to infection in the joint itself or may occur as a result of a reactive joint effusion from nearby long bone infection. *Brucellosis* is transmitted by unpasteurized milk from cows infected with *Brucella abortus*. Classic symptoms are undulant fever, weakness and pain in limbs and joints. Although virtually eradicated in the UK, treatment is with tetracycline and rifampicin.

2.3 **A.**F **B.**T **C.**T **D.**F **E.**F
The underlying cause of perioperative hypertension must be identified and treated appropriately. Common causes include inadequate depth of anaesthesia for the current stimulus (e.g. intubation), inadequate paralysis and underlying hypertensive disease. Increasing anaesthetic vapour concentration, ensuring adequate muscle relaxation and anticipating nociceptive stimuli with opiates are all important initial manoeuvres. Appropriate drugs to control blood pressure need to be rapid in onset, easily titratable and have a short duration of action. They include labetolol, hydralazine, nifedipine, glyceryl trinitrate and sodium nitroprusside. Phenoxybenzamine forms a covalent linkage with α adrenoceptors which results in both a slow onset and a prolonged (several days) action. It is best reserved for the preoperative management of phaeochromocytoma or hypertensive crises with sudden withdrawal of monoamine oxidase inhibitors (MAOIs). A rise in VMA excretion is found with a phaeochromocytoma. As it is a very rare cause of hypertension, routine measurement cannot be recommended for all cases of intraoperative hypertension. A 'fit' patient assumes a normal blood pressure and, as such, abandonment of the procedure is unnecessary as blood pressure can be brought under control by the means suggested above without adverse consequences.

2.4 **A.**T **B.**T **C.**T **D.**F **E.**T
A cystic hygroma is a benign congenital tumour of lymphatic origin, most commonly found in the neck. Embryonically sequestered lymph vessels penetrate normal tissue to produce large multiloculated cysts filled with serous secretions. Transillumination is normally brilliant. Bladder malignancies are nearly all derived from transitional cells with only about 7% squamous cells and 1% adenocarcinomas. They are uncommon under 50 years of age. Testicular maldescent is found in 0.3% of 1-year-old boys. The testes can be found at any point on their path of descent from the posterior abdominal wall to the

scrotum, but most are palpable in the groin at the superficial inguinal pouch outside the external inguinal ring; only rarely are they found in the perineum. The appendix arises from the caecum just distal to the ileocaecal junction. It is retrocaecal in 74% of cases, pelvic in 21% and paracaecal in the rest. The scaphoid bone accounts for 60–70% of all wrist bone fractures. This is often mistaken for a sprain owing to the paucity of clinical and radiological signs. If the diagnosis is in doubt, treatment should be as for a fracture and the wrist immobilized to prevent the complications of non-union (10%) or avascular necrosis.

2.5   A.F   B.T   C.F   D.T   E.T
These ABGs are found with type II respiratory or 'ventilatory' failure, i.e. insufficient alveolar ventilation to excrete the CO_2 produced by metabolism. The accompanying polycythaemia suggests compensation for a long-standing respiratory problem. This combination can be found with chronic obstructive pulmonary disease (COPD) or severe chest wall deformities (scoliosis). The coexisting confusion suggests central depression of respiration, which can occur with acute decompensation of COPD secondary to infection or cardiac failure. Central cyanosis occurs with COPD and can be detected when arterial oxygen saturation falls below 80–85%, as long as more than $5\,g/dl$ of reduced haemoglobin is present. Reference to oxyhaemoglobin dissociation curve reveals a P_aO_2 of $7.5\,kPa$ corresponds to a saturation in excess of 85%. If this patient is dependent on hypoxic drive, then oxygen therapy may precipitate acute decompensation. In practice, these patients should never be denied oxygen therapy but this must initially be at low concentrations (F_iO_2 <28%) with ABGs repeated to ensure that P_aCO_2 does not rise. Type I or acute hypoxaemic respiratory failure is typified by a decrease in both P_aO_2 and P_aCO_2. Common causes include pulmonary oedema, pneumonia, pulmonary emboli and fibrosing alveolitis. Hypocarbia is usually due to tachypnoea.

2.6   A.T   B.T   C.T   D.T   E.T
Cytokines are low molecular-weight proteins and glycoproteins (e.g. TNF-α, interleukin-2, IL-6) whose release from leukocytes, macrophages and endothelial cells is stimulated by a wide variety of insults including infection, trauma and surgery. They act as intercellular mediators in an autocrine (on the producer cell) or paracrine (neighbouring cell) manner to activate the

inflammatory and immune systems in order to combat the insult. Some patients develop an excessive or prolonged response manifesting clinically as SIRS. Cytokine activity has a genetic component and some suggest it is possible to predict individual cytokine responses and outcome. General anaesthesia modulates cytokine activity. (See: Masterson GR (1996) Immunomodulation. *British Journal of Anaesthesia* **77**, 569–571. Also: Yentis SM (1995) Cytokines and sepsis: time for reappraisal. *British Journal of Anaesthesia* **74**, 119–120.)

2.7 **A.**F **B.**T **C.**F **D.**T **E.**F
Most drugs are poorly absorbed through intact skin because of their high molecular weight and low lipid solubility. Drugs that are absorbed transcutaneously to produce systemic effects tend to have high lipid solubility; they include glyceryl trinitrate, hyoscine, ethinyloestradiol and fentanyl. (See: Berti JJ, Lipsky JJ (1995) Transcutaneous drug delivery: a practical view. *Mayo Clinic Proceedings* **70**, 581–586.)

2.8 **A.**T **B.**F **C.**F **D.**F **E.**T
The Goldman cardiac risk index is a scoring system devised to identify preoperatively patients at risk from major perioperative cardiovascular complications. Retrospective analysis of patients undergoing non-cardiac surgery identified nine variables and each were given a score as follows:

third heart sound, increased jugular venous pressure (JVP)	– 11
previous MI within 6 months	– 10
premature ventricular contractions	– 5
non-sinus rhythm	– 7
age over 70 years	– 5
emergency surgery	– 4
severe aortic stenosis	– 3
poor general condition	– 3
abdominal or thoracic surgery	– 3

Points	% Morbidity	% Mortality
0–5	0.7	0.2
6–12	5	2
13–25	11	2
>26	22	56

Unfortunately, its clinical usefulness is limited owing to its low sensitivity. It does not make allowance for particular patient subgroups nor operations that place the patient at particular risk of cardiac morbidity and mortality. Recent research has shown it to be of greater predictive value when used in combination with ASA (American Society of Anesthesiologists) grading. (See: Goldman L *et al.* (1977) Multifactorial index of cardiac risk in non-cardiac surgical procedures. *New England Journal of Medicine* **297**, 845–850. Also: Goldman L (1994) Assessment of perioperative cardiac risk. *New England Journal of Medicine* **330**, 707–711. And: Prause G *et al.* (1997) Can ASA grade or Goldman's cardiac risk index predict peri-operative mortality? *Anaesthesia* **52**, 203–206.)

2.9   A.T   **B.**F   **C.**F   **D.**F   **E.**F

The adult trachea is approximately 11 cm in length and 1.5–2.0 cm wide in adults. It commences at C6, with a bifurcation at T4–5. It is lined with columnar ciliated epithelium containing many mucus-secreting goblet cells. The blood supply comes mainly from the inferior thyroid arteries, but the bronchial arteries supply the lower end of the trachea.

2.10   A.T   **B.**T   **C.**F   **D.**F   **E.**F

Carcinoid tumours arise from argentaffin-producing cells commonly found in the appendix, terminal ileum and rectum. Most are asymptomatic but about 5% develop carcinoid syndrome as a result of liver metastases. Clinical features mainly affect skin, heart and gastrointestinal tract and are due to release of biologically active amines and peptides including 5-hydroxytryptamine, prostaglandins, histamine, kinins, and rarely adrenocorticotrophic hormone (ACTH). The commonest symptoms are facial flushing, tachycardia and hypotension, abdominal pain, intestinal hypermotility, diarrhoea and malabsorption. Cardiac abnormalities affect about 50% of patients due to formation of fibrous tissue on valvular cusps and cardiac chambers leading to stenosis or regurgitation, or both. Diagnosis is by increased urinary excretion of 5-hydroxyindoleacetic acid (5-HIAA). Excision is the best treatment, including isolated hepatic metastases. If this is not possible, treatment with octreotide is useful as it inhibits release of many gut hormones and may inhibit tumour growth. Often this is the only drug needed, but H_1 and H_2 antagonists can also provide symptomatic relief. Without a curative excision, mean survival is 5–10 years. Urine turns pink on standing with some of the porphyrias.

2.11 A.F B.T C.T D.T E.F
The Mapleson A (Magill) is efficient for spontaneous ventilation because exhaled dead space gas is reused at the next inspiration whilst exhaled alveolar gases pass out through the valve. Thus, FGF can equal alveolar minute volume (70 ml/kg/min). Mapleson B and C are really used for resuscitation only and require an FGF 2–3 times the minute volume. Mapleson D (Bain) also requires an FGF in excess of minute volume (about 150–250 ml/kg/min) because the exhaled gases pass into the reservoir bag and may be rebreathed unless the FGF is high enough to displace them. Mapleson E (Ayre's T-piece) and F (Jackson Rees modification) work on the same principle as Mapleson D and similarly require an FGF 2–3 times the minute ventilation. The universal breathing system/Humphrey ADE functions as a Mapleson A for spontaneous ventilation.

2.12 A.F B.F C.T D.T E.T
The sciatic nerve is the largest nerve in the body. Derived from the lumbosacral plexus (L4, L5, S1, S2, S3), it supplies the hip and knee joints, the hamstrings and part of the adductor magnus before dividing at the knee to form the tibial and peroneal nerves. It supplies sensation over most of the lower leg apart from the medial calf, which is innervated by the saphenous branch of the femoral nerve. The knee jerk is supplied by the femoral nerve, the ankle jerk by the sciatic nerve. Peroneal nerve damage can cause a foot drop. Conservative treatment is best, with 90% of cases recovering within 6 weeks after 1–2 weeks' bedrest and analgesics; about 10% come to surgery. Delay does not affect long-term outcome unless there is significant neurological deficit requiring immediate intervention (e.g. urinary retention, cauda equina syndrome).

2.13 A.T B.F C.T D.T E.F
A low cardiac output has many causes but when it is fixed there is either physical restriction to cardiac filling or obstruction to cardiac emptying. Constrictive pericarditis normally limits ventricular filling in late diastole secondary to thickening and fibrosis of the pericardium. Cardiac tamponade does the same by the presence of blood or serous fluid between the pericardium and the myocardium. Aortic stenosis physically

limits the amount of blood ejected in systole. The low cardiac output seen with heart failure from any cause including cor pulmonale is not fixed as it is due to a reduction in myocardial contractility causing a decrease in ejection fraction and not a fixed physical impediment. It also has the potential to be increased by appropriate drug therapy, unlike fixed conditions. Aortic regurgitation increases cardiac output.

2.14 A.T B.F C.F D.T E.F

Ondansetron is a potent and selective antagonist at 5-hydroxytryptamine$_3$ (5-HT$_3$) receptors found both centrally (medulla, chemotactic trigger zone and tractus solitarius) and peripherally (intestinal wall). Used initially for chemotherapy-induced nausea and vomiting, it is now commonly employed for the prophylaxis and management of postoperative nausea and vomiting. It is available in both tablet and injection form. It is moderately bound to plasma proteins, has a relatively large volume of distribution and a relatively short half-life of 3 hours. It is metabolized to inactive metabolites in the liver with less than 5% excreted unchanged in the urine. It increases bowel transit time, and constipation is a common side-effect. Head-aches, dizziness, flushing, chest pain, cardiac arrhythmias and hypersensitivity reactions have also been reported. Other 5-HT$_3$ antagonists include donesitron, granisetron and tropisetron. There appears to be little to choose between them as regards their efficacy. Extrapyramidal effects and sedation are not seen with ondansetron as with other antiemetic agents. As it has little effect on opioid-induced emesis or motion sickness, it cannot be completely effective given the multifactorial nature of postoperative nausea and vomiting.

2.15 A.T B.T C.F D.F E.F

Pregnanolone is a steroid metabolite of progesterone with similar actions to propofol. It is currently undergoing clinical trials as an intravenous anaesthetic induction agent. It is insoluble in water and formulated as an isotonic emulsion of soya bean oil, triglycerides, egg phosphatide and glycerol with a pH of about 7.5. Induction is associated with minor involuntary movements and hypertonus. It has less cardiovascular effects than propofol, with a small reduction in blood pressure and a slight increase in heart rate (about 10% for both). Pain on injection is minimal and anaphylactoid reactions are rare, although there have been some reports of skin rashes and urticaria. Loss of eyelash reflex is not a reliable sign of loss of consciousness. Dose required is 0.5–0.6 mg/kg making it more potent than propofol. (See: Powell H *et al.* (1992) Pregnanolone: a new steroid intravenous anaesthetic. A dose finding study. *Anaesthesia* **47**, 287–290.)

2.16 A.F **B.**T **C.**T **D.**T **E.**T

Long-term complications of IDDM occur as a result of large or small vessel vascular disease. The former is typified by atherosclerosis causing stroke or myocardial infarction. The latter is known as 'diabetic microangiopathy' and is due to capillary basement membrane thickening with an associated increase in vascular permeability. This principally affects three main sites causing:

> **Retinopathy** – Microaneurysms, haemorrhages, exudates, retinal infarcts and new vessel formation.
> **Nephropathy** – Glomerulosclerosis leading to proteinuria and renal failure; renal papillary necrosis is a rare complication of urinary tract infections which are more frequent in diabetics.
> **Neuropathy** – Symmetrical distal sensory neuropathy with numbness and tingling, proximal motor neuropathy and autonomic neuropathy with postural hypotension and impotence.

Good glycaemic control decreases the incidence of complications. Insulin requirements increase in pregnancy.

2.17 A.F **B.**T **C.**T **D.**F **E.**T

Most cases of abdominal pain in children have no definable aetiology. If anything, it is most likely to be constipation or school refusal. Most patients with acute pancreatitis are over 45 years of age, with a peak incidence between 50 and 60 years. Carcinoma of the breast is found mainly in the upper outer quadrant. The testes are normally anchored by the spermatic cord with attachment to the posterior wall of the scrotum. Torsion is more likely when the spermatic cord is longer than normal thus allowing the testis to become twisted around its long axis, and thereby threatening its blood supply. Ophthalmic Graves' disease produces proptosis resulting in conjunctival oedema, lid lag and corneal scarring and ultimately limitation of eye movements. Surgery or radioiodine to control hyperthyroidism does not control progression of eye signs.

Following thyroidectomy hypothyroidism must be prevented as it may exacerbate the eye signs. Treatment includes methylcellulose eye drops, systemic steroids, lateral tarsorrhapy, surgical decompression and corrective eye muscle surgery.

2.18 A.T B.F C.F D.T E.T

The ranges of normal values are:

protein	– 100–400 mg/l
glucose	– 2.5–4 mmol/l
chloride	– 120–170 mmol/l
pressure	– 7–15 cm H_2O
cells	– <5 lymphocytes per mm^3
	(or $10^6/l$ in SI units)

CSF is formed in the choroid plexuses, around vertebral vessels and along ventricular walls. Its composition is dependent on filtration and diffusion from blood. Total volume is 100–150 ml, of which one-third comprises spinal fluid. Glucose concentration is lower in CSF than in plasma while chloride is higher. Sodium and potassium mirror blood levels. White cell count can increase with systemic infection. Other values include:

specific gravity	– 1007
osmolality	– 306 mosmol/kg
calcium	– 1–1.5 mmol/l
pH	– 7.3–7.35 (50–54 nmol/l)

2.19 A.F B.T C.F D.T E.T

Excess salicylate directly stimulates the respiratory centre to cause hyperventilation and respiratory alkalosis. To compensate, bicarbonate is excreted in the urine. As this is accompanied by Na, K and water, dehydration and hypokalaemia result. Bicarbonate loss diminishes buffering capacity and so allows a metabolic acidosis to develop. Salicylates uncouple oxidative phosphorylation so that energy normally used for conversion of inorganic phosphate to adenosine triphosphate (ATP) is dissipated as heat, resulting in hyperpyrexia, sweating and further dehydration. Nausea and vomiting arise from stimulation of the chemoreceptor trigger zone (CTZ). Other features include epigastric pain, tinnitus, deafness, tremor, irritability, hypoprothrombinaemia, pulmonary oedema and hypo- or hyperglycaemia. Drowsiness and confusion can occur but coma is very rare. As absorption is slow plasma salicylate should be measured at least 6 hours after ingestion. A salicylate level of >750 mg/l indicates severe toxicity and requires ingestion of 10–20 g of aspirin. Treatment is essentially supportive. Gastric lavage and activated charcoal may limit drug absorption if given early enough. Haemodialysis is reserved for severe cases as it is effective in removing salicylate. Approximately 200 die in the UK each year from overdose.

2.20 A.F B.T C.F D.F E.F
Sarcoidosis is a multisystem, non-caseating granulomatous disease. The aetiology is unknown but genetic, environmental and infective factors have been implicated. It commonly presents with bilateral hilar lymphadenopathy with or without pulmonary involvement. Extrapulmonary granulomata are found most commonly in the skin (erythema nodosum, lupus pernio) and the eye (anterior uveitis), but can cause potentially severe problems elsewhere. Examples include cardiac conduction defects, cranial nerve palsies and hypercalcaemia. Diagnosis is clinical and by exclusion of other granulomatous diseases, particularly tuberculosis (TB). Delayed hypersensitivity reaction is depressed. Transbronchial biopsy is the most useful diagnostic test, along with demonstration of a restrictive defect on spirometry. The Kveim test (intradermal injection of sarcoid with histological examination for granulomata after 4–6 weeks) is used less and less because of the superiority of other tests and the potential danger of infection. There is no cure. One-third to two-thirds of patients remit spontaneously. A small minority proceed to progressive pulmonary fibrosis and cor pulmonale.

2.21 A.T B.F C.T D.F E.T
Cricoid pressure aims to prevent passive regurgitation of gastric and oesophageal contents. It does so by compressing the oesophagus between the vertebrae and the cricoid cartilage – this being the only complete cartilaginous ring supporting the airway. Sellick suggested that the neck should be extended (as for tonsillectomy) without a supporting hand, and NG tubes removed to allow closure of the oesophagus and maintain efficacy of the lower oesophageal sphincter. This is probably the correct answer as regards the MCQ but there is little evidence to suggest that the presence of an NG tube promotes regurgitation. In addition, neck extension can make laryngoscopy difficult and Magill's technique of using a pillow is now

commonly accepted, as is a supporting hand, to prevent flexion of the neck during cricoid pressure. It must be released during active vomiting to prevent oesophageal rupture. Preoxygenation should be for 3 minutes but, although essential for safe rapid sequence induction, it is not required for cricoid pressure to be effective. (See: Sellick BA (1961) Cricoid pressure to control regurgitation of stomach contents during induction of anaesthesia. *Lancet* **2**, 404–406.)

2.22 A.F B.T C.F D.T E.F
C. tetani is a spore-bearing, Gram-positive bacillus found in soil and in animal and human faeces. It gains access into tissues mainly through trivial puncture wounds and lacerations which cannot be found in 20% of cases. Tetanus can also follow burns, surgery, chronic ulcers, abortion and childbirth. It is an obligate anaerobe and germination of spores occurs in necrotic anaerobic tissue to produce the exotoxin tetanospasmin. This acts at motor endplates to inhibit release of acetylcholine, causing paralysis. It also acts on the spinal cord and brain to cause seizures and cortical inhibition. Diagnosis is clinical as there are no reliable laboratory tests and culture of the wound reveals *C. tetani* in only about one-third of cases. The incubation period is 2–60 days, with 90% occurring within 15 days. Presenting symptoms commonly include trismus with pain, rigidity and spasms. A worse outcome is associated with a short incubation period and greater frequency and severity of spasms. Autonomic dysfunction from episodic increases in catecholamines can occur in severe cases, and death from arrhythmias, hypertensive crises and cardiac failure may occur. Treatment is supportive: wound debridement, antibiotics *and* immunization as natural immunity does not occur. Intrathecal antitetanus toxin is not widely available and is considered by many to be ineffective. Mortality is high at extremes of age: about 10% with intensive care unit (ICU) facilities, 80% without. (See: Benson CA, Harris AA (1986) Acute neurologic infections. *Medical Clinics of North America* **70**, 1001–1002.)

2.23 A.F B.F C.F D.F E.T
Acute appendicitis is the commonest emergency operation with 1 in 7 of the UK population having had an appendicectomy. Children classically present with periumbilical pain that may localize to the RIF. Anorexia, nausea and vomiting can occur which can lead to significant dehydration. Progression of

the inflammatory process can lead to pain being referred back to the RIF on palpation of other areas of the abdomen, including the left iliac fossa (Rovsing's sign). Diarrhoea with abdominal pain can mimic or be associated with appendicitis owing to the inflamed appendix irritating the neighbouring rectum. A low-grade fever, rarely above 38°C, is common. Tachycardia rarely occurs until the appendix has perforated. Surgery should be prompt but should not take precedence over correction of dehydration and electrolyte disturbance. Laparoscopy is becoming popular for both diagnosis and surgery as conventional surgery leads to females having a normal appendix removed in about 22% of cases (9% in males). The presence of 10 or more white cells/mm^3 in a urine sample indicates a urinary tract infection.

2.24 A.T **B.**T **C.**T **D.**T **E.**T

Aspiration is a potential risk for all unconscious and anaesthetized patients as lower oesophageal sphincter tone decreases and laryngeal reflexes are depressed. Preoperative fasting for elective procedures should be in the order of 6 hours for food and 2–3 hours for clear fluids in adults. Factors predisposing to aspiration include:

> **Full stomach** – not starved, trauma, ileus, gastrointestinal bleeding, opioid drugs, pregnancy.
> **Impaired lower oesophageal sphincter activity** – hiatus hernia, opioids, atropine, nasogastric tube, pregnancy with heartburn.
> **Raised intra-abdominal pressure** – pregnancy (especially with polyhydramnios), lithotomy position, obesity.
> **Oesophageal problems** – achalasia, strictures, pharyngeal pouch.

(See: Strunin L (1993) Editorial: How long should patients fast before surgery? Time for new guidelines. *British Journal of Anaesthesia* **70**, 1–3.)

2.25 A.F **B.**T **C.**T **D.**F **E.**F

PLP is common after amputation (up to 85% in some trials). Predisposing factors include age (PLP is uncommon in children), pre-existing limb pain and proximal amputation. The aetiology is uncertain but central mechanisms have been suggested whereby sustained nociceptive impulses produce morphological changes in the spinal cord/brain to produce a memoi y of the pain which persists after amputation. Inhibiting nociceptive impulses to abolish the memory of pain has been attempted using extradural blockade prior to amputation, with some success; further studies are needed to confirm this. Spinal anaesthesia can aggravate symptoms although some success in treatment has been achieved with intrathecal opioid via an indwelling catheter. Physiotherapy, transcutaneous electrical nerve stimulation (TENS), anticonvulsants, antidepressants, NSAIDs, nerve blocks and destructive techniques such as cordotomy have all been employed. None has been consistently successful. In a significant number the pain is intractable.

2.26 A.F B.T C.T D.F E.T
DC cardioversion aims to restore sinus rhythm by applying current across the chest. It is synchronized with the R wave of the ECG since delivery during ventricular repolarization could produce VF. It is used to treat atrial flutter or fibrillation, supraventricular tachycardia and non-pulseless VT, particularly if refractory to drug therapy or associated with angina, heart failure or low cardiac output. Serum electrolytes must be checked and digoxin toxicity excluded. Energy levels of 20–200 J are used. It restores sinus rhythm in 70–95% of patients depending on the tachyarrhythmia. Non-synchronized ventricular defibrillation is used to treat pulseless VT or VF as there is no organized rhythm.

2.27 A.T B.T C.T D.T E.F
Porphyrias arise from enzymatic defects in synthesis of haem, resulting in overproduction and accumulation of intermediates known as 'porphyrins'. Although there are erythropoietic porphyrias, it is only hepatic porphyrias that pose anaesthetic problems. The hepatic porphyrias include AIP, variegate porphyria, coproporphyria and porphyria cutanea tarda. All have autosomal dominant inheritance with variable penetrance and therefore a spectrum of manifestations. AIP is caused by reduced activity of porphobilinogen deaminase which results in increased amounts of porphobilinogen and δ-aminolaevulinic acid during attacks. The urine turns brown on standing. Faecal porphyrins are usually normal in AIP but are very high with variegate porphyria. Attacks may be triggered by drugs, pregnancy, alcohol, stress, infections and starvation but not every exposure results in an attack. The condition often presents in early adulthood, with females affected more

frequently than males. Symptoms during an attack include abdominal pain, tachycardia and hypertension, anxiety or frank psychosis, and motor or sensory polyneuropathies. Heterozygotes are rarely symptomatic but they are at increased risk when exposed to potent triggering agents. Treatment includes withdrawing offending drugs, high carbohydrate intake (reduces overproduction of porphyrins) with 10% glucose, haematin to suppress δ-aminolaevulinic acid activity, analgesia and adequate hydration. (See: Ashley EMC (1996) Anaesthesia for porphyria. *British Journal of Hospital Medicine* **56**, 37–42.)

2.28 A.F B.T C.T D.F E.F
PONV complicates about 30% of all anaesthetics. The incidence is higher in children than in adults (with peak incidence at age 11–14 years), in females and obese patients, and also in those with excessive anxiety, delayed gastric emptying (e.g. diabetes mellitus (DM)) and a history of motion sickness or PONV. Other causes include gastric distension from mask ventilation prior to intubation, prolonged surgery, nitrous oxide, opioids, etomidate and ketamine. Abdominal laparoscopic procedures have the highest incidence but eye and ear, nose and throat (ENT) procedures in children, dental extractions and neurosurgery are also potent stimulants. Spinal and epidural anaesthesia have a reported incidence of about 20%, mainly due to hypotension. The inhalational agents (except ether) tend not to cause PONV. Propofol has been used as an antiemetic in its own right. The CTZ is postulated to lie in the area postrema of the medulla. As dopamine is an important stimulant in this area, drugs with antidopaminergic activity (e.g. droperidol, metoclopramide) will have antiemetic activity. Central anticholinergic activity is also associated with antiemetic activity. This is the basis for the efficacy of cyclizine, atropine and hyoscine. (See: Broomhead CJ (1995) Physiology of PONV and reducing the incidence of PONV. *British Journal of Hospital Medicine* **53**, 327–328, 511–512.)

2.29 A.T B.T C.T D.F E.T
The incidence of asthma is 2–4% of the population and rising. It causes approximately 2000 deaths each year in the UK. Clinical features indicating a severe attack include:

1. Inability to speak or complete a sentence in a single breath.
2. Respiratory rate >25 breaths per min with use of accessory muscles.
3. Tachycardia >110 beats per min, pulsus paradoxus >10 mmHg.
4. Peak expiratory flow <40% of normal, high $P_a co_2$, low $P_a o_2$, low pH.

Treatment should be prompt and aggressive, and includes:

1. Highest possible inspired oxygen concentration by facemask.
2. Large i.v. cannula and fluids as dehydration is common.
3. Nebulized or intravenous β_2-adrenoceptor agonists (e.g. salbutamol). Ipratropium bromide is an anticholinergic agent which inhibits parasympathetically mediated broncho-motor tone and may also be of value.
4. Corticosteroids should be given immediately. Their peak action is at 6–12 hours but they ameliorate an attack and may even abort an attack if given at the earliest sign of an exacerbation.
5. Aminophylline is a useful bronchodilator but it has a narrow therapeutic index and so requires careful monitoring.
6. Ventilation should be instituted if the patient is exhausted, there is no improvement in clinical signs, or there is a deterioration in blood gases ($P_a co_2$ >8 kPa, $P_a o_2$ <8 kPa, respiratory acidosis).

Sodium chromoglycate is a mast cell stabilizer more often used for prophylaxis. (See: Keeley D, Rees J (1997) New guidelines on asthma management. *British Medical Journal* **314**, 315–316.)

2.30   A.T   B.T   C.F   D.F   E.F
Fallot's tetralogy is pulmonary stenosis, ventricular septal defect (VSD), overriding of the VSD by the aorta and right ventricular hypertrophy. It is the commonest cause of cyanotic heart disease (incidence 1 in 2000). Cyanosis occurs when right ventricular pressure exceeds left ventricular pressure and blood is shunted from right to left across the VSD. This can be influenced by adrenergic stimulation or after feeding and crying causing hypoxic pulmonary vasoconstriction. Cyanosis becomes increasingly apparent in older children along with associated growth retardation, polycythaemia and clubbing. Relief is sometimes achieved by adopting a squatting position

after exertion (this raises afterload, reversing the flow through the VSD). The ECG shows right ventricular hypertrophy and right axis deviation. A chest radiograph (CXR) shows a boot-shaped heart, an abnormally small pulmonary artery and, if anything, pulmonary oligaemia. Correction before 5 years of age has excellent results unless the pulmonary arteries are very hypoplastic; in this situation a shunt between pulmonary and subclavian arteries may be performed to improve pulmonary blood flow and facilitate definitive correction later.

2.31 A.F B.T C.F D.T E.T
Electromyogram (EMG) studies suggest that postoperative shivering from hypothermia differs from that from anaesthesia. Whereas the former can be suppressed by peripheral warming, the latter cannot. It has been proposed that general anaesthetics suppress the descending pathways which normally inhibit spinal reflexes. This is found with all inhalational agents but particularly with halothane. Shivering with extradural anaesthesia is also common and is thought to be caused by differential nerve blockade, either suppressing descending inhibition of spinal reflexes or allowing selective transmission of cold sensation. It is rare with spinal anaesthesia as neural blockade is more dense. Shivering increases metabolic rate and oxygen consumption, which results in hypoxaemia and a respiratory alkalosis as it promotes hyperventilation. Supplementary oxygen therapy is often required. Pethidine and fentanyl have been used with some success to ameliorate shivering, as has doxapram. (See: Editorial (1991) Perioperative shivering. *Lancet* **338**, 547–548. Also: Crossley AWA (1992) Postoperative shivering. *Anaesthesia* **47**, 193–195.)

2.32 A.F B.T C.F D.T E.T
The Severinghaus electrode consists of glass sensitive to hydrogen ions in contact with a thin layer of sodium bicarbonate buffer separated from the liquid being tested (usually arterial blood) by a thin Teflon or silicone membrane which is permeable to CO_2. The CO_2 and hydrogen ions are in equilibrium according to the equation:

$$CO_2 + H_2O \rightleftharpoons H_2CO_3 \rightleftharpoons H^+ + HCO_3{}^-$$

Thus CO_2 diffuses from the blood into the buffer and the change in hydrogen ion concentration is measured and converted into P_{CO_2}. The process is temperature-dependent and the electrode should be maintained at 37°C. Before use it requires calibration with standard gas mixtures containing known concentrations of carbon dioxide. The accuracy is to about 130 Pa (1 mmHg). It measures only CO_2 dissolved in solution, not CO_2 combined with bicarbonate or haemoglobin. It is considered to be a direct method, unlike capnography, the Siggard–Anderson nomogram or the van Slyke apparatus.

2.33 A.F   B.F   C.T   D.T   E.T

Since there is a continuous column of blood from the pulmonary vessels to the left atrium in normal subjects PAOP will be a reasonable estimate of left atrial pressure (LAP), and thus of left ventricular end-diastolic pressure or preload. It is a more useful measurement than central venous pressure (CVP) when right atrial pressures do not reflect left heart function, as with LV failure, myocardial infarction, severe bundle branch block, pulmonary hypertension, cardiac tamponade and constrictive pericarditis. It is *not* reliable in the following situations:

1. When the position of the catheter tip is outside West's zone III (i.e. pulmonary artery pressure (PAP) > LAP > alveolar pressure: flow independent of the alveolar pressure).
2. Pulmonary venous obstruction, e.g. atrial myxoma and pulmonary fibrosis.
3. Valvular heart disease, e.g. mitral stenosis and regurgitation and aortic regurgitation.
4. After considerable loss of the pulmonary bed, e.g. pneumonectomy or a large pulmonary embolus.

2.34 A.T   B.T   C.F   D.F   E.T

Cor pulmonale is right heart failure due to chronic lung disease, principally chronic bronchitis and emphysema but can also be associated with recurrent pulmonary emboli, sleep apnoea syndrome and pulmonary fibrosis. The underlying mechanism is an increase in pulmonary vascular resistance by a combination of pulmonary vascular bed destruction and pulmonary vasoconstriction from the coexisting hypoxia and acidosis. This increases pressure in the right side of the heart, which initially compensates by hypertrophy before failing. The classic triad of signs consists of raised jugular venous pressure, hepatomegaly and peripheral oedema which can result in ascites or pleural effusion when severe. A third heart sound coincides with the end of ventricular diastolic filling; this is physiological in young adults but in middle age or later indicates impaired ventricular function and a raised end-diastolic pressure. It can originate from either ventricle and is heard as a gallop rhythm. A third heart sound is often associated with tricuspid and pulmonary incompetence. HPOA causes joint pain, finger clubbing and subperiosteal new bone formation and is associated with lung cancer.

2.35 A.F B.F C.T D.F E.F
MRI produces images by detecting induced changes in hydrogen using a strong magnetic force measured in tesla (0.05–2 T normally). One T = 10 000 gauss (earth's magnetic field = 0.5–1.0 G). The magnetic field needs to be protected from radiofrequency waves by a Faraday cage. Safe distances from the magnet are measured as the 5 gauss and 50 gauss lines. These are variable distances measured in metres and need to be ascertained prior to use as the attractive force exerts a substantial pull on ferromagnetic objects nearby and can distort the image. Cardiac pacemakers should not pass the 5 gauss line. Many implanted prostheses are safe (e.g. cardiac valves, joints) but care needs to be taken with cerebral aneurysm clips and metal intraocular foreign bodies. The procedure is anaesthetically challenging, but initial difficulties with monitoring have since been resolved using non-ferromagnetic equipment. Ferromagnetic gas cylinders should be behind the 50 gauss line. Metal detectors are too insensitive to be of value. (See: Menon DK *et al.* (1992) Magnetic resonance imaging. *Anaesthesia* **47**, 240–255, 508–517.)

2.36 A.T B.T C.T D.T E.T
Central venous cannulation should ideally place the catheter in the superior vena cava. The incidence of failed cannulation and complications mainly depends on operator experience rather than the approach used: 10% if experienced, 20% if inexperienced. Relatively frequent complications include sepsis (>50% from skin around the puncture), pneumothorax, vascular perforation, thrombosis, arterial puncture and air embolism. Less common ones include cardiac tamponade from myocardial wall rupture, hydrothorax, haemothorax, brachial plexus and phrenic nerve injury and damage to the thoracic duct. Horner's syndrome arises from damage to the sympathetic chain.

2.37 A.T   B.F   C.T   D.F   E.T

The use of hypotensive anaesthesia is controversial but its aims are to reduce blood loss (some estimate up to 50% less during major surgery) and to improve the surgical field, particularly in middle ear and neurosurgery. Hypotensive anaesthesia is normally defined as lowering blood pressure (BP) more than 30% from its resting level. In a previously normotensive patient a mean arterial pressure of 50–60 mmHg is considered safe. A drop to a mean BP of 35 mmHg has been used with minimal adverse effects but invasive monitoring is desirable (cerebral function monitor, jugular bulb oxygen content, for example). As hypotension decreases organ perfusion a further reduction in oxygen delivery due to anaemia can only worsen cerebral damage. BP at the head is 15–20 mmHg lower than mean systemic blood pressure, thus an extreme head-up position may compromise cerebral blood flow further. If necessary, a tilt of 15–20° is usually sufficient. It is routine in open-heart surgery to maintain a low perfusion pressure of between 30 and 50 mmHg. Cerebral consequences of open-heart surgery have been documented in up to 60% of patients. They are thought to be partly due to air-bubble embolization and blood aggregate formation from cardiopulmonary bypass rather than the hypotension. Isoflurane confers some cerebral protection compared with halothane and enflurane as it is better at preserving cerebral autoregulation and reducing cerebral metabolic rate. Moderate hyperventilation is used for cerebral protection in the management of head injuries. (See: McDowall DG (1985) Induced hypotension and brain ischaemia. *British Journal of Anaesthesia* **57**, 110–119.)

2.38 A.F   B.T   C.T   D.T   E.F

A cataract is a lens opacity usually associated with ageing (and exposure to ultraviolet light). It is found in 50% of the population over the age of 65 years. Systemic diseases which cause cataracts include DM, hypoparathyroidism, myotonic dystrophy, atopic dermatitis, galactosaemia and the syndromes of Werner's, Lowe's and Down's. Other causes are congenital (e.g. maternal rubella infection), traumatic, inflammatory, and vitamin deficiencies. Marfan's syndrome is associated with either upwards or sideways lens dislocation (homocysteinuria is downwards!) along with increased height, hypermobility, high arched palate, scoliosis and dilatation of the ascending aorta.

2.39 A.F **B.**T **C.**F **D.**F **E.**F

Therapeutic interventions for a severe head injury include elective hyperventilation in the first 24 hours to reduce $P_a CO_2$ to 3.5–4.0 kpa. It aims to induce cerebral vasoconstriction, thereby reducing blood volume and improving cerebral acidosis. Lowering the $P_a CO_2$ below 3.5 kPa must be avoided as it can lead to lactic acidosis and cerebral infarction. Hypothermia of 32–33°C is thought to be of value. It was initially assumed to be due to a reduction in energy requirements and prevention of build-up of toxic metabolites. However, it may be more subtle, instead involving improvement in cell membrane and ion channel integrity, with amelioration of the adverse effects of free oxygen radicals. Pharmacological reduction of cerebral metabolism with thiopentone and etomidate has not been found to be of value unless given prior to cerebral insult. A combination of hyperglycaemia, salt and water retention, and an increased incidence of infectious complications induced by steroids, is probably responsible for the poorer outcome associated with their use. Calcium channel antagonists (e.g. nimodipine) are selective cerebral vasodilators and are useful in the management of cerebral vasospasm after subarachnoid haemorrhage. Unfortunately, no improvement in clinical outcome has been demonstrated with their use in severe head injuries.

2.40 A.F **B.**T **C.**F **D.**F **E.**F

The PT measures the extrinsic pathway of the coagulation cascade. It is prolonged with deficiency of factor VII and clotting factors common to both pathways (X, V, prothrombin and fibrinogen). Haemophilia A is a sex-linked recessive disease due to lack of factor VIII. PT and bleeding time are normal in haemophilia A but the partial thromboplastin time (PTT) is prolonged. Von Willebrand's disease is an autosomal dominant condition which results in reduced synthesis of von Willebrand factor. This protein promotes platelet adhesion and as a carrier molecule for factor VIII protects it from premature destruction, which explains the low levels of factor VIII also seen. Platelet count is normal, as is PT, but the bleeding time is prolonged and the PTT may be normal or prolonged. Christmas disease (haemophilia B) is due to factor IX deficiency and has the same effects and results as haemophilia A.

2.41 A.T B.T C.F D.T E.T

MI most often occurs as a result of coronary artery thrombosis from atherosclerotic plaque rupture. It is the commonest cause of death in developed countries and old age, stress and social isolation increase mortality. Pulmonary oedema may arise from heart failure due to extensive infarction or rupture of the ventricular septum/mitral valve papillary muscle and is associated with a high mortality. Similarly, complete heart block with an anterior MI indicates involvement of the bundle of His and occurs as a result of extensive myocardial necrosis. Primary VF occurring within 24–48 hours of an MI has no effect on prognosis if treated promptly. However, delayed VF after more than 48 hours is associated with large infarcts, heart failure and a much poorer prognosis. Diabetics are more likely to have heart disease and to die from its complications.

2.42 A.F B.F C.F D.F E.T

	Sevoflurane	Desflurane
MAC	2	6
Blood : gas coefficient	0.65	0.45
% metabolized	3	0.0002

Sevoflurane is a non-flammable, polyfluorinated methyl isopropyl ether. Its blood : gas partition coefficient is lower than that of isoflurane (which is 1.4), suggesting faster induction and emergence. It is non-irritant to the respiratory tract. It is metabolized by cytochrome P-450 to fluoride ions (no renal effects found) and hexafluorisopropanol, which undergoes rapid glucuronidation, preventing any potential liver damage by hapten formation. In combination with dried-out baralyme and possibly soda lime it has been implicated in the production of toxic vinyl derivatives (compound A), lethal to rats. It is not considered clinically important. *Desflurane* is a polyfluorinated methyl ethyl ether. It differs from isoflurane by substitution of a fluoride ion for a chloride ion. Its blood : gas partition coefficient is low but as it is irritant to the airways at more than 1 MAC it limits speed of induction. It is stable with soda lime. As expected from the small amount metabolized serum fluoride ion concentration does not increase. As desflurane has a boiling point of 23.5°C, a temperature-controlled, pressurized vaporizer is required. Both have analgesic properties. Desflurane is probably more emetogenic than sevoflurane. (See: Merrett KL, Jones RM (1994) Inhalational anaesthetic agents. *British Journal of Hospital Medicine* **52**, 260–263.)

2.43 A.T B.F C.T D.T E.T
In starvation, the body initially relies on breakdown of hepatic glycogen to glucose for energy. As liver stores are small, increased gluconeogenesis is necessary to maintain glucose levels. Suitable substrates include glycerol from lipolysis and amino acids from protein catabolism. Non-esterified fatty acids are also produced by lipolysis and are either used directly as a fuel or oxidized in the liver to ketone bodies where they soon replace glucose as the main source of energy. Insulin levels fall, which is useful in as much as it normally inhibits lipolysis. Growth hormone secretion is increased by hypoglycaemia, stress (including starvation) and exercise. As it stimulates protein synthesis, lipolysis and gluconeogenesis, trials of growth factor in enteral feeds have shown it consistently to improve nitrogen balance and the rate of protein synthesis. However, it is expensive and has yet to be validated in terms of reduced hospital stay or mortality.

2.44 A.F B.T C.T D.T E.F
Syndrome of inappropriate antidiuretic hormone secretion (SIADH) results in a dilutional hyponatraemia and a low plasma osmolality owing to excessive water retention. Clinical signs include confusion, nausea and irritability and, later, fits and coma, particularly if sodium falls below 120 mmol/l. Causes are many and include:

Tumours	– small-cell lung, prostate, thymus, pancreas, lymphomas.
Pulmonary	– pneumonia, tuberculosis, lung abscess.
CNS	– meningitis, tumours, head injury, subdural, abscess, systemic lupus erythematosis (SLE) vasculitis.
Metabolic	– alcohol withdrawal, acute intermittent porphyria.
Drugs	– chlorpropamide, carbamezapine, cyclophosphamide.

Treatment includes correcting the underlying cause, and fluid restriction. If severe, hypertonic saline and frusemide can be given, although reported complications include congestive cardiac failure and central pontine myelinolysis.

2.45 A.F B.F C.T D.F E.F

The dissociation constant, pK_a, of a drug is the pH at which ionized (water-soluble) and non-ionized (lipid-soluble) forms are equal. As pK_a increases, the amount of drug available in the non-ionized form at physiological pH decreases. As the cell membrane is impermeable to the ionized form of a drug, a slower onset of action will be seen. Thus, lignocaine with a pK_a of 7.7 has a faster onset of action than bupivacaine with a pK_a of 8.1. The stronger the acid, the lower its pK_a. Equally, the stronger the base the higher its pK_a, and a drug with a pK_a of 9.4 is therefore alkaline. Such a drug is thus unlikely to be a gastric irritant (antacids are alkaline), but will have increased excretion with acidic urine. pK_a has little effect on protein binding, although as a general rule acidic drugs tend to bind to albumin, whereas basic drugs tend to bind to glycoproteins.

2.46 A.T B.T C.T D.F E.T

The parotid is the commonest site for tumours of the salivary gland. Of these about 75% are benign. Despite treatment, they often recur and occasionally manifest as metastatic disease. They are more common in women (1.7 : 1), with a peak incidence at age 60–70 years. Most present as a slow-growing, painless mass visible on opening the mouth. Palpation alone cannot distinguish whether the mass is benign, malignant or inflammatory. Prognostic indicators of malignant change include sudden and rapid acceleration of growth, facial, lingual or hypoglossal nerve involvement, local pain, enlarged lymph nodes or the presence of distant metastases (rare). Malignant disease tends to be aggressive and 5-year survival is <50%. Staging is important but open biopsy is contraindicated as local seeding of the tumour can occur. Treatment is surgical excision with or without adjuvent radiotherapy.

2.47 A.F B.F C.F D.T E.F

Cushing's disease is due to excess glucocorticoids from inappropriate pituitary secretion of ACTH. Cushing's syndrome, however, is the general term used to refer to elevated glucocorticoid levels from other causes, the most common of which is chronic steroid therapy. The end-result is the same: patients are truncally obese with moon facies and a plethoric complexion. Hypertension is common. Cortisol is catabolic and breaks down protein resulting in thin, easily bruised skin, striae, proximal myopathy and osteoporosis. Increased gluconeogenesis results in impaired glucose tolerance. Increased susceptibility to infections occurs but is normally asymptomatic due to suppression of the normal inflammatory response. Androgen levels are raised, resulting in hirsutism and acne. Gonadal function is frequently abnormal with oligomenorrhoea in women and impotence in men. Many present with psychiatric problems (e.g. depression and overt psychosis). In 80%, a cure can be achieved with surgical excision of the adenoma.

2.48 A.F **B.**T **C.**F **D.**T **E.**T

Double lumen tubes are used for one-lung ventilation (OLV). The lumens of the tracheal tube can lie behind or at the side of each other, depending on the make. The Carlen's tube has a carinal hook, the Robertshaw does not. Left-sided tubes are more difficult to insert but are preferred even for right-sided surgery as the origin of the right upper lobe bronchus is variable and may lead to inadequate ventilation and right upper lung collapse if the opening is blocked. Overinflation of the bronchial cuff can lead to bronchial rupture. The smallest double lumen tube is comparable to a size 7.0 mm tracheal tube which limits its use to those aged 8 years and over. If OLV is required in a younger child, bronchial placement of a tracheal tube can be achieved using fibreoptic bronchoscopy. (See: Vaughan RS (1993) Editorial: double lumen tubes. *British Journal of Anaesthesia* **70**, 497–498. Also: Hurford *et al.* (1992) Placement and complications of double lumen endobronchial tubes. *Anesthesia and Analgesia* **74**, S141.)

2.49 A.T **B.**F **C.**F **D.**T **E.**F

ICP is normally 7–15 mmHg; this can be increased by tumours, abscesses, haematomas and cerebral oedema. Clinical features are initially non-specific and include headache, often worse in the morning and exacerbated by stooping or straining, nausea and vomiting, and confusion. As ICP continues to rise papilloedema, impaired consciousness, hypertension and bradycardia (Cushing's reflex) occur. When severe, hypotension, coma, irregular respiration or apnoea with fixed dilated pupils indicate impending brainstem death. Rhinorrhoea is suggestive of a base-of-skull fracture.

2.50 **A**.F **B**.F **C**.T **D**.T **E**.F

Pulmonary contusion after blunt chest injury can be present even in the absence of superficial signs of injury. Auscultation is initially normal. Chest radiograph changes usually occur within 6 hours to show hazy shadowing and diffuse opacities. This was initially thought to be due to interstitial lung damage producing consolidation and collapse but computerized tomography (CT) scanning has confirmed it to be the result of a pulmonary laceration surrounded by intra-alveolar haemorrhage, without significant interstitial injury. Within 12–24 hours the damaged part of the lung becomes increasingly oedematous, and lung compliance falls. This is compounded by significant hypoventilation and impaired cough as a result of pain. Short-term ventilation may be required. However, contusion results in few long-term respiratory problems even though it is followed by superimposed infection in over 50% of cases. (See: Wagner RB, Jamieson PM (1989) Pulmonary contusion. Evaluation and classification by computed technology. *Surgical Clinics of North America* **69**, 31–40. Also: Allen GS, Coates NE (1996) Pulmonary contusion: a collective review. *American Surgeon* **62**, 895–900.)

2.51 **A**.F **B**.F **C**.F **D**.T **E**.F

An explosion is like a fire in that a combustible substance, a gas to support combustion and a source of ignition are required. The difference is that in an explosion the speed of the reaction is so fast that large amounts of heat, light and sound are given out. Combustible substances of importance in clinical practice include alcohol used to clean skin and methane and hydrogen found in the patient's gastrointestinal tract. The modern inhalational agents (e.g. halothane, enflurane, isoflurane) are non-flammable as they have resistant C–F bonds. Oxygen is not explosive but it supports combustion. Nitrous oxide rapidly breaks down to oxygen and nitrogen in the presence of heat. As such, it can also prolong or increase the extent of a fire or explosion. Similarly, the most violent reactions occur in stoichiometric mixtures, i.e. where the concentrations of combustible vapour (e.g. cyclopropane) and oxidizing agent (e.g. oxygen) are in exact proportion so that if an explosion occurs the combustible vapour and the oxidizing agent will be completely used up. The source of ignition can be a spark from a laser, naked flame or from a build-up of static electricity in electrical equipment (e.g. diathermy machines, monitors, switches). As static electricity is worse in a dry environment, relative humidity in the operating theatre is maintained above 50%. (*See* MacDonald AG (1994) A short history of fires and explosions caused by anaesthetic agents. *British Journal of Anaesthesia* **72**, 710–722.)

2.52 A.F B.F C.T D.T E.F
Blood supply to the nose is from branches of the internal and external carotid arteries (mainly ophthalmic and maxillary arteries). A number of these meet and anastomose with each other in Little's area found medially, at the lower part of the nasal septum. The lateral wall of the nose consists of the superior, medial and inferior conchae which guard the meatal openings of the paranasal sinuses. Epistaxis is common, and can be venous or arterial; the former is more common in the young, the latter in older age groups. A sudden rise of vascular pressure from coughing, sneezing, sinusitis, nose-blowing, etc. has been implicated. Hypertension does not increase the incidence of epistaxis in the general population but if nose-bleeding occurs in a person with hypertension then the bleeding tends to be more severe and persistent, which explains why many admitted to hospital have high blood pressure. Treatment is by nose-pinching (for venous bleeding), topical anaesthesia and cauterization if the bleeding point is visible, or anterior packing or postnasal packing if not. If bleeding persists over 4–5 days or after removal of packs, external carotid artery ligation may be required (as this supplies >90% of the nasal mucosa). Vincent's angina is malaise and pyrexia with lymphadenopathy and throat ulcers due to bacterial infection, probably *Borrelia vincenti*. Treatment is with penicillin.

2.53 A.T B.F C.T D.F E.T
Streptokinase is produced by Lancefield group C β-haemolytic streptococci. It promotes fibrinolysis by activating conversion of plasminogen to plasmin. Its use has been shown to reduce hospital and 1-year mortality after a MI by re-establishing blood flow through the occluded coronary artery in 50–70% of patients (although 30% recanalize without any treatment). It is best given within the first 6 hours, but is still clinically effective for up to 24 hours after a MI. Concurrent aspirin therapy reduces mortality further, unlike heparin. The rise in plasmin can increase the risk of bleeding complications. It is also

associated with allergic and anaphylactic reactions, the incidence of which can be reduced by slow infusion rates and steroid cover. Although antibody-mediated inhibition of plasminogen activation precludes repeated use, as does a recent stroke and surgery within the previous 14 days, diabetes does not.

2.54 A.T **B.**T **C.**T **D.**T **E.**F
Raised ICP in adults is primarily associated with erosion of the dorsum sellae. In young children suture diastasis occurs instead. Craniopharyngiomas present mainly in children as calcified tumours above the sella, but some are located in the sella leading to distortion. Chiasmatic gliomas, also more common in children, are associated with an odd-shaped sella. Cushing's disease is pituitary-dependent adrenal hyperplasia from a pituitary adenoma. Primary hyperaldosteronism (Conn's syndrome) arises from the adrenal gland.

2.55 A.T **B.**T **C.**F **D.**F **E.**F
Developed in 1971, etomidate is a carboxylated imidazole induction agent, structurally related to the imidazole antifungals (e.g. ketaconazole). It is soluble in water but is presented in solution with 35% propylene glycol at a pH of 4.2 and a pK_a of 4.1. Elimination half-life is short at 75 min, and it undergoes rapid hydrolysis by hepatic esterases before renal excretion as glucuronide conjugates (2% is excreted unchanged). Etomidate produces minimal ventilatory depression, confers cerebral protection and is thought to produce greater haemodynamic stability by having less cardiodepressant effect than other agents. Cardiac output and blood pressure fall by about 10%. Despite recent doubts, it is probably still the preferred agent for induction in those at risk of cardiovascular depression. In addition, it does not routinely provoke histamine release and is very rarely associated with adverse drug reactions making it useful for atopic individuals. The most serious adverse effect is blocking of 17α-hydroxylase and 11β-hydroxylase enzymes, thereby inhibiting production of steroids including cortisol. Following a single dose, the rise in plasma cortisol normally seen after surgery is delayed. As such, it is no longer used by infusion for sedation in ICUs. Although non-irritant to the tissues, about 10% of patients suffer local thrombophlebitis and pain on injection, which can be reduced with concomitant use of lignocaine. Approximately one-third of patients develop

myoclonic movements on induction. This is not associated with EEG changes and, in fact, etomidate is an effective anti-convulsant. The incidence of nausea and vomiting is increased. It has a mild depressing effect on plasma cholinesterase and may slightly prolong the action of suxamethonium.

2.56 A.T B.F C.F D.F E.F

Gas chromatography separates a mixture into its components by injecting a sample of the mixture into a stream of inert gas such as argon, nitrogen or helium (mobile phase). This is then passed through a long, coiled glass column filled with material such as polyethylene glycol or silicone-coated silica-alumina (stationary phase). The components separate owing to their relative solubilities in the two phases. A detector then monitors the appearance of the components at the outlet. The most commonly employed method is the flame ionization detector. Suitable alternatives include the thermal conductivity detector (best for analysis of inorganic gases, e.g. N_2O and O_2) or the electron capture detector (best for halogenated compounds). The method is used for volatile anaesthetics, barbiturates, benzodiazepines, catecholamines and steroids. It is sensitive to minute concentrations but requires calibration to quantify each substance. Continuous analysis is not possible.

2.57 A.F B.F C.T D.T E.F

Myoglobin is an iron-containing pigment found in skeletal and heart muscle. It resembles haemoglobin but reversibly binds 1 rather than 4 molecules of oxygen per molecule of myoglobin. Its dissociation curve is a rectangular hyperbola which lies to the left of that for haemoglobin; this allows it to take up oxygen from haemoglobin in the blood. It releases oxygen at low partial pressures (<1 kPa) and acts as a reservoir for actively contracting muscle where the partial pressure of oxygen is near to zero. The Bohr effect (a decrease in the O_2 affinity of haemoglobin when the pH of blood falls – this shifts the oxyhaemoglobin dissociation curve to the right) does not occur and it does not bind with CO_2. The molecular weight of myoglobin is 17 000 whilst that of haemoglobin is 64 500.

2.58 A.T B.F C.T D.F E.T

Disequilibrium syndrome is a relatively common problem associated with haemodialysis. The pathogenesis is thought to be the 'reverse urea hypothesis' whereby haemodialysis removes urea more slowly from the brain than from the plasma, thus creating an osmotic gradient resulting in cerebral oedema. The syndrome is more often seen with very rapid haemodialysis. Symptoms include headache, nausea, vomiting, cramps, restlessness, hypotension and, when severe, seizures and coma. It occurs with acetate dialysate and only very rarely with bicarbonate dialysate. As both peritoneal dialysis and haemofiltration are continuous processes, toxins and excess fluid are removed slowly and disequilibrium syndrome rarely, if ever, occurs. Autonomic neuropathy, a known complication of chronic renal failure, plays no part in the pathogenesis of disequilibrium syndrome. (See: Arieff AI (1994) Dialysis disequilibrium syndrome: current concepts in pathogenesis and prevention. *Kidney International* **45**, 619–635.)

2.59 A.T   B.F   C.T   D.T   E.F
Suction involves generating a vacuum, the efficiency of which is determined by the degree of subatmospheric pressure generated and the volume of air that can be moved in unit time (displacement). Anaesthesia requires suction to be of high displacement with a high negative pressure to be able to clear vomit and secretions, etc. This can be achieved by a variety of methods including using the Venturi principle from a high flow of compressed gas. Surgery requires suction of high displacement with low pressure whilst drainage (e.g. thoracic drains) requires low pressure and low displacement. For standard use in anaesthetic practice, minimal flows and pressures in the order of 25 l/min and 60–80 kPa have been suggested. Active scavenging of waste anaesthetic gases should have its own dedicated system separate from the normal hospital vacuum system to prevent excessive vacuum applied to the patient and contamination from anaesthetic gases.

2.60 A.F   B.T   C.F   D.T   E.T
Body weight depends on energy balance between intake and demand. In diabetes, energy intake may be adequate but nutrients fail to reach the cells where they are needed so weight is lost. This is because insulin is required for passage of glucose from blood into the cells. As insulin is reduced or absent in untreated DM, blood glucose is high but intracellular glucose is low so cells must catabolize fat and protein. Thyrotoxicosis increases metabolic rate and thus energy demand which is rarely compensated by increased food intake. Tuberculosis, like

all chronic infective diseases, increases catabolic demand, resulting in weight loss. Underlying malignancy is probably the most common cause of weight loss despite in the initial stages a normal or increased appetite. The pain of gastric ulcer may be so severe as to prevent eating and weight loss is the norm (the opposite is said to be true for duodenal ulcers). Similarly hypoadrenalism – Addison's disease – also causes weight loss as a result of anorexia.

2.61 A.T B.T C.F D.T E.F

The femoral nerve arises from the anterior primary divisions of L2, L3, L4. The femoral artery lying medially is the landmark for the block. Obturator nerve block is also necessary for knee surgery but femoral nerve block alone can provide adequate analgesia for a fractured femur and postoperative analgesia following an arthroscopy or reconstructive knee surgery. The saphenous branch of the femoral nerve supplies sensation over the medial side of the calf; the lateral side is supplied by the lateral cutaneous nerve from the common peroneal nerve. (See: Banssillon V (1988) Femoral nerve block for postoperative analgesia after open knee surgery. *Canadian Journal of Anaesthesia* **35**, 439.)

2.62 A.T B.F C.T D.F E.T

The Fick principle states that the amount of substance taken up by an organ per unit time is equal to the arterial level of the substance minus the venous level multiplied by the blood flow. This can be rearranged to measure blood flow to an organ, i.e.

$$\text{Blood flow to an organ in unit time} = \frac{\text{amount of marker taken up by the organ in unit time}}{\text{concentration difference of the substance between the vessels supplying and draining the organ}}$$

Applying this principle to the measurement of cardiac output, either oxygen or carbon dioxide can be employed as the 'marker' substance. Thus with oxygen:

$$\text{Cardiac output} = \frac{\text{oxygen consumption (ml/min)}}{\text{arterial} - \text{mixed venous oxygen content (ml/l)}}$$

Substituting normal (i.e. expected) values:

$$\text{Cardiac output} = \frac{250\,\text{ml/min}}{200 - 150\,\text{ml/l}} = 5\,\text{l/min}$$

Calculating cardiac output with carbon dioxide uses the formula:

$$\text{Cardiac output} = \frac{\text{carbon dioxide produced (ml/min)}}{\text{mixed venous} - \text{arterial carbon dioxide}}$$
$$\text{concentration (ml/l)}$$

Again substituting normal (i.e. expected) values:

$$\text{Cardiac output} = \frac{200}{540 - 500\,\text{ml/l}} = 5\,\text{l/min}$$

The same principle can also be used to determine blood flow to other organs, e.g. cerebral (Kety–Schmidt technique) and renal blood flow.

2.63 A.F   B.T   C.F   D.T   E.F
Heatstroke tends to occur in young fit people during fun runs and short-duration events. A very high temperature ($>42°C$ core) can lead to cardiovascular collpase due to release of endotoxins, interleukin-1 and TNF from a relatively ischaemic bowel. Treatment must be aggressive and immediate. It includes rapid rehydration with intravenous crystalloid and cool packs over the large vessels of the axillae, neck and groin. The most effective way of achieving rapid cooling while preserving dilatation of the skin is to spray the naked patient with warm water whilst also fanning warm air over the skin. If the temperature does not fall below $40°C$ within 30 min peritoneal lavage with iced saline or rarely extracorporeal cooling using cardiopulmonary bypass can be instituted. Active cooling can be stopped when the core temperature reaches $39°C$. Steroids and prophylactic antibiotics are not recommended. Salicylates are implicated in precipitating hyperthermia as they uncouple oxidative phosphorylation. Dantrolene is effective in malignant hyperthermia (MH) and neuroleptic malignant syndrome (NMS) but is not useful in heatstroke.

2.64 A.T   B.F   C.F   D.T   E.T
H_1-receptor blockers such as chlorpheniramine have various clinical uses. They have a palliative function in mild allergic reactions such as hay fever and urticaria although they are ineffective in more severe conditions (e.g. asthma and acute anaphylaxis) where autocoids such as leukotrienes or bradykinin are produced. Although nausea and vomiting have been

reported with their use, some (e.g. cyclizine, promethazine) are effective antiemetics for motion sickness, labyrinthine disorders, chemotherapy and after surgery. This is probably mediated through central antagonism of acetylcholine. The newer drugs (e.g. terfenadine) which do not cross the blood–brain barrier are not effective antiemetics. H_1-receptor blockers can both stimulate and depress the CNS, which makes them unpredictable as premedicants in children (e.g. trimeprazine). They often have significant peripheral anticholinergic effects which may result in a dry mouth and urinary retention but are without adrenergic effects. Haemolytic anaemia, leukopenia and agranulocytosis are very rare side-effects.

2.65 A.F **B.**F **C.**F **D.**T **E.**F
The approximate male : female ratios are:

SLE	– 1 : 9
primary adrenocortical deficiency	– 1 : 2
primary biliary cirrhosis	– 1 : 6
congenital hypertrophic pyloric stenosis	– 5 : 1
Parkinson's disease	– 1 : 1

2.66 A.F **B.**T **C.**F **D.**F **E.**F
Carbon dioxide may be present in the stomach but sustained levels in repeated expirations indicate correct tracheal tube placement and capnography is the monitoring method of choice. Preoxygenation may delay hypoxaemia, thus significantly delaying detection of oesophageal intubation if pulse oximetry is relied upon. Condensation on the tracheal tube has been demonstrated with both oesophageal and tracheal intubation. Chest expansion and auscultation are not reliable in the very young (inflating the stomach can cause similar signs), the obese or patients with hyperexpanded chests (e.g. chronic obstructive pulmonary disease). Carbon dioxide indicators giving breath-by-breath colour changes have been advocated, as has the aspiration test of Wee, but to be certain direct visualization with a fibreoptic bronchoscope is required. The light wand is used to aid blind nasal intubation. (See: Wee MYK (1988) The oesophageal detector device. *Anaesthesia* **43**, 27–29. Also: Birmingham PK *et al.* (1986) Esophageal intubation: a review of detection techniques. *Anesthesia and Analgesia* **65**, 886–891.)

2.67 A.F B.F C.F D.T E.F

PCA, described in 1971, is a widely used method of administering analgesia for surgery and cancer-related pain, amongst others. Possible routes of administration include intravenous, intramuscular, subcutaneous, extradural and intrathecal. Self-administration allows a predetermined bolus of painkiller (most opiates, including fentanyl, local anaesthetics (LAs), clonidine, etc.) to be given in a preset time period with or without a background infusion. It has been successfully used in children as young as 4 years of age. There is no upper age limit although postoperative confusion in the elderly may limit its use. The incidence of side-effects is often no less with PCA compared with the intramuscular route. This includes all the typical side-effects including respiratory depression, prolonged postoperative ileus, urinary retention and nausea and vomiting. Concomitant use of NSAIDs reduces analgesic demand, as does oral clonidine. Overall patient satisfaction is high (>90%), although this is an insensitive indicator of analgesic efficacy. (See: Ballantyne JC *et al.* (1993) Postoperative patient controlled analgesia: metanalysis of randomised control trials. *Journal of Clinical Anesthesia* **5**, 182–193. Also: Hall GM, Salmon P (1997) Editorial: patient-controlled analgesia – who benefits? *Anaesthesia* **52**, 401–402.)

2.68 A.T B.F C.T D.T E.F

Hydroxyethyl starch (hetastarch) is synthesized from amylopectin, a starch derived from maize or sorghum. The size of molecules is heterogeneous with a mean molecular weight (MW) of 450 000. About 40% remains in the intravascular compartment after 24 hours, the remainder being eliminated by renal excretion or extravasated into the interstitial space. Adverse effects include mild-to-moderate anaphylactoid reactions (1 in 1200), increase in serum amylase and pruritus. Although studies are conflicting, it does seem to affect coagulation adversely, possibly through precipitation of factor VIII and fibrinogen. It does not interfere with cross-matching. *Dextrans* are polysaccharides derived from bacterial action on sucrose. There are three types, classified according to MW (40, 70 and 110 kDa). Side-effects include anaphylactic reactions (urticaria, hypotension, bronchospasm possibly from previous cross-immunization against bacterial antigens) and interference with cross-matching. A coagulopathy resulting in increased bleeding time occurs from impaired fibrin polymerization and reduced platelet function. *Gelatin* solutions include Gelofusin (succiny-lated) and Haemaccel (urea-linked). Average MW is about 35 000 Da with an intravascular half-life of 3–5 hours. Both, but particularly Haemaccel, have been responsible for anaphylac-toid reactions (0.15%), which are occasionally severe. Renal function, cross-matching and coagulation are not affected by their use. (See: Warren BB, Durieux ME (1997) Hydroxyethyl starch: safe or not? *Anesthesia and Analgesia* **84**, 206–212. Also: Cone A (1995) The use of colloids in clinical practice. *British Journal of Hospital Medicine* **54**, 155–159.)

2.69 A.F B.F C.T D.F E.T
The T wave represents ventricular repolarization. It follows the direction of the QRS complex and is normally less than 5 mm in height in the standard leads and less than 10 mm in the chest leads. It is inverted with myocardial ischaemia. Hyperkalaemia produces tall-peaked Ts, absent Ps, wide QRS complexes and ultimately complete heart block, VT or VF. Hypokalaemia shows a prominent U wave and T wave flattening. ECG changes with digoxin are non-specific: ST depression (reverse tick), U waves and QT shortening can occur but the amplitude of the T wave does not increase. Atrial fibrillation (AF) results in the loss of P waves but has no effect on T waves.

2.70 A.T B.F C.T D.T E.F
Digoxin is a highly protein-bound cardiac glycoside with inotropic and antiarrhythmic actions. Its inotropic actions are due to competitive inhibition of the Na^+K^+ ATPase pump resulting in high levels of intracellular Na^+. This, in turn, is exchanged for extracellular Ca^+ which enhances myocardial contractility. This was the basis for using digoxin for congestive cardiac failure, although it has now largely been replaced with safer drugs which have a higher therapeutic index. Its antiarrhythmic actions arise from a combination of increased vagal activity and prolongation of the refractory period of the atrioventricular (AV) node. It is thus useful in controlling AF and converting atrial flutter to AF. Digoxin's toxic effects include nausea and vomiting, anorexia, abdominal pain and diarrhoea. Adverse cardiac effects include all types of arrhyth-mias and varying degrees of AV block. Other features include fatigue, weakness and visual disturbances (abnormal red-green colour perception). Hypokalaemia enhances toxicity (adjuvant effect with digoxin by increasing phase 4 depolarization and

thus myocardial automaticity). Digoxin antibodies (Fab) are a useful antidote for life-threatening toxicity. Digoxin is contra-indicated in WPW syndrome as the AV block may encourage conduction through the accessory pathway with resultant arrhythmia.

2.71 A.F **B.**T **C.**T **D.**T **E.**T

Data which are not normally distributed can be analysed by non-parametric statistical tests. The chi-squared test and the Mann–Whitney rank sum test are used for nominal and ordinal data, respectively, when the data are in two groups (i.e. different subjects, different treatments). The McNemar test and the Wilcoxon rank sum test can be used for nominal and ordinal data, respectively, when the data are derived from one group (i.e. data from the same subjects before and after a treatment). Others non-parametric tests include Fischer's exact test, contingency coefficients and the Spear-mann rank correlation test; these compare two variables for association using nominal and ordinal data, respectively. Data can occasionally be 'normalized' by mathematical means to allow use of the more sensitive parametric tests, e.g. Student's *t*-test.

2.72 A.T **B.**T **C.**F **D.**F **E.**F

Both heart rate and stroke volume increase to contribute to an increase in cardiac output. Haematological changes include a 40% increase in blood volume with a 20% increase in red cell mass, resulting in a dilutional anaemia. The rise in GFR is mirrored by a rise in creatinine clearance; the tubular reabsorption of glucose universally declines. Pregnancy acti-vates the clotting system. All clotting factors bar XI and XIII increase, particularly VII, VIII, X and fibrinogen. Progesterone lowers oesophageal sphincter tone and there will be a tendency to develop heartburn and oesophagitis. Gastric emptying has long been thought to be delayed but recent research suggests it is not affected until late in labour.

2.73 A.T **B.**F **C.**T **D.**T **E.**T

Hydatidiform moles are part of a spectrum of gestational trophoblastic abnormalities associated with pregnancy. They tend to occur in older women and the 'mole' consists of the trophoblastic lining of the placental villi. Principal symptoms are vaginal bleeding, larger uterus than expected for dates, increased incidence of nausea and vomiting and abdominal pain. Pre-eclampsia with hypertension in the first trimester is almost pathognomonic. Diagnosis is by an excessively large increase in HCG and ultrasonography demonstrating multiple echoes but no gestational sac or fetus. Initial treatment with suction curettage results in a cure in 80–85% of cases. Serial HCG measurements are required to ensure complete elimination of trophoblastic tissue. Twenty per cent proceed to choriocarcinoma with or without metastatic disease which can be found in the gastrointestinal tract, genitourinary tract, liver, lung and brain. It does not cause a coagulopathy but is often associated with haemorrhage because of the propensity of trophoblastic disease to invade blood vessels. It is invariably fatal without treatment and chemotherapy and hysterectomy may be required. There is an increased incidence of recurrence in subsequent pregnancies.

2.74 A.F **B.**F **C.**T **D.**F **E.**T

Acute anaphylaxis arises from an antigen–antibody reaction producing mast cell degranulation and release of vasoactive kinins, which results in urticaria, angio-oedema, bronchospasm and cardiovascular collapse. Most anaesthetic drugs have been implicated in causing anaphylaxis; suxamethonium is the commonest trigger followed by thiopentone, atracurium and Haemaccel. The incidence in anaesthesia is about 1 in 6000. Immediate management is 100% oxygen, intubation and ventilation and external cardiac compression if the patient is pulseless. Adrenaline is the drug of choice. Combined with fluid expansion its use counteracts hypotension and hypovolaemia resulting from vasodilatation and increased vascular permeability. It also ameliorates bronchospasm (although bronchodilators, e.g. salbutamol and aminophylline, may also be of value) and limits angio-oedema. Noradrenaline may be required if hypotension is unresponsive to adrenaline. Isoprenaline will be ineffective as it principally has a chronotropic – not an inotropic – action. Although isoprenaline is also an effective bronchodilator, its use has been associated with significant arrhythmias which further precludes its use. Steroids have no proven benefit. H_1 blockers such as chlopheniramine are indicated only when anaphylaxis is protracted or if angio-oedema is a problem. There have been a few reports suggesting improvement in protracted anaphylaxis with H_2 blockers. It is not easy to decide which fluid is the best. Colloids are probably superior in the acute phase as they remain in the intravascular space for longer, but 0.9% saline is a valid option.

2.75 A.T **B**.T **C**.T **D**.T **E**.T

Mass spectrometry passes a gas sample through an ionizing chamber to be bombarded by an electron beam. Some gas molecules are hit, become charged and exit the chamber to pass through a strong magnetic field. The amount deflected depends on their mass and can be detected and displayed. *Raman spectrometry* employs the Raman effect: when light interacts with a gas molecule, the change in rotational and vibrational energy of the molecule during the interaction is characteristic of the molecule concerned. *Photoacoustic spectroscopy* exposes a gas sample to three beams of radiation which are absorbed by components of the mixture. Audio signals generated by the expansion and contraction of the gases are detected by microphone, filtered and recorded as breath-by-breath changes in gas composition. The *piezoelectric effect* is the change in the resonant frequency of a crystal of quartz in the presence of anaesthetic agents dissolved in an oily coating on the surface of the crystal. As the quantity of vapour dissolved is proportional to the partial pressure of the vapour present (Henry's Law), electronic measurement of the extent of the change in resonant frequency allows the amount of volatile anaesthetic to be determined. *Ultraviolet light* from a mercury lamp is absorbed by halothane and is the basis for a photocell. Infrared analysers and refractometers are also suitable.

2.76 A.T **B**.F **C**.F **D**.F **E**.T

Trigeminal neuralgia – tic douloureux – is a rare episodic, recurrent, unilateral facial pain within the distribution of the trigeminal nerve (44% mandibular, 36% maxillary, 20% ophthalmic). The electric shock-like pain has an abrupt onset and termination which can last a few seconds to minutes. The frequency of attacks is variable, ranging from few to many times a day. The condition can also remit for many years. It is triggered by non-noxious ipsilateral stimulation, such as rubbing, chewing, talking, etc. Neurological examination is normal unless associated with underlying pathology (1–5% are associated with e.g. multiple sclerosis, tumour). Aetiology is uncertain although abnormal vascular compression of the nerve is a possible cause. 70% of cases respond to pharmacological therapy alone, notably with carbamazepine, baclofen or phenytoin but not chlorpromazine. More invasive treatment, reserved for failed medical treatment, involves radiofrequency thermocoagulation or surgical microvascular decompression of the Gasserian ganglion. As a last resort, a peripheral neurectomy of the affected branch of the trigeminal nerve by cryotherapy or avulsion can denervate the trigger area but can result in anaesthesia dolorosa – pain far worse and intractable than the original. (See: Walchenbach R, Voormolen JHC (1996) Editorial: surgical treatment for trigeminal neuralgia. *British Medical Journal* **313**, 1027–1028.)

2.77 A.T **B.**F **C.**T **D.**F **E.**T
The three branches (femoral, obturator and lateral cutaneous nerves) of the lumbar plexus can be blocked with a single injection of a large volume of LA in the fascial sheath that accompanies the femoral nerve to the inguinal ligament. The needle is inserted as for a femoral nerve block but is directed obliquely cephalad. Paraesthesia ensures correct placement. Firm pressure distally encourages the local anaesthetic to spread upwards between the psoas and quadratus lumborum. Continuous infusion is possible using a catheter. The obturator nerve is frequently missed. (See: Winnie AP *et al.* (1973) The inguinal paravascular technique of lumbar plexus anesthesia: 'the 3 in 1 block'. *Anesthesia and Analgesia* **52**, 989–996. Also: Parkinson SK *et al.* (1989) Extent of blockade with various approaches to the lumbar plexus. *Anesthesia and Analgesia* **68**, 243.)

2.78 A.F **B.**T **C.**T **D.**T **E.**F
Specific gravity of urine is the measure of the number of particles in urine and their molecular weight. When urine principally consists of urea and sodium chloride it can be an approximate measure of urine osmolality and the kidney's ability to concentrate urine. A specific gravity of 1.030 suggests normal renal function and, as such, will be found in pre-renal failure and dehydration. Diabetes insipidus produces dilute urine in excessive quantities. In chronic renal failure, concentration of the urine is not possible and therefore specific gravity will be low.

2.79 A.F   B.T   C.T   D.T   E.F

Mixed venous blood is found only in the right ventricle or pulmonary artery. Blood in the inferior and superior vena cavae is different in composition and mixes only with passage through the heart. Mixed venous oxygen saturation reflects the amount of oxygen left after perfusion of the capillary beds in the systemic circulation and, as such, can be regarded as the oxygen reserve. It is a function of oxygen content [(Hb × S_aO_2 × 1.34 × 10)+ dissolved oxygen], oxygen consumption and cardiac output. Decreasing oxygen content and cardiac output and increasing oxygen consumption all lead to decreased mixed venous saturation. Mixed oxygen saturation is used clinically as an indicator of oxygen supply/demand in the critically ill. Serial recordings are best but a value below 50% (normal 75%) suggests haemodynamic failure. It should not be used in isolation as it can rise if oxygen delivery exceeds oxygen consumption, as seen with hypothermia and cyanide toxicity. In sepsis, tissue hypoxia is partly due to impaired utilization of oxygen and the value can be normal or high. Another source of error arises because the mixed venous oxygen saturation is the value for the mixture of blood draining from all the various vascular beds. Thus, localized hypoxia in one region may be masked by luxury perfusion in another. Mixed venous oxygen saturation can also be elevated as a result of a left-to-right intracardiac shunt. Measurement can be performed photometrically with the aid of a pulmonary artery flotation catheter.

2.80 A.F   B.T   C.F   D.F   E.F

Nutritional status is an important factor in survival and recovery from a critical illness. Unfortunately, there is no definitive test of nutritional status. Weight loss is too crude an indicator as it can be attributable to several factors such as loss of fat or lean body mass and changes in fluid status. Anthropometric tests, such as skinfold thickness, estimate body fat but are of little use in the critically ill as the relationship between subcutaneous and total body fat is no longer predictable. Plasma proteins have been described as nutritional indicators because they have been thought to reflect amino acid availability for hepatic protein synthesis. Albumin is a valuable test for predicting outcome but its long plasma half-life (20 days), insensitivity to pure nutritional depletion and need for albumin infusions in some patients make it unsuitable. Measuring nitrogen excretion is difficult and time-consuming but improvement in nitrogen balance is the single nutritional parameter associated with good outcomes and, as such, is useful. Changes in lymphocyte count are too non-specific to be of value. Other techniques for measuring body composition include bioelectrical impedance, neutron activation analysis and MRI but these are mainly used as research tools. (See: Murray MJ *et al.* (1988) Nutritional assessment of intensive care unit patients. *Mayo Clinic Proceedings* **63**, 1105–1115.)

2.81 A.F B.T C.F D.T E.T

In one-lung ventilation it is important to minimize hypoxaemia by reducing blood flow to the non-ventilated lung, i.e. the one being operated upon. This is facilitated by a combination of mechanical and physiological mechanisms which increase pulmonary vascular resistance to the non-ventilated lung, thereby shifting blood flow to the ventilated lung. These include gravity (lateral decubitus position), pathological distortion and altered vascular architecture (from chronic pulmonary vascular disease, tumour), the effects of opening the chest and creating a pneumothorax and hypoxic pulmonary vasoconstriction (HPV). Nevertheless, the non-ventilated lung will still have some blood flow and many studies have shown this can be up to 50% of normal. Although it has been suggested to be of theoretical rather than practical importance, a suggested cause is inhibition of HPV by hypocapnia and by the use of vasodilators such as volatile anaesthetics and glyceral trinitrate. Intravenous induction agents such as propofol do not inhibit HPV. It has also been shown that excessive PEEP to the ventilated lung impairs oxygenation by diverting blood to the non-ventilated one. However, clonidine has been shown to enhance HPV, probably through reduced sympathetic activity. Perioperatively clinical practice tends to focus less on decreasing blood flow to the ventilated lung and more on mimimizing ventilation–perfusion mismatch and alveolar hypoventilation in the ventilated lung. This may be achieved by increasing the F_iO_2, limiting surgical trauma and increasing tidal volume to the amount normally used for both lungs. In addition insufflation of oxygen to the non-ventilated lung may reduce hypoxaemia. If all these methods fail, occluding the pulmonary artery to the non-ventilated lung, extracorporeal membrane oxygenation (ECMO) and cardiopulmonary bypass are all possible options to help provide adequate oxygenation. (See:

Benumof JL (1985) One lung ventilation and hypoxic pulmonary vasoconstriction. Implications for anaesthetic management. *Anesthesia and Analgesia* **64**, 821–833.)

2.82 A.T **B.**T **C.**F **D.**T **E.**T

Phenytoin is an anticonvulsant which both reduces and limits seizure activity by membrane stabilization. It is absorbed slowly and is extensively bound to plasma proteins. It is metabolized in the liver to inactive compounds, before being excreted in bile and urine. Cardiac arrhythmias and hypotension occur when given rapidly by the intravenous route. Chronic oral administration can result in cerebellar–vestibular effects (nystagmus, diplopia, vertigo and ataxia), hirsutism, osteomalacia, megaloblastic anaemia, rashes, gingival hyperplasia, behavioural changes (particularly in children) and gastrointestinal problems (nausea, anorexia, pain). Like phenytoin, all the major anticonvulsants have been associated with fetal abnormalities (cleft lip, spina bifida, cardiac defects), although carbamazepine is the least likely to cause these. The greatest risk occurs with administration in the first trimester of pregnancy.

2.83 A.F **B.**T **C.**T **D.**T **E.**T

DVT is found in 25–30% of all postsurgical patients. Orthopaedic patients are at greatest risk with up to 70% developing a DVT after hip or knee surgery. Predisposing factors include obesity, age greater than 40 years, varicose veins, malignancy (e.g. pancreas), heart failure, oral contraceptive pill, prolonged surgery, dehydration and hypotensive anaesthesia but not sickle cell anaemia. Inherited thrombophilic conditions (antithrombin III, protein C and S deficiencies) are also a possibility, particularly if there is a history of recurrent DVTs. Diagnosis based solely on clinical signs and symptoms is often incorrect and venography is one of the best diagnostic tools available. It is superior to radiolabelled [^{125}I]fibrinogen uptake scans which can miss thrombi in the pelvis and upper thigh. Prevention of postoperative DVT is best achieved with a combination of graduated compression stockings and subcutaneous heparin. The value of low-molecular-weight heparin compared with unfractionated heparin is uncertain, although it may increase the risk of postoperative bleeding but has the advantage of once-daily administration. Intermittent pneumatic compression boots are less effective but still useful. A study assessing benefits of prophylactic oral low-dose warfarin is currently underway. The initial treatment of choice for a proven DVT is intravenous heparin infusion. Aspirin has not been proven to be useful either for prophylaxis or for treatment of DVT. (See: Wheatley T, Veitch PS (1997) Editorial: recent advances in prophylaxis against deep vein thrombosis. *British Journal of Anaesthesia* **78**, 118–120.)

2.84 A.T B.T C.T D.F E.F

Lower motor lesions arise when there is neuronal interruption from and including the anterior horn cells of the spinal cord to the periphery. Classic signs include weakness, hypotonia, reduced or absent tension reflexes, and wasting and fasciculation. Examples include polio and Guillain–Barré syndrome. Joint position sense, vibration, light touch and two-point discrimination are carried by the dorsal columns and will therefore be preserved in lower motor neurone lesions. Similarly the spinothalamic tracts, which carry pain, temperature and poorly localized touch sensation, will be unaffected.

2.85 A.T B.T C.T D.T E.T

The signs and symptoms of oxygen toxicity are wide ranging. Pulmonary symptoms include retrosternal pain, chest tightness, an increasingly severe cough and dyspnoea. There is a reduction in residual volume due to atelectasis secondary to both loss of surfactant and nitrogen washout. In adults visual disturbances include potentially reversible peripheral field constriction and loss of vision. Other symptoms include nausea and vomiting, dizziness, confusion, tremors and convulsions. These changes are probably bought about by excess presence of oxygen free radicals which overwhelm the normal intracellular scavenging process. Premature neonates requiring high oxygen concentrations ($Fio_2 > 0.6$) differ in as much as they are in danger of permanent blindness from constriction of retinal vessels causing retrolental fibroplasia.

2.86 A.T B.T C.T D.T E.T

No one will fail the final FRCA for not knowing the historical landmarks of anaesthesia, but it has been asked in the viva so it is probably worth having a vague idea of what has happened in the past. As such, all the stems are correct!

2.87   A.T **B.**T **C.**F **D.**F **E.**T

Casts are microscopic glycoprotein cylindrical structures formed in renal tubules. Their composition can vary depending on the associated cellular elements such as red, white or epithelial cells. Haematuria with red cell casts indicates a glomerular lesion as do epithelial casts characteristically seen with acute glomerulonephritis. Hyaline casts are without cellular elements and can be found in normal urine, during febrile illnesses or after administration of loop diuretics. Deformed red cells occur with bleeding from the upper tract but if morphology is normal this suggests ureteric, bladder, prostatic or urethral bleeding. Heavy proteinuria invariably indicates glomerular disease.

2.88   A.T **B.**T **C.**T **D.**F **E.**F

Atropine is short-acting (1–2 h) with both peripheral and central actions. These include tachycardia (may be initial bradycardia from central vagal stimulation), bronchodilatation which increases physiological dead space, and a reduction in sweating, salivation, gastrointestinal secretion and motility. *Hyoscine* also has a short duration of action but a greater effect on the brain, sweating, salivation and the pupils (mydriasis) than atropine. It is extensively metabolized by liver esterases with about 1% eliminated unchanged in the urine. *Glycopyrrolate* is an ionized quaternary amine which does not readily cross the blood–brain barrier, thus limiting central actions. It is a more effective antisialogogue than atropine but has less effect on the heart. It is also longer-acting, with a similar duration of action to neostigmine (6 h).

2.89   A.T **B.**T **C.**T **D.**F **E.**T

Platelets are cytoplasmic fragments of megakaryocytes. As they are anucleate, platelets age quickly and if not involved in the clotting process survive in the blood for about 10 days. Their production is under the control of thrombopoietin. Following a break in the endothelium, platelets adhere to collagen. They change shape from disc to spiny sheres to form a haemostatic plug; help to initiate the coagulation cascade; and release both adenosine diphosphate (ADP), which is a potent platelet aggregating substance, and thromboxane A_2, which stimulates local vasoconstriction. Platelets are also helped in the clotting process by the presence of coagulation factors (factor V, fibrinogen, von Willebrand factor) in cytoplasmic granules and on their surface. Plug size is limited by prostacyclin produced by surrounding endothelial cells. In time, the plug becomes stable by the addition of fibrin and platelet-induced clot retraction. Platelets play no part in fibrinolysis by plasmin.

2.90 A.F B.T C.T D.T E.T

Motor and sensory innervation of the legs arises from L1–S3 spinal segments. L1–L4 form the lumbar plexus which divides into the lateral femoral cutaneous, femoral and obturator nerves. These supply the upper leg, with only a branch of the femoral nerve (saphenous nerve) extending medially below the knee. L4–S3 form the sciatic nerve which divides into the tibial and common peroneal nerves providing innervation below the knee. The sciatic nerve also supplies some muscles in the upper thigh. The genitofemoral nerve provides cutaneous innervation of the scrotum, adjacent thigh and femoral triangle.

Exam 3

Questions

3.1 **The following are compatible with a diagnosis of acute respiratory distress syndrome (ARDS):**
- **A.** an increase in lung compliance.
- **B.** an arterial P_aO_2 of 10 kPa in air.
- **C.** a pulmonary capillary wedge pressure (PCWP) of 12 mmHg.
- **D.** bilateral diffuse infiltrates on chest radiograph.
- **E.** rapid resolution of chest radiograph changes following intravenous frusemide.

3.2 **Mitral stenosis causes:**
- **A.** a displaced apex beat.
- **B.** systemic thromboembolism.
- **C.** haemoptysis.
- **D.** a loud first heart sound.
- **E.** an early diastolic murmur.

3.3 **Remifentanil:**
- **A.** has a larger volume of distribution than alfentanil.
- **B.** is broken down by plasma esterases.
- **C.** should be avoided in the presence of cholinesterase deficiency.
- **D.** can be used intrathecally.
- **E.** accumulates with repeated dosage.

3.4 **Appropriate criteria for extubation after long-term ventilation include:**
- **A.** a minute ventilation of 15 l/min.
- **B.** a tidal volume of 7 ml/kg.
- **C.** a respiratory rate of 20 breaths per min.
- **D.** functional residual capacity (FRC) of less than 50% of predicted.
- **E.** clinical judgement.

3.5   After failed intubation for an emergency Caesarean section the following actions are acceptable:
   A.   wake patient up and perform spinal anaesthesia.
   B.   continue by maintaining anaesthesia with a facemask, cricoid pressure and intermittent ventilation.
   C.   continue by maintaining anaesthesia with a facemask, cricoid pressure and spontaneous ventilation.
   D.   call for senior help and, when present, attempt a further intubation.
   E.   continue by maintaining anaesthesia and cricoid pressure, insert laryngeal mask and allow to breathe spontaneously.

3.6   Transoesophageal echocardiography (TOE):
   A.   can detect myocardial ischaemia.
   B.   can detect aortic dissection.
   C.   is contraindicated with oesophageal varices.
   D.   can evaluate left ventricular function.
   E.   can cause cardiac arrhythmias.

3.7   Likely blood chemistry findings in a previously fit 25-year-old man vomiting for 2 weeks include:
   A.   raised blood urea.
   B.   potassium   –   3.0 mmol/l.
   C.   bicarbonate   –   18 mmol/l.
   D.   sodium   –   150 mmol/l.
   E.   chloride   –   110 mmol/l.

3.8   Appropriate treatment of established ARDS includes:
   A.   inverse ratio ventilation.
   B.   steroids.
   C.   diuretics.
   D.   positive end-expiratory pressure (PEEP).
   E.   nitric oxide.

3.9   Extradural anaesthesia for an elective Caesarean section:
   A.   is an indication for using ergometrine instead of syntocinon.
   B.   rarely requires more than 20 ml of 0.5% bupivacaine.
   C.   requires a sensory block up to T4 when tested using a cold stimulus.
   D.   requires a fluid preload.
   E.   is associated with prolonged backache postoperatively.

3.10 Spontaneous pneumothorax:
- A. is commonly associated with emphysema.
- B. is found equally in men and women.
- C. requires surgical repair in more than 50% of cases.
- D. requires oxygen therapy.
- E. more commonly affects the right lung.

3.11 The following exceed the maximum safe amount for a 70 kg individual:
- A. 40 mg of amethocaine.
- B. 10 ml of 2% lignocaine.
- C. 60 ml of 1% prilocaine with adrenaline.
- D. 100 mg of cocaine.
- E. 30 ml of 0.75% bupivacaine.

3.12 Intracranial calcification on plain skull radiograph can be seen with:
- A. congenital hydrocephalus.
- B. Sturge–Weber syndrome.
- C. meningioma.
- D. cysticercosis.
- E. cytomegalovirus (CMV).

3.13 In myasthenia gravis:
- A. there is increased sensitivity to depolarizing muscle relaxants.
- B. a cholinergic crisis can occur with edrophonium.
- C. there is fade on electromyelogram (EMG) after repetitive stimulation.
- D. thymectomy may be useful in the young patient.
- E. extradural anaesthesia is contraindicated.

3.14 Patient safety can be compromised by:
- A. exposure to a current of 100 mA.
- B. use of transformers.
- C. space blankets.
- D. use of contact breakers.
- E. earth leakage current less than 2 mA.

3.15 Acute epiglottitis in a small child:
  A. is commonly due to *Haemophilus influenzae.*
  B. is associated with parainfluenza type 2 virus.
  C. frequently requires treatment with hydrocortisone.
  D. rarely causes stridor.
  E. nebulized adrenaline is the first line of management.

3.16 Infections transmissible by blood transfusion include:
  A. malaria.
  B. Chagas disease.
  C. hepatitis A.
  D. syphilis.
  E. CMV.

3.17 Contraindications to suxamethonium include:
  A. grand mal epilepsy.
  B. perforating eye injury with a full stomach.
  C. chronic renal failure on dialysis.
  D. motor neurone disease.
  E. delayed skin grafting of burns covering 15% of the body surface area (BSA).

3.18 A patient with an arterial bicarbonate of 12 mmol/l may have a:
  A. metabolic acidosis.
  B. compensated metabolic acidosis.
  C. compensated metabolic alkalosis.
  D. compensated respiratory alkalosis.
  E. respiratory acidosis.

3.19 Dopamine:
  A. is a physiological neurotransmitter.
  B. must be administered through a central venous catheter.
  C. interferes with the release of thyroid-stimulating hormone (TSH) from the pituitary gland.
  D. has diuretic effects.
  E. action is antagonized by droperidol.

3.20 Mivacurium:
  A. does not cross the blood–brain barrier.
  B. is broken down by Hoffman elimination.
  C. has minimal cardiovascular effects.
  D. can block ganglionic nicotinic receptors.
  E. releases histamine.

3.21 Oesophageal varices may be caused by:
A. portal vein thrombosis.
B. cirrhosis of the liver.
C. achalasia of the cardia.
D. hepatic vein thrombosis.
E. linitis plastica.

3.22 A jaundiced male drug addict has a fever and a pansystolic murmur. The following may be true:
A. he has a viral infection.
B. he has a bacterial infection.
C. diagnosis and treatment of the viral infection, if present, is more important.
D. the murmur could be due to tricuspid regurgitation.
E. suitable treatment would initially be with oral antibiotics.

3.23 Vitamin B$_{12}$:
A. supplements are required in pregnancy.
B. is commonly deficient in vegetarians.
C. is routinely given to postgastrectomy patients.
D. can be required in Crohn's disease.
E. may be needed in conjunction with phenytoin therapy.

3.24 Complications of epidural anaesthesia include:
A. cauda equina syndrome.
B. meningitis.
C. Brown–Séquard syndrome.
D. epidural haematoma.
E. anterior spinal artery occlusion.

3.25 Baroreceptor activity is:
A. mediated via the IXth cranial nerve.
B. responsive to oxygen concentration.
C. located primarily in the carotid body.
D. increased in response to increased venous pressure.
E. minimally suppressed by isoflurane.

3.26 Regarding a permanent pacemaker:
A. the use of bipolar diathermy is contraindicated.
B. it is a risk for microshock.
C. it should be inactivated intraoperatively.
D. the use of pancuronium is contraindicated.
E. it has a normal life span of 3–5 years.

3.27 The extradural space in an adult:
   A. extends from the foramen magnum to the sacral hiatus.
   B. is triangular in shape with an average depth of 6–7 mm.
   C. contains valveless veins.
   D. is widest in the lumbar region.
   E. reliably lies 5 cm from the skin in the lumbar region.

3.28 A 6-year-old boy with a sore throat responds initially to antibiotics. He worsens, develops a rash on his legs, haematuria, a puffy face and looks very unwell. The following may occur:
   A. haematuria.
   B. raised blood pressure.
   C. non-specific arthritis.
   D. deafness.
   E. chronic renal failure.

3.29 Regarding treatment of fungal infections:
   A. miconazole interferes with cell wall synthesis.
   B. nystatin can be useful in systemic infections.
   C. griseofulvin is suitable for systemic infections.
   D. fluconazole is hepatotoxic.
   E. polyene antibiotics have antifungal activity.

3.30 A massive pulmonary embolus (PE) commonly results in:
   A. haemoptysis
   B. pyrexia
   C. increase in blood pressure.
   D. pleuritic chest pain.
   E. a gallop rhythm.

3.31 The Mallampati test for difficult intubation:
   A. is extremely reliable.
   B. requires the tongue to be inside the mouth.
   C. takes into account head and neck movement.
   D. is superior to the Wilson criteria.
   E. has considerable interobserver variability.

3.32 Dopexamine:
   A. has significant α-adrenergic agonist action.
   B. is structurally similar to dopamine.
   C. has an inotropic action.
   D. increases renal blood flow.
   E. decreases splanchnic blood flow.

3.33 The following are true:
- **A.** phenoxybenzamine causes non-specific adrenoceptor blockade.
- **B.** metaraminol causes presynaptic sympathetic blockade.
- **C.** sodium nitroprusside works by direct action on blood vessels.
- **D.** methyldopa is a sympathetic ganglion blocker.
- **E.** hydralazine is an α_1 adrenoceptor blocker.

3.34 Carcinoma of the prostate:
- **A.** is normally an adenocarcinoma.
- **B.** can increase serum alkaline phosphatase.
- **C.** gives rise to osteoblastic bone deposits.
- **D.** presents early with urinary retention.
- **E.** can be beneficially treated with androgens.

3.35 Selection of patients for randomized trials may be done:
- **A.** by tossing a coin.
- **B.** by random number tables.
- **C.** as they arrive.
- **D.** by Bartlett's test.
- **E.** by the therapeutic index.

3.36 Fresh-frozen plasma (FFP):
- **A.** is suitable for use as a plasma volume expander.
- **B.** contains all the coagulation factors.
- **C.** can be used to reverse the action of warfarin.
- **D.** is a source of cholinesterase.
- **E.** is treated to prevent viral transmission.

3.37 Appropriate postoperative analgesia for a thoracotomy includes:
- **A.** intrapleural bupivacaine.
- **B.** transcutaneous electrical nerve stimulation (TENS).
- **C.** lumbar extradural anaesthesia.
- **D.** NSAIDs.
- **E.** intercostal cryoanalgesia.

3.38 A patient with hyperparathyroidism requires an urgent laparotomy. Serum calcium is 4.0 mmol/l. Appropriate treatment includes:
A. disodium etidronate.
B. intravenous frusemide.
C. infusion of normal saline.
D. oral sodium phosphate.
E. intravenous corticosteroids.

3.39 As regards pollution:
A. inhalational agents contribute to nearly 1% of the yearly global release of chlorofluorocarbons (CFCs).
B. the upper recommended limit for isoflurane in the UK is 75 ppm.
C. the upper recommended limit for halothane in the UK is 10 ppm.
D. the upper recommended limit for nitrous oxide in the UK is 150 ppm.
E. scavenging systems have 30 mm connectors.

3.40 Pulseless electrical activity (PEA):
A. is always fatal.
B. can be due to a pulmonary embolus.
C. is an indication for intravenous calcium.
D. is an indication for temporary pacing.
E. can result from cardiac tamponade.

3.41 In leptospirosis:
A. the onset is slow and insidious.
B. myalgia is an early sign.
C. splenomegaly can occur.
D. meningitis can occur.
E. the diagnosis can be confirmed by blood culture.

3.42 Normal daily requirements for total parenteral nutrition (TPN) in an adult include:
A. insulin.
B. phosphate.
C. 30–35 ml/kg of water per day.
D. D-amino acids.
E. basal energy requirements of 30 kcal/kg/day.

3.43 Postoperative pain relief in children:
- A. is normally unnecessary in premature neonates.
- B. cannot be safely treated with a continuous morphine infusion.
- C. can be measured using the 'oucher' scale.
- D. should not be treated with aspirin.
- E. with opiates is associated with a greater incidence of respiratory depression than in adults.

3.44 Hypokalaemia occurring during anaesthesia and surgery can be due to:
- A. mannitol administration.
- B. hypocapnia due to intermittent positive-pressure ventilation (IPPV).
- C. intravenous digoxin.
- D. presence of a metabolic acidosis.
- E. intravenous frusemide.

3.45 Carcinoma of the larynx:
- A. incidence is equally distributed between males and females.
- B. metastasizes early.
- C. commonly presents as hoarseness.
- D. is often painful on presentation.
- E. usually causes haemoptysis.

3.46 HFJV:
- A. uses a frequency greater than 1 Hz.
- B. may be beneficial in the management of a bronchopleural fistula.
- C. needs an I : E ratio of at least 1 : 3.
- D. can be beneficial for a severe asthmatic requiring ventilation.
- E. allows for humidification.

3.47 Cystic fibrosis (CF):
- A. is an autosomal dominant condition.
- B. is diagnosed by decreased chloride in the sweat.
- C. can present with cirrhosis of the liver and portal hypertension.
- D. has an incidence of 1 in 1000 live births.
- E. may cause diabetes mellitus (DM).

3.48 Clonidine:
  A. is contraindicated in pregnancy.
  B. has intravenous analgesic properties.
  C. can produce significant postural hypotension.
  D. reduces the MAC of isoflurane.
  E. can result in rebound hypertension on withdrawal.

3.49 Bundle branch block (BBB) on the ECG:
  A. will show a prolonged PR interval.
  B. is represented with widening of the QRS complex.
  C. will show ST depression over the blocked ventricle.
  D. will show T wave inversion over the ventricle with normal conduction.
  E. is always pathological.

3.50 Peribulbar block for cataract extraction:
  A. is not as safe as retrobulbar blocks.
  B. can result in subarachnoid injection.
  C. results in enophthalmos.
  D. reduces intraocular pressure.
  E. is best performed with the eye looking 'up and in'.

3.51 Profound hypothermia is associated with:
  A. loss of tendon reflexes.
  B. a metabolic alkalosis.
  C. shivering.
  D. hyperglycaemia.
  E. a diuresis.

3.52 With peripheral nerve stimulation:
  A. a train of four (TOF) is delivered at 5 Hz for 2 s.
  B. post-tetanic stimulation can be reliably repeated every 2–3 min.
  C. a single twitch following a TOF stimulus implies over 95% neuromuscular block.
  D. double-burst stimulation is more sensitive than a TOF.
  E. a dual block can be reversed with neostigmine.

3.53 Renal clearance of a drug:
   A. is proportional to its lipid solubility.
   B. has no relationship to creatinine clearance.
   C. is normally constant for any given drug.
   D. varies with pH.
   E. may exceed renal blood flow.

3.54 Apgar scoring:
   A. is a sensitive indicator of the physiological status of a neonate.
   B. has a maximum score of 8.
   C. is first taken at 1 min after delivery of the baby.
   D. is of little value after birth by Caesarean section.
   E. heart rate is a better indicator than colour.

3.55 Causes of overdamping in a transducer system include:
   A. blood clots.
   B. wide tubing.
   C. saline as a priming fluid.
   D. short manometer tubing.
   E. air bubbles.

3.56 Phaeochromocytoma:
   A. is bilateral in 30% of cases.
   B. metastases, if they occur, will commonly be to the liver.
   C. is usually associated with hypoglycaemia.
   D. may be associated with carcinoma of the thyroid.
   E. increases urinary excretion of 5-hydroxyindoleacetic acid (5-HIAA).

3.57 Propofol:
   A. has no effect on intraocular pressure.
   B. has no cardiovascular depressant effects.
   C. can turn urine green.
   D. has antiemetic properties.
   E. occurs as a 10% solution.

3.58 The liver:
   A. is the largest organ in the body.
   B. is mainly supplied by the hepatic artery.
   C. is the sole site for the production of albumin.
   D. synthesizes vitamin K.
   E. is normally just palpable below the rib margin.

3.59 Ropivacaine:
  A. is less cardiotoxic than bupivacaine.
  B. lasts longer than bupivacaine for extradural blockade.
  C. is more potent than bupivacaine.
  D. is useful for spinal anaesthesia.
  E. has the same pK_a as bupivacaine.

3.60 Pulse oximetry:
  A. is reliable in the presence of hyperbilirubinaemia.
  B. compensates for ambient light.
  C. requires pulsatile flow to work.
  D. is accurate in the presence of carboxyhaemoglobin.
  E. has a faster response time than a transcutaneous oxygen electrode.

3.61 An amniotic fluid embolus is associated with:
  A. abdominal pain.
  B. respiratory depression.
  C. permanent neurological sequelae.
  D. a coagulopathy.
  E. considerable mortality.

3.62 When a patient presents with a femoro-popliteal thrombosis:
  A. limb survival is usually 2 years.
  B. anticoagulation is indicated.
  C. pain is a late feature.
  D. paralysis is an early feature.
  E. early treatment with thrombolytic agents improves prognosis.

3.63 Advantages of low-flow anaesthesia with the circle system include:
  A. economy of fresh gas flow.
  B. minimal risk of rebreathing.
  C. reduced need for capnography.
  D. low resistance to breathing.
  E. simplicity of design.

3.64 A normal haemoglobin value does not exclude the diagnosis of:
  A. sickle cell trait.
  B. haemoglobin C (HbC) trait.
  C. glucose 6 phosphate dehydrogenase (G6PD) deficiency.
  D. thalassaemia minor.
  E. pernicious anaemia.

3.65 Complications within 24 hours of having a tracheostomy include:
   A. subcutaneouos emphysema.
   B. inominate artery erosion.
   C. apnoea.
   D. tracheal stenosis.
   E. occult haemorrhage.

3.66 Low serum acetylcholinesterase levels may be found in:
   A. a farmer using high-phosphate feeds.
   B. pilocarpine eye drops.
   C. physostigmine eye drops.
   D. liver failure.
   E. pregnancy at term.

3.67 Blood group A antigens:
   A. occur in all red blood cells of the population with blood group A.
   B. are the commonest antigens in Caucasians.
   C. would not cause problems if given to patients of blood group O.
   D. may be detected in saliva.
   E. are the commonest cause of haemolytic disease of the newborn.

3.68 A haemoglobin 8.0 g/dl and a reticulocyte count 10% could be due to:
   A. aplastic anaemia.
   B. untreated pernicious anaemia.
   C. haemolytic anaemia.
   D. acute leukaemia.
   E. polycythaemia.

3.69 Intrathecal opioids:
   A. act on kappa receptors.
   B. cause piloerection.
   C. have a lower incidence of nausea and vomiting than systemic opioids.
   D. cause delayed respiratory depression.
   E. can have all their side-effects reversed with naloxone.

3.70 Contraindications to ambulatory (day case) surgery include:
   A. age less than 6 months.
   B. DM.
   C. procedures longer than 3 hours.
   D. intermittent positive pressure ventilation.
   E. use of spinal anaesthesia.

3.71 Humidity can be measured by:
   A. a wet and dry bulb thermometer.
   B. a hair hygrometer.
   C. a mass spectrometer.
   D. measurement of the dew point.
   E. absorption of water by silica gel.

3.72 Tidal volume may be characteristically large in:
   A. cerebral haemorrhage.
   B. diabetic ketoacidosis.
   C. acute tubular necrosis.
   D. emphysema.
   E. ankylosing spondylitis.

3.73 The oculocardiac reflex can be reliably obtunded by:
   A. atropine given as a premedicant.
   B. deepening anaesthesia.
   C. asking the surgeon to stop.
   D. retrobulbar block.
   E. glycopyrrolate at time of stimulation.

3.74 Appropriate findings in a 3.5 kg neonate 24 hours old are:
   A. haemoglobin 18 g/dl.
   B. tidal volume of 60 ml.
   C. cardiac output of 1.5 l/min.
   D. blood volume of approximately 65 ml/kg.
   E. spinal cord terminating at L3.

3.75 Difficult intubation can be anticipated in:
   A. Marfan's syndrome.
   B. cleft lip and palate.
   C. Treacher Collins syndrome.
   D. Ludwig's angina.
   E. acromegaly.

3.76 Adult polycystic kidney disease (APKD):
   A. is an autosomal recessive disorder.
   B. is not an indication for renal transplant.
   C. rarely causes hypertension.
   D. is rarely associated with survival beyond 40 years of age.
   E. can involve the liver.

3.77 Internal haemorrhoids:
   A. are usually seen at 3, 6, 10 o'clock on proctoscopy in the lithotomy position.
   B. can usually be felt on rectal examination.
   C. are often painful.
   D. can cause malaena.
   E. can cause perianal irritation.

3.78 Nitrous oxide (N$_2$O):
   A. induces nausea and vomiting.
   B. increases myocardial sensitivity to catecholamines.
   C. has a high blood : gas partition coefficient.
   D. potentiates non-depolarizing neuromuscular blocking agents.
   E. increases serum folate.

3.79 Ankylosing spondylitis is usually associated with:
   A. the female sex.
   B. morning stiffness.
   C. urethritis.
   D. aortic incompetence.
   E. involvement of peripheral joints.

3.80 Signs of fulminant hepatic failure commonly include:
   A. ascites.
   B. encephalopathy.
   C. massive hepatomegaly.
   D. rapidly progressive jaundice.
   E. splenomegaly.

3.81 Sensory impairment occurs in:
   A. amyotrophic lateral sclerosis.
   B. Friedrich's ataxia.
   C. syringomyelia.
   D. Paterson–Brown–Kelly syndrome.
   E. vitamin B$_1$ deficiency.

3.82 The elderly have:
   A. a less sensitive autonomic nervous system.
   B. decreased GFR.
   C. higher MAC requirement.
   D. reduced FRC.
   E. a greater volume of distribution for water-soluble drugs.

3.83 Indications for dialysis in acute renal failure in the ICU include:
   A. potassium of 6.5 mmol/l.
   B. pulmonary oedema.
   C. urea in excess of 30 mmol/l.
   D. severe anaemia.
   E. hypoproteinaemia.

3.84 TEC6 vaporizers:
   A. require an electrical supply.
   B. can be used for sevoflurane.
   C. are accurate with flow rates of up to 10 l/min.
   D. cannot be filled when in use.
   E. are calibrated up to 18% of volatile agent.

3.85 Hyponatraemia is a feature of:
   A. decompensated hepatic failure.
   B. oat (small) cell carcinoma of the lung.
   C. inappropriate ADH secretion.
   D. Conn's syndrome.
   E. nephrotic syndrome.

3.86 Bilateral facial pain is commonly associated with:
   A. glaucoma.
   B. temporomandibular joint dysfunction (TMJD).
   C. multiple sclerosis (MS).
   D. Guillain–Barré syndrome.
   E. maxillary sinusitis.

3.87 A patient develops a bronchopleural fistula after a pneumonectomy. He is ventilated but has an air leak of 1.5 l/min through the fistula. This can be reduced by:
  A. subtracting 1.5 l from the minute volume.
  B. adding 10 cm PEEP.
  C. decreasing respiratory rate.
  D. decreasing inflation pressure.
  E. increasing flow rate.

3.88 Appropriate management of an elderly woman found collapsed at home with a core temperature of 32°C includes:
  A. rapid rewarming.
  B. intubation and ventilation.
  C. prophylactic intravenous lignocaine.
  D. warmed intravenous fluids.
  E. steroid therapy.

3.89 Sickle cell trait:
  A. is a homozygous condition.
  B. is commoner in males.
  C. cannot occur simultaneously with thalassaemia trait.
  D. is sometimes associated with a negative sickling test.
  E. does not prevent the use of a tourniquet.

3.90 The erythrocyte sedimentation rate (ESR):
  A. is often higher in men than in women.
  B. is normally less than 15 mm.
  C. is considerably elevated in temporal arteritis.
  D. is decreased in the presence of anaemia.
  E. increases with age.

Answers

3.1 A.T B.F C.T D.T E.F

ARDS is the most severe manifestation of acute lung injury. It can occur at any age and may arise from a number of diverse insults. Sepsis is the commonest cause but aspiration, trauma, burns and pancreatitis are also important precipitants. The lung damage results from the action of inflammatory mediators such as cytokines, free oxygen radicals, proteolytic enzymes (collagenase, trypsin) and activated neutrophils. Surfactant production is reduced and vascular permeability is increased, resulting in non-cardiogenic pulmonary oedema. This is followed by production of a haemorrhagic intra-alveolar exudate rich in platelets, fibrin, clotting factors and cellular debris. This is responsible for hyaline membrane formation and the clinical picture of pulmonary fibrosis. Lung compliance decreases, and an increased shunt often leads to a refractory hypoxaemia of 8 kPa or less in air. Diffuse infiltrates are found on chest radiograph and signs of respiratory failure (tachypnoea, dyspnoea and respiratory distress) develop. ARDS can be distinguished from cardiogenic pulmonary oedema by a PCWP less than 18 mmHg. Rapid resolution of chest radiograph changes with diuretics is seen with cardiogenic pulmonary oedema.

3.2 A.F B.T C.T D.T E.F

Mitral stenosis is almost invariably a result of rheumatic fever. Patients are often asymptomatic until the stenosis is moderately severe, i.e. when the surface area of the mitral orifice is halved (<2 cm). Cardiac output can then be maintained only by a rise in left atrial pressure. The transmitted back pressure to the lungs eventually leads to pulmonary hypertension and, ultimately, right heart failure. The dilated left atrium is prone to fibrillate, thus promoting thromboembolism. The onset of atrial fibrillation often causes a dramatic clinical deterioration with the associated fall in cardiac output leading to left ventricular failure and pulmonary oedema. The main symptoms are cough with haemoptysis and exertional dyspnoea. The main signs are malar flush, a palpable ('tapping') first heart sound, left parasternal heave, loud first heart sound, an opening snap and a delayed low-pitched, mid-diastolic murmur. As the left ventricle is not involved, the apex tends not to be displaced. The murmur becomes longer and moves closer to the second heart sound with increasing stenosis. If medical treatment fails, surgery is required to perform a valvuloplasty or valve replacement.

3.3 **A.**T **B.**T **C.**F **D.**F **E.**F
Remifentanil is a mu receptor agonist with a rapid action of short duration, and a potency similar to fentanyl. It has a half-life of 9–11 min, making alfentanil its closest rival. Unlike alfentanil, remifentanil does not accumulate as it is broken down by plasma and tissue esterases. As it does not specifically require butyryl-cholinesterases, its clearance will not be affected by cholinesterase deficiency. It has minimally active metabolites. Its haemodynamic effects are similar to other opiates, causing a mild bradycardia and a 15–20% drop in blood pressure. Remifentanil can cause respiratory depression but this wears off quickly as the drug is broken down. It does not release histamine, nor does it have any effect on intraocular pressure. It blocks the stress hormone response to surgery in a dose-dependent fashion and reduces the minimum alveolar concentration (MAC) of inhalational agents. Side-effects include the typical adverse effects of all mu receptor agonists – nausea, vomiting, pruritus and muscle rigidity – with a similar incidence to other opioids. The short-acting analgesic action makes other forms of analgesia essential for adequate postoperative pain relief. (See: Burkle H *et al.* (1996) Remifentanil: a novel, short acting, mu opioid. *Anesthesia and Analgesia* **83**, 646–651. Also: Smith MA, Morgan M (1997) Remifentanil. *Anaesthesia* **52**, 291–293.)

3.4 **A.**F **B.**T **C.**T **D.**F **E.**T
Criteria for weaning have long been controversial. Ultimately, clinical judgement is best. Patients should have a good nutritional status, normal electrolyte and fluid balance, minimal sedation and have no major organ failure or infection. Respiratory values needed for extubation are less clear-cut and no single factor has been shown to be universally applicable. Reasonable suggestions include:

arterial blood gases near premorbid values on F_iO_2 <0.3–0.4
respiratory rate under 25 breaths per min
maximum negative inspiratory airway pressure $>-25\,\text{cm}\,H_2O$
minute ventilation under 10 l/min
tidal volume >5 ml/kg
functional residual capacity >50% of predicted value

Up to 20% of patients need to be reintubated despite fulfilling the chosen criteria. Techniques to facilitate weaning include sitting the patient up to increase FRC and diaphragmatic efficiency, adequate humidification, gradually increasing the periods of spontaneous ventilation in between intermittent ventilation, low-resistance ventilators to decrease the work of breathing, and continuous positive airway pressure (CPAP) with or without a T-piece. (See: Coates NE, Weigelt JA (1991) Weaning from mechanical ventilation. *Surgical Clinics of North America* **71**, 859–876. Also: Shneerson JM (1997) Editorial: Are there new solutions to old problems with weaning? *British Journal of Anaesthesia* **78**, 238–240.)

3.5 A.T **B**.T **C**.T **D**.T **E**.T

This is a nightmare question as 'expert' opinion seems to be polarized as to what is best. It is safe to say that the mother comes first and it is vital to maintain oxygenation without aspiration. No one approach is ideal and although all of the stems have been suggested as both appropriate and justifiable, they each have their own limitations. In the 1991–1993 confidential enquiries into maternal death, 8 deaths were attributed to anaesthesia and a further 7 to substandard care (accounting for 6.5% of all deaths). Hypoxia and airway obstruction were responsible for 5 (2 failed reintubations after the initial procedure), ARDS for 2 and 'failure of tissue perfusion' for 1. There were no deaths attributed to failed intubation for the initial operation. Overall, criticism was directed at poor monitoring and lack of senior help, usually because they were not informed: there is a lesson to be learned. (See: HMSO report on Confidential Enquiries into Maternal Deaths in the UK, 1991–1993. Also: Harmer M (1997) Difficult and failed intubation in obstetrics. *International Journal of Obstetric Anesthesia* **6**, 25–31).

3.6 A.T **B**.T **C**.F **D**.T **E**.T

TOE consists of an ultrasound probe attached to the end of a flexible endoscope. Placed in mid-oesophagus it gives high-quality imaging of the heart without the interference from lungs and ribs found with conventional echocardiography. It is excellent for evaluating valvular function, particularly aortic and mitral valves, whether prosthetic or native, and for identifying the vegetations of endocarditis and the presence of intracardiac thrombi. It is particularly good for visualizing the aorta, e.g. acute dissecting thoracic aneurysms from blunt trauma. It can also be used to evaluate left ventricular function, with assessment of wall thickness, contraction, relaxation and change in chamber size. In myocardial ischaemia a TOE can detect segmental wall motion abnormalities earlier than ECG changes. Combined with Doppler colour flow imaging it can determine direction and velocity of blood flow and thus estimate cardiac output. Appropriate uses for TOE include cardiac assessment of critically ill and high-risk patients either in the intensive care unit (ICU) or perioperatively for cardiac and non-cardiac surgery in adults and children. Absolute contraindications include oesophageal strictures, active gastrointestinal bleeding and severe cervical spine instability. Caution is required with oesophageal varices and cervical spine arthritis. The incidence of complications is low at less than 0.5%. Common problems include difficulty in insertion, nausea and vomiting in awake patients. Rare complications include transient vocal cord paralysis, gastro-oesophageal perforation, persistent swallowing dysfunction and cardiac arrhythmias (bradycardia, atrial fibrillation). (See: Seward JB *et al.* (1994) Transoesophageal echocardiography. *Mayo Clinic Proceedings* **63**, 649–666.)

3.7   A.T   B.T   C.F   D.F   E.F
The clinical picture suggests pyloric stenosis probably due to chronic duodenal ulceration, or rarely in this age group gastric carcinoma. Chronic vomiting causes dehydration which leads to an increase in serum urea. It also causes a metabolic alkalosis from loss of gastric juices rich in hydrogen and chloride and to a lesser extent sodium and potassium. Renal compensation preserves sodium at the expense of potassium and hydrogen so their serum concentration should be low. However, as this compensatory mechanism for preserving sodium is never complete, serum sodium is likely to remain on the low side. Hydrogen ions, in turn, are preferentially preserved at the expense of potassium. Chloride deficit increases bicarbonate reabsorption, maintaining the metabolic alkalosis. Overall a hypochloraemic, hypokalaemic metabolic alkalosis with a paradoxical acid urine occurs. Treatment is rehydration, electrolyte correction and surgery.

3.8   A.T   B.F   C.T   D.T   E.T
Conventional ventilation can exacerbate ARDS due to the large minute volumes and high peak inspiratory pressures needed to maintain oxygenation. PEEP is added to reduce small airway closure and allow a decrease in F_iO_2. Inverse ratio inspiration : expiration and pressure-controlled ventilation may improve oxygenation. High-frequency jet ventilation (HFJV), extracorporeal membrane oxygenation (ECMO) and intravascular oxygenation device (IVOX) have also been employed with limited success. A negative fluid balance is preferred and is achieved by fluid restriction, diuretics or haemofiltration. Fluid therapy in ARDS is controversial and there are valid arguments for using crystalloid, colloid or a combination of both. Inhaled nitric oxide has been used to reduce the often elevated pulmonary artery pressure in an attempt to reduce ventilation/perfusion mismatching without systemic vasodilatation. The benefits are variable. High-dose corticosteroids are currently not considered of value; nor is inhaled surfactant. Superimposed infection must be treated but prophylactic antibiotics are not indicated. The outcome depends on the aetiology. For example, mortality is over 90% where the underlying cause is sepsis but under 10% when due to a fat embolus. The cause of death is usually multiorgan failure. (See: Wenstone R, Wilkes RG (1994) Editorial: Clinical management of ARDS. *British Journal of Anaesthesia* **72**, 617–618.)

3.9   A.F   B.F   C.T   D.F   E.F
Extradural anaesthesia for Caesarean section requires a block up to T4. Assuming 1.0–1.5 ml of 0.5% bupivacaine per segment, the 18 segments needed to be blocked require about 18–27 ml. Fluid preloading to prevent hypotension is controversial. Many studies have found it ineffective with both crystalloid and colloid, and there is also a risk of pulmonary oedema. Prompt use of ephedrine is advocated for both spinal and extradural anaesthesia. It has long been suggested that epidurals for pain relief in labour (but not for Caesarean section) were a source of chronic backache. However, current research has disproved this notion as backache is common in pregnancy (about 44%), particularly in those who are of short stature and obese. (See: Jackson R *et al.* (1995) Volume preloading is not essential to prevent spinal induced hypotension at Caesarean section. *British Journal of Anaesthesia* **75**, 262–265. Also: Breen TW *et al.* (1994) Factors associated with

backpain after childbirth. *Anesthesiology* **81**, 29–34. And: Buggy D, MacEvilly M (1996) Do epidurals cause back pain? *British Journal of Hospital Medicine* **56**, 99–100.)

3.10 A.T **B.**F **C.**F **D.**F **E.**F

Spontaneous pneumothorax is more common in young men, especially those who are tall and thin. It often arises from rupture of an apical pleural bleb caused by a congenital defect in the connective tissues of the alveolar walls, although AIDS is rapidly becoming a significant cause. In patients over 40 years of age the usual cause is chronic bronchitis and emphysema. Rarer causes include asthma, carcinoma, pulmonary fibrosis and lung abscess. Both lungs may be affected equally. A simple pneumothorax, even with complete collapse of one lung, is not an immediate threat to life, although it may be uncomfortable with pleuritic pain and dyspnoea. Oxygen and carbon dioxide exchange remains relatively unimpaired and, although it may be given, oxygen therapy is not essential. Treatment depends on the degree of lung collapse. If <20%, then observation is all that is required; pneumothorax >20% requires needle aspiration. If it recurs a chest drain should be inserted for 2–3 days. If it fails to re-expand or recurs more than twice (20% recur in the first year), surgery is indicated. This can be either pleurectomy (recurrence rates close to zero) or talc pleurodesis (associated with some recurrences).

3.11 A.F **B.**F **C.**F **D.**F **E.**T

Drug	Plain (mg/kg)	with adrenaline (mg/kg)
Amethocaine	1.5	–
Lignocaine	4	7
Prilocaine	6	9
Cocaine	3	–
Bupivacaine	2–3	3–4

3.12 A.F **B.**T **C.**T **D.**T **E.**T

Calcification can be a normal finding in the pineal gland, choroid plexuses, pituitary and basal ganglia. Pathologically it can arise from:

Neoplasms – meningioma, glioma, ependymoma, dermoid, hamartoma.

Vascular	– atheroma, aneurysms, angioma, subdural haematoma.
Infections	– cysticercosis, CMV, rubella, toxoplasmosis, hydatid cysts.
Miscellaneous	– Sturge–Weber syndrome, neurofibromatosis, tuberous sclerosis, lead poisoning.

Meningioma shows ball-like amorphous calcification in 10% of cases. Sturge–Weber syndrome produces tramline calcification in the occipital cortex, facial port wine stain and epilepsy. Cysticercosis is seen as scattered calcified nodules due to infestation of tapeworm *Taenia solium*, endemic in Mexico, parts of Asia and South Africa. Congenital CMV produces widespread periventricular, stippled, symmetrical calcification with microcephaly.

3.13 A.F B.F C.T D.T E.F
Myasthenia gravis is due to production of IgG antibodies against acetylcholine receptors on the muscle end-plate. The antibodies have been suggested to reduce the number of active receptors by a number of mechanisms including functional block of the receptors, increased rate of receptor degradation or complement-mediated lysis. It commonly presents with muscle weakness, mainly extraocular, with ptosis. The degree of weakness and fatigability vary and are worse after exercise. The condition may be associated with thymic hyperplasia in the young (<40 years), and with thymic tumours in the elderly. Edrophonium is used in the 'tensilon' test for diagnosis of myasthenia gravis: it will cause a marked but temporary improvement in muscle power in patients with the disease. Longer-acting anticholinesterases (e.g. pyridostigmine) are the mainstay of treatment; these improve the muscle weakness but not the progression of the disease. In excess they can cause a cholinergic crisis with generalized depolarization of muscle end-plate and muscarinic cholinergic receptor overstimulation. Atropine reduces the muscarinic side-effects which include miosis, salivation, colic and diarrhoea. Steroids and antimitotics, e.g. azathioprine and cyclophosphamide, are used in severe cases. Thymectomy may be useful in the young but the outcome is inconsistent. Myasthenics are extremely sensitive to non-depolarizing muscle relaxants. Atracurium and vecuronium are safe in small doses, but mivacurium may be a better choice, although in any case intubation is often possible without the use of muscle relaxant. EMG studies show fade

after repetitive stimulation even in the absence of muscle relaxants. The response to suxamethonium is unpredictable but myasthenics are usually resistant to it unless taking anticholinesterases. Extradural anaesthesia is an acceptable technique but may require a reduced dose of local anaesthetic (LA). (See: Baraka A (1992) Anaesthesia and myasthenia gravis. *Canadian Journal of Anaesthesia* **39**, 476–486.)

3.14 A.T B.F C.T D.T E.T
There are stringent guidelines on standards of electrical safety for protection of patients and staff. These centre on over-current protection, insulation and isolation. All equipment is classified into 1 of 3 classes and must satisfy British Standard 5724 (safety of medical electrical equipment) requirements. Class I equipment has the metal casing connected to an earth wire; class II has double insulation; class III has its own independent power source such as batteries with transformers to reduce voltage. Space blankets are often metal-coated and may become a hazard if in contact with earthed apparatus such as diathermy. Contact breakers switch off current when excessive leakages are detected. Although popular in some countries, they have the potential disadvantage of depriving the patient of crucial monitoring or life-support equipment. Exposure to currents greater than 100 mA is potentially lethal. Earth leakage currents should be less than 0.5 mA. (See: Litt L, Ehrenwerth J (1994) Electrical safety in the operating room: important old wine, disguised new bottles. *Anesthesia and Analgesia* **78**, 417–419.)

3.15 A.T B.F C.F D.F E.F
Acute epiglottitis is most often due to *H. influenzae* type B. It causes acute upper airway obstruction from massive inflammatory oedema of the epiglottis and surrounding area. It is most commonly seen between the ages of 2 and 6 years. Onset is acute with fever, toxaemia and difficulty in breathing and talking. Children are exhausted and extremely frightened. They often adopt a characteristic posture of sitting forward with an open mouth dribbling saliva. Stridor may be loud or very quiet and absence of coughing is a well-recognized feature. Airway compromise may be rapid and is often provoked by stressful events such as pharyngeal examination and intravenous cannulation. Lateral radiographs of the neck may reveal epiglottic enlargement but are not required for diagnosis,

which should be based on clinical findings. Treatment should be immediate and usually requires careful intubation following inhalational induction in 100% oxygen. Difficult intubation should be anticipated and all the necessary equipment should be to hand prior to starting. Intubation is usually required for 1–2 days or until a leak occurs around the tube. Adequate rehydration and humidification are essential. Sedation is only required to prevent self-extubation. Tracheostomy is rarely necessary but facilities must be present before intubation is attempted. Ampicillin has been replaced by cefotaxime as antibiotic of choice owing to the emergence of resistant strains. Nebulized adrenaline is mainly of value in the management of laryngotracheobronchitis (croup).

3.16 A.T **B.**T **C.**T **D.**T **E.**T
Any disease in which microbes circulate in the blood may be transmitted by transfusion. All four species of *Plasmodium* survive in refrigerated blood but most cases are attributable to *P. malariae*. Asymptomatic carriers of the parasite *Trypanosoma cruzi* can transmit Chagas disease (megacolon, heart failure). Hepatitis A transmission is possible if the blood is donated during the few days of viraemia before symptoms develop. CMV is a serious viral pathogen to the immunodeficient. Transmission of HTLV-1, syphilis, toxoplasmosis, leishmaniasis and parovirus is rare. The greatest threat is from hepatitis B and C and HIV, all of which still occur despite screening. HIV transmission from transfusion is estimated at 1 in 225 000, largely due to the interval between acquiring HIV and antibody development (6–12 weeks). Lyme disease (rash, fever, cardiac or neurological symptoms with or without arthritis) from tick-borne spirochaetes *Borrelia burgdorferi* can survive in stored blood for 45 days, but infection following transfusion has not yet been reported.

3.17 A.F **B.**F **C.**F **D.**F **E.**T
Fasciculation of the extraocular muscles by suxamethonium leads to an increase in intraocular pressure (IOP) of about 8 mmHg. Although it is not currently recommended for perforating eye injuries, recent literature suggests this is an unfounded worry, particularly as a blink increases IOP by 10–15 mmHg and coughing by 40 mmHg! Suxamethonium normally increases plasma potassium by 0.5 mmol/l from a combination of leakage of potassium from muscle cells either

at the neuromuscular junction or from trauma during the fasciculations. Any increase is dangerous when potassium levels are high, but renal failure with normal serum potassium is not an exclusion unless there is a coexisting neuropathy. Severe burns (more than 10% BSA), spinal cord damage, tetanus and extensive muscle trauma result in a large increase in acetylcholine receptors throughout the surface of muscle fibres. Subsequent depolarization can then cause massive hyperkalaemia (4–9 mmol/l increase), leading to cardiac arrhythmias and arrest. As this denervation hypersensitivity takes some time to develop, suxamethonium is probably safe to be given up to 1 week after injury. Motor neurone disease results in degeneration of anterior horn cells and the spinal pyramidal tracts. An exaggerated hyperkalaemic response is theoretically possible when the disease is advanced and there is considerable muscle wasting. As such it is not contraindicted but is probably best avoided. Suxamethonium can be safely used in epilepsy. (See: McGoldrick KE (1996) Challenges in anesthesia for ophthalmic surgery. American Society of Anesthesiologists' annual refresher course lectures No. 173.)

3.18 A.T B.F C.F D.T E.F
Normal arterial bicarbonate is 26 mmol/l. Expected changes resulting from a primary acid–base disorder are:

	Disturbance	Compensation
Metabolic acidosis	Decrease HCO_3^-	Hyperventilation, CO_2 falls
Metabolic alkalosis	Increase HCO_3^-	Hypoventilation, CO_2 increases
Respiratory acidosis	Increase $P{CO_2}$	Increase HCO_3^-
Respiratory alkalosis	Decrease $P{CO_2}$	Decrease HCO_3^-

As a primary disturbance it can be only metabolic acidosis. HCO_3^- is very low for a compensated respiratory alkalosis but on the information available it cannot be excluded as these two acid–base states are the only ones where a reduced bicarbonate would be expected. Compensatory mechanisms never overcorrect.

3.19 A.T B.F C.T D.T E.T
Dopamine is a naturally occurring catecholamine and neurotransmitter found in postganglionic sympathetic nerve endings and in the adrenal medulla. It is a precursor of adrenaline and

noradrenaline. At low dose ($1-2\,\mu g/kg/min$) it is thought to act on D_1 receptors in the kidney to improve renal blood flow thereby preserving urine output. This protective action has been questioned as an increase in urine flow is not thought to be due to renal vasodilatation but to inhibition of proximal tubular sodium reabsorption. Thus, dopamine is simply acting as a diuretic. Equal and better improvements in renal function have been demonstrated with both dobutamine and noradrenaline, and the current weight of evidence suggests that dopamine does not preserve renal function. Higher doses ($2-10\,\mu g/kg/min$) stimulate β and α adrenoceptors to improve cardiac output but at the expense of a higher incidence of cardiac arrhythmias. It has a half-life of $1-2\,min$ before being metabolized by monoamine oxidase (MAO) (dose must be reduced in patients on MAO inhibitors). It can be given via a large peripheral vein but central vein administration is preferred because of the problems with vasoconstriction and tissue necrosis after accidental extravasation. Dopamine suppresses the pituitary axis and production of prolactin, TSH and growth hormone. This may adversely affect the stress response of the critically ill. Droperidol is a butyrphenone which is antagonistic to dopamine. (See: Duke GJ *et al.* (1994) Renal support in critically ill patients: low dose dopamine or low dose dobutamine. *Critical Care Medicine* **22**, 1919–1925. Also: McCrory C, Cunningham AJ (1997) Editorial II: Low-dose dopamine: will there ever be a scientific rationale? *British Journal of Anaesthesia* **78**, 350–351.)

3.20 A.T B.F C.T D.F E.T
Mivacurium is a non-depolarizing muscle relaxant, structurally similar to atracurium in that it is a benzylisoquinolinium diester. However, it has a shorter duration of action because it is broken down by plasma cholinesterase rather than by Hoffman elimination. Its effects are dose-related in that a larger dose produces a faster onset, but at the expense of a more prolonged effect. Recovery generally occurs twice as quickly as with atracurium or vecuronium, at about 16–17 min with a dose of 0.15 mg/kg. Mivacurium has negligible effects on the cardiovascular system but weakly stimulates histamine release. The only non-depolarizing muscle relaxant with significant effects on the sympathetic ganglia is tubocurarine; mivacurium has no such effects. In common with all muscle relaxants, mivacurium does not cross the blood–brain barrier.

3.21 **A.**T **B.**T **C.**F **D.**T **E.**F

Oesophageal varices develop secondary to portal hypertension from pre-, intra- or post-hepatic obstruction. They allow portal blood to bypass the liver and enter the systemic circulation directly. *Prehepatic* portal vein thrombosis may occur as a complication of neonatal umbilical artery catheterization. *Intrahepatic* causes are responsible for the vast majority of cases (>90%). Causes of cirrhosis include alcohol, drugs and myeloproliferative conditions, and in developing countries schistosomiasis. *Post-hepatic* causes include Budd–Chiari syndrome (hepatic vein thrombosis), veno-occlusive diseases (e.g. Tahayasu's) and right heart failure. Achalasia of the cardia is due to progressive loss of ganglion cells in Auerbach's plexus resulting in loss of normal oesophageal peristalsis and failure of the lower oesophageal sphincter to open; 10% of cases will develop carcinoma of the oesophagus, regardless of treatment. Linitis plastica ('leather bottle stomach') is the name given to a diffuse infiltrating scirrhous carcinoma of the stomach that spreads submucosally.

3.22 **A.**T **B.**T **C.**F **D.**T **E.**F

Hepatitis B and bacterial endocarditis are common in drug addicts and the presence of both may reasonably be assumed from the history. Hepatitis B is a DNA virus that is spread mainly by blood and blood products and is commonly found in intravenous drug abusers. *Staphylococcus aureus* is a highly virulent and invasive organism and is the commonest cause of acute endocarditis in drug addicts, arising from skin infections at injection sites. Acute endocarditis can present as a severe febrile illness with prominent and changing heart sounds due to florid vegetations on the heart valves. Petechiae and embolic events are common, and cardiac and renal failure may develop rapidly. For this reason the bacterial infection is more important than the viral, and diagnosis (blood culture, echocardiography) must be confirmed and appropriate antibiotic therapy instituted as soon as possible for 6 weeks: starting intravenously for the first 2 weeks, then continuing orally. Flucloxacillin is best, or vancomycin and rifampicin if there is resistance. Severe heart failure and deterioration in renal function require valve replacement.

3.23 **A**.F **B**.F **C**.T **D**.T **E**.F

Vitamin B_{12} is principally found in animal sources (meat, fish, eggs). Vegetarians, unlike strict vegans, rarely require B_{12} supplements. B_{12} binds to intrinsic factor in the stomach before traversing the gut and is absorbed at the terminal ileum. It is then stored in the liver in amounts sufficient to last for 2–3 years. The main cause of B_{12} deficiency is pernicious anaemia due to gastric atrophy and autoantibody destruction of intrinsic factor. B_{12} deficiency is also found in pancreatitis, coeliac disease, Crohn's disease with involvement of the terminal ileum and metformin administration. Pregnant women and patients taking phenytoin often require folic acid, not B_{12}, supplements. The growing fetus increases folic acid requirements by 50%, whilst phenytoin decreases folic acid absorption from the gastrointestinal tract.

3.24 **A**.T **B**.T **C**.F **D**.T **E**.T

Complications of epidural anaesthesia are fortunately rare. An epidural haematoma (incidence 1 in 190 000) presents with neurological deficits due to cord compression. Most occur spontaneously but anticoagulation therapy, including the use of non-steroidal anti-inflammatory drugs (NSAIDs) and prophylactic low-dose heparin, has been implicated. It is best to avoid central neural blockade within 12 hours of heparin having been given. If a haematoma is suspected, immediate decompressive laminectomy is required as neurological recovery is unlikely if this is delayed for more than 8–12 hours. Meningitis is extremely rare and often associated with underlying generalized sepsis. Abscess formation is also ususual and more often occurs with long-term placement of an epidural catheter. Clinical signs include severe back pain, local tenderness, fever and evidence of cord compression. Chronic adhesive arachnoiditis resulting in cauda equina syndrome can be caused by a variety of factors including bacterial infection, direct cord trauma, distilled water, blood, ischaemia or direct LA toxicity. Anterior spinal artery thrombosis causes a lower extremity paresis with a variable sensory deficit. The aetiology is uncertain. Direct trauma to the artery and ischaemia secondary to hypotension and vasoconstrictor agents may be causative factors, as well as advanced age and pre-existing peripheral vascular disease. It can be difficult to distinguish from other causes of cord compression. There is no treatment. Brown–Séquard syndrome results in ipsilateral motor loss and contralateral loss of pain and temperature sensation, usually from a tumour of the spinal canal. (See: Wildsmith JAW, Lee JA (1989) Editorial: Neurological sequelae of spinal anaesthesia. *British Journal of Anaesthesia* **63**, 505–507. Also: Wulf H (1996) Epidural anaesthesia and spinal haematoma. *Canadian Journal of Anaesthesia* **43**, 1260–1271.)

3.25 A.T B.F C.F D.T E.T
Baroreceptors are stretch receptors found in the carotid sinus, aortic arch and the heart. They are important for short-term control of arterial blood pressure. The carotid sinus is a small dilatation of the internal carotid artery, and should not be confused with the carotid body, a separate entity located nearby which responds to chemical, not mechanical, changes (Po_2, Pco_2, H^+ concentration). When blood pressure rises baroreceptors are directly stimulated by mechanical stretching as a result of vessel distension. This inhibits tonic discharge of vasoconstrictor nerves and excites the cardioinhibitory centre in the medulla to produce vasodilatation, bradycardia and reduced cardiac output via the IXth (glossopharyngeal) and Xth (vagus) nerves. Isoflurane has minimal effects on baroreceptor function unlike, for example, halothane.

3.26 A.F B.T C.F D.F E.F
Pacemakers are the treatment of choice for symptomatic arrhythmias arising from either sick sinus syndrome or complete heart block. They are powered by a lithium battery and have a life span of 4–10 years. All pacemakers have a five-letter code to explain their function and, in sequence, this is:

1. Chamber being paced: A, V, D, O, S for atrium, ventricle, dual, off, single chamber.
2. Chamber being sensed: as above.
3. Sensing mode: inhibition, triggering, dual (inhibition and triggering), neither.
4. Programmability: none, simple, multiprogrammability, communication, rate-adaptive.
5. Antitachycardia function: none, overdrive pacing, shock (implantable defibrillator) or dual function (overdrive and shock).

Whenever possible regional anaesthesia or LA is preferable to general anaesthesia for surgery. Intraoperatively a 'demand' pacemaker may be converted to fixed rate by placing a magnet over the pulse generator and switching off the rate response, but this is not recommended as it can lead to 'phantom reprogramming'. The metal contacts of the pacing wires are insulated to reduce the risk of conduction of small currents to the heart, resulting in microshock. Bipolar diathermy should be used if diathermy cannot be avoided as it reduces the risk of electrical interference which may lead to triggering of arrhythmias or pacemaker damage. The use of pancuronium, like all the other neuromuscular blocking drugs, is not contraindicated. (See: Bloomfield P, Bowler GMR (1989) Anaesthetic implication of the patient with a permanent pacemaker. *Anaesthesia* **44**, 42–46.)

3.27 A.T B.F C.T D.T E.F
The extradural space lies between the spinal dura and the 3–5 mm thick ligamentum flavum. It is circular at cervical level, becoming triangular and wider as it descends to the thoracic and lumbar regions. It lies 3.5–5 cm below the skin in the lumbar region of patients of average build. Extradural valveless veins are connected to cerebrospinal fluid (CSF) by bulbs of arachnoid mater protruding through the dura. This allows drainage of CSF to the vascular system as well as helping to facilitate the spread of LA into the subarachnoid space.

3.28 A.T B.T C.T D.F E.T
This scenario suggests Henoch–Schönlein purpura, an IgA-mediated autoimmune disease that causes widespread small vessel vasculitis. It is commoner in boys (3 : 1). Characteristic features include purpura on extensor surfaces, particularly the legs and buttocks, abdominal pain, arthritis, frank haematuria, proteinuria, oedema and glomerulonephritis (with hypertension). It is often preceded by an acute upper respiratory tract infection (haemolytic streptococcus is isolated in 30% of cases). Some antibiotics (e.g. sulphonamides, penicillins, cefuroxime) have been implicated as initiating agents. The prognosis is better in children than adults with spontaneous and complete recovery in 50%. The remainder may have persisting urinary abnormalities which may proceed to renal failure after 10 years or more. There is no known effective treatment and use of anti-inflammatory and immunosupressive agents has been disappointing. (See: Szer IS (1996) Henoch–Schönlein purpura. *Journal of Rheumatology* **23**, 1661–1665.)

3.29 A.T **B.**F **C.**F **D.**F **E.**T

Fungal infections in man can be divided into moulds (e.g. aspergillus), true yeasts (e.g. cryptococcus) or yeast-like fungi (e.g. candida). Infections can be superficial or systemic, the latter usually found in the immunocompromised. The broad-spectrum imidazoles (miconazole, ketoconazole) act by destroying fungal cell membranes whilst the newer triazoles (fluconazole, flucytosine, griseofulvin) inhibit fungal micro-tubular function. Nystatin is too toxic for intravenous use. Amphotericin is reserved for life-threatening systemic infections and for intrathecal use. Ketoconazole can cause hepatic necrosis and adrenal suppression. Griseofulvin is used for superficial infections (ringworm, athlete's foot). Many anti-biotics, including the polyenes nystatin and amphotericin, have antifungal properties.

3.30 A.F **B.**F **C.**F **D.**F **E.**T

Symptomatic PE occurs in up to 1% of all postoperative patients but is found at autopsy in 10–25%; it is probably responsible for death in one-third of these. Clinical features depend on size. A massive PE classically presents several days after a major operation with central chest pain, acute dyspnoea and circulatory collapse. This is accompanied by a tachycardia (commonly a gallop rhythm), hypotension, central cyanosis and an elevated central venous pressure (CVP). A small-to-medium PE is more likely to cause pleuritic chest pain, pyrexia and haemoptysis.

3.31 A.F **B.**F **C.**F **D.**F **E.**T

The Mallampati score is based on the pharyngeal structures seen when the patient is sitting upright, mouth open and tongue maximally extruded. Grade 1 is when the fauces, soft palate and uvula are visible; grade 2 when the uvula is hidden by the tongue; grade 3 when only the soft palate is visible; and grade 4 when the soft palate is not visible. Unfortunately, it predicts only about 50% of difficult airways (similar to the Wilson criteria), has considerable interobserver variability and a high incidence of false positive results. Other tests devised include:

> **Cormack** } – best view at laryngoscopy. Grade 1: glottis
> **Lehane** } visible; grade 2: anterior glottis not visible; grade 3: epiglottis seen but no glottis; grade 4: epiglottis not seen.

Wilson — score based on patient characteristics including weight, head and neck movements, jaw mobility, mandibular recession and presence of buck teeth.

Patil — thyromental distance <6.5 cm with neck extended suggests difficult intubation.

Frerck — Mallampati and Patil combined. This gives a higher specificity and sensitivity than each individually.

Savva — sternomental distance plus Mallampati, Patil, jaw protrusion and interincisor gap.

The incidence of difficult intubation in the general population is about 1% and this is likely to increase from inexperience as fewer intubations are carried out in current anaesthetic practice. No test is ideal. (See: Mallampati SR *et al.* (1985) A clinical sign to predict difficult intubation: a prospective study. *Canadian Anaesthetists Society Journal* **32**, 429–434. Also: Editorial (1993) *British Journal of Anaesthesia* **71**, 333–334.)

3.32 A.F B.T C.T D.T E.F
Dopexamine is a synthetic structural analogue of dopamine which itself is a precursor of noradrenaline. It acts on β_2, DA_1 and DA_2 receptors to cause renal, splanchnic and systemic vasodilatation with the aim of reducing afterload and improving blood flow to vital organs. It is an effective natriuretic and diuretic agent, and studies are awaited to confirm its efficacy in preserving renal function in the critically ill. It is a weakly positive inotrope and this effect, in combination with a decrease in systemic vascular resistance (SVR), increases cardiac output with minimal increase in myocardial oxygen consumption. Unlike dopamine, dopexamine has no clinically significant β_1 or α adrenergic activity and is unlikely to cause arrhythmias. Dosage is 0.5–0.6 µg/kg/min. Half-life is 5–7 min. It is extensively metabolized in the liver, and renally excreted. Studies have shown tolerance with progressive attenuation of haemodynamic response with prolonged infusion (72 hours). Side-effects include mild tachycardia, nausea, vomiting and tremor.

3.33 A.T B.F C.T D.F E.F
Phenoxybenzamine is useful for treatment of secondary hypertension, e.g. phaeochromocytoma. *Metaraminol* is an α receptor agonist used in the management of hypotension resulting from

unintentional vasodilatation, e.g. after extradural blockade. *Sodium nitroprusside* relaxes the smooth muscles of arterioles and venules. It has a rapid onset and a short duration of action and must be given intravenously. Its metabolism can produce cyanide ions which are normally converted to non-toxic thiocyanate by hepatic rhodanase. In excess the system can be overwhelmed, leading to toxicity. *Methyldopa* crosses the blood–brain barrier and is converted in adrenergic nerve endings to a false neurotransmitter, α-methylnoradrenaline, which stimulates α_2 receptors in the medulla to reduce sympathetic outflow. A positive antiglobulin (Coombs') test occurs in 10–20% but few proceed to haemolytic anaemia. *Hydralazine* directly relaxes arteriolar smooth muscle in a way similar to nitrates by increasing intracellular cyclic guanosine monophosphate (cGMP). Reflex tachycardia, fluid retention and a lupus-like syndrome can occur in slow acetylators.

3.34 A.T **B.**T **C.**T **D.**F **E.**T
Prostate cancer is common after the fifth decade. Most are well-differentiated adenocarcinomas, which tend to arise in peripheral prostatic tissue. At first they slowly invade adjacent prostatic tissue, bladder neck, etc., before reaching the pelvic lymph nodes and blood vessels from where they spread to bone and other organs, most commonly the lungs. Survival with metastatic disease is about 3 years. Unless picked up incidentally, only advanced cases give rise to symptoms, which include urinary retention, haematuria, pelvic and bone pain, anaemia or renal failure. Diagnosis is by rectal examination, prostate-specific antigen (which has superseded serum acid phosphatase), transrectal ultrasonography and biopsy. Alkaline phosphatase can be elevated from bone or liver involvement. Treatment depends on the staging and ranges from a curative prostatectomy for localized disease to radiotherapy and reduction of serum testosterone (by orchidectomy, luteinizing hormone-releasing hormone or androgens) for disseminated disease. Bone metastases are principally osteoblastic but osteolytic lesions are also found.

3.35 A.T **B.**T **C.**T **D.**F **E.**F
Fisher in the 1920s advocated randomization for clinical trials. Tossing a coin and random number tables (computer-generated nowadays) are simple and acceptable, although they can lead to uncertainty concerning the numbers in each group.

Serial entry – as they arrive – is possible since many patients become available for a trial only after it has started but it is open to allocator bias. Bartlett's test is useful for comparing variances, and the therapeutic index indicates the safety margin of a drug.

3.36 A.F **B**.T **C**.T **D**.T **E**.F

FFP is prepared from whole blood by separating the plasma within 6–8 hours of donation and freezing to $-18°C$. This preserves all the components of the coagulation, fibrinolytic and complement systems as well as the proteins that maintain oncotic pressure and modulate immunity. It should be used within 6 hours of thawing to obtain adequate coagulation levels of factor V and VIII, as they start to diminish after 1–2 hours. Overuse of FFP is common and may be attributed to excessive reliance on its haemostatic properties and an underestimation of the incidence and magnitude of complications including viral transmission (higher than for blood transfusion owing to pooling). Suggested indications include multiple coagulation defects, e.g. disseminated intravascular coagulation (DIC), emergency reversal of warfarin and possibly suxamethonium (FFP is a source of cholinesterase), vitamin K deficiency when combined factor concentrates are unavailable, and treatment of thrombotic thrombocytopaenic purpura. As there are more suitable replacements available it should not be used as a plasma volume expander, as a source of nutritional protein nor for replacement of immunoglobulins. Neither is it of benefit in the coagulopathy of cardiopulmonary bypass, as bleeding is due to disordered platelet function not lack of coagulation factors, nor after small blood transfusions (less than 1 whole blood volume). Its value in massive transfusions is also disputed as bleeding is associated with the duration of volume deficit rather than the volume transfused. (See: Thompson A, Napier JAF, Wood JK (1992) Editorial II: Use and abuse of fresh frozen plasma. *British Journal of Anaesthesia* **68**, 237–238.)

3.37 A.F **B**.F **C**.T **D**.F **E**.T

Infusion of intrapleural bupivacaine via an epidural catheter placed above the incision is technically simple but analgesia is inconsistent as the LA can exit through the drains. TENS is extremely unlikely to be helpful. There is no difference between thoracic and lumbar extradural analgesia using opiates (sufentanyl, fentanyl, morphine, etc.), although the use of LAs via the lumbar route can cause significant hypotension. Use of NSAIDs on their own does not provide adequate analgesia; however, they have a substantial opiate-sparing effect and, barring contraindications to their use, should be given in combination. Cryoanalgesia topically freezes the intercostal nerve; although useful, numbness persists until the nerve regrows (6–8 weeks). (See: Brodner G (1997) Pain management in patients undergoing thoracic surgery. *Current Opinion in Anaesthesiology* **10**, 54–59. Also: Sabanathan S *et al.* (1993) Management of pain in thoracic surgery. *British Journal of Hospital Medicine* **50**, 114–120.)

3.38 A.T B.T C.T D.F E.F
Hypercalcaemia greater than 3.5 mmol/l is a medical emergency. Symptoms may include nausea and vomiting, nocturia, polyuria, drowsiness and altered consciousness. Disodium etidronate gives an immediate reduction in serum level by chelating calcium to form a stable complex which is then excreted by the kidney. Its use is reserved for life-threatening emergencies as it can lower calcium too quickly, resulting in hypocalcaemic tetany, seizures, arrhythmias and respiratory arrest. Large doses are associated with renal failure. If laparotomy can be delayed for several hours, rehydration with normal saline and frusemide is appropriate. Frusemide promotes calcium loss by increasing glomerular filtration rate (GFR) and decreasing tubular resorption of Ca^{2+}. However, a urine output of at least 6 l daily is needed. With this technique, electrolyte replacement and prevention of dehydration are essential. Corticosteroids, such as prednisolone, act by inhibiting bone resorption and increasing renal loss but take several days to work. They tend to be more effective for conditions such as myeloma, sarcoidosis and vitamin D excess. Oral or intravenous phosphates are no longer recommended as they may increase ectopic calcification.

3.39 A.F B.F C.T D.F E.T
Anaesthetic volatile agents may contribute up to 0.01% of the yearly global release of CFCs (chemicals which promote ozone destruction as a result of photolytic release of chlorine ions). Nitrous oxide is also a significant pollutant as it reacts with oxygen in the atmosphere to produce nitric oxide, which not only contributes to ozone layer destruction but is also found in acid rain. Scavenging tubing has 30 mm connectors to prevent

connection with the breathing systems. Recommendations on safe levels of inhalational agents vary between countries, but in the UK the Control of Substances Hazardous to Health (COSHH) regulations have made it a legal requirement to limit occupational exposure (over an 8-hour reference period) of inhalational agents as follows:

Inhalational agent	UK	Range from other countries
Nitrous oxide	100 ppm	100–500 ppm
Halothane	10 ppm	10 ppm
Enflurane	50 ppm	4–20 ppm
Isoflurane	50 ppm	4–20 ppm

There are currently no published recommended levels for sevoflurane or desflurane. An often unrecognized source of pollution in the operating theatre is sidestream gas sampling with some capnographs. Upwards of 250 ml/min of gas may be extracted from the breathing circuit which, after analysis, is then vented without scavenging. (See: Barker JP, Abdelatti MO (1997) Anaesthetic pollution, potential sources, their identification and control. *Anaesthesia* **52**, 1077–1083.)

3.40 A.F **B.**T **C.**T **D.**F **E.**T
Previously known as 'electromechanical dissociation', PEA describes absent cardiac output with normal ventricular electrical activity. It can be primary due to failure of the myocardium to respond to depolarization, or secondary from mechanical problems with the passage of blood from the heart, e.g. cardiac tamponade, pulmonary embolism, tension pneumothorax and hypovolaemia. It also occurs in hypothermia, electrolyte abnormalities and drug overdose. It is seldom amenable to treatment unless an underlying, easily identifiable cause can be treated promptly. If this is not possible, management should be with adrenaline, intubation and cardiopulmonary resuscitation. Calcium is recommended for PEA only in the presence of hyperkalaemia, hypocalcaemia or an overdose of calcium channel-blocking drugs. An endocardial pacing wire would be inappropriate as there is no problem with initiation of electrical activity.

3.41 **A**.F **B**.T **C**.T **D**.T **E**.F

Also known as Weil's disease, leptospirosis is transmitted via infected urine of rats and rodents containing spirochaetes, which penetrate human skin and mucosa. Abattoir and farm workers are most at risk. The onset is abrupt with headache, severe myalgia, pyrexia, conjunctival suffusion, vomiting and a petechial rash. Splenomegaly and hepatomegaly are likely. In severe cases hepatitis leading to acute liver necrosis, renal failure, myocarditis and meningitis can occur. The mortality rate is 15–20% but those who recover do so completely, usually within a month. Diagnosis is confirmed by rising titre of leptospiral antibodies.

3.42 **A**.F **B**.T **C**.T **D**.F **E**.T

The aim of TPN is to provide protein, energy (carbohydrates, fats), electrolytes, water, vitamins and trace elements. Basal energy requirements are about 30 kcal/kg/day, increasing by 50% or more in critically ill patients. Protein requirements in the form of essential and non-essential L-amino acids is in the order of 1.25 g/kg (0.2 g/kg nitrogen) per day. Glucose is the carbohydrate of choice but high levels of stress hormones in critically ill patients mean that insulin is usually, but not always, required. Fat as soya bean emulsion supplies about 30–40% of the energy as well as providing cholesterol and preventing essential fatty acid deficiency. Phosphate is also essential as deficiency leads to muscle weakness, cardiac arrhythmias and reduced 2,3-diphosphoglyceride, which results in increased oxygen affinity of haemoglobin. Critically ill patients who lose in excess of 30% of their initial body weight are unlikely to survive without nutritional support. TPN has not been found to be of value preoperatively in the absence of severe malnutrition or within 48–72 hours of a non-surgical critical illness. (See: Willatts SM (1986) Nutrition. *British Journal of Anaesthesia* **58**, 201–222.)

3.43 **A**.F **B**.F **C**.T **D**.T **E**.F

Neonates, premature or not, are now known to feel pain as they show hormonal, metabolic and autonomic responses following surgery which can be attenuated by opiates. Pain measurement is difficult in young children: their general responses such as crying or motor withdrawal are non-specific. From 3 years of age simple scales using pictures (e.g. oucher) or colours to represent pain have been validated. Children over 5 years of age can use a visual analogue scale. Children do not have a higher pain threshold than adults but are often given less analgesia because of the fear of respiratory depression. Methods of administration are the same as with adults. Morphine remains the best opioid for pain relief and can be given by continuous intravenous infusion, particularly as studies suggest children over 3 months of age are no more susceptible to respiratory depression than adults. Other ingenious methods of pain relief administration include fentanyl either as a dermal patch or as a 'lollipop', tramadol, and caudal injection of clonidine and ketamine. Aspirin has been associated with Reye's syndrome and is not recommended. (See: Lloyd Thomas A (1995) Editorial: Assessment and control of pain in children. *Anaesthesia* **50**, 753–755. Also: Ball AJ, Ferguson S (1996) Analgesia and analgesic drugs in paediatrics. *British Journal of Hospital Medicine* **55**, 586–590.)

3.44   A.F   B.T   C.F   D.F   E.T
Hypokalaemia is defined as a potassium level of under 3.5 mmol/l. As it is principally an intracellular ion, the deficit can be substantial (>500 mmol) before significant changes occur in the serum level. Perioperatively, intravascular expansion due to large amounts of normal saline or colloid can induce a dilutional hypokalaemia. Diuretic therapy, particularly with frusemide, is also a potent cause of hypokalaemia. An acute respiratory or metabolic alkalosis induces hypokalaemia by promoting transfer of potassium into the cells in exchange for hydrogen ions. This intracellular increase in potassium also causes a favourable gradient within the distal tubule cell of the nephron to induce a kaliuresis. IPPV can similarly induce hypokalaemia from a respiratory alkalosis arising from hypocapnia. Metabolic acidosis has the opposite effect. Digoxin has no effect on potassium levels, although the incidence of side-effects and toxicity of digoxin increases with hypokalaemia. Mannitol, like hypertonic saline, increases serum potassium independent of any effect on acid–base balance. The exact mechanism is unclear but it has been postulated that the hypertonic solution causes an efflux of free intracellular water down a concentration gradient. This, in effect, increases the potassium gradient and promotes migration of potassium out of the cell. On a more practical note, it has always been assumed that a potassium level greater than 3.0 mmol/l is required before anaesthesia. Many reports now suggest that it is

possible to anaesthetize patients below that level if the hypokalaemia is chronic (e.g. diuretic therapy). If the low potassium has occurred acutely (e.g. vomiting, diarrhoea, bowel preps), physiological compensation has yet to occur and replacement therapy is needed. (See: Wong KC *et al.* (1993) Hypokalaemia and anesthetic implications. *Anesthesia and Analgesia* **77**, 1238–1260.)

3.45 A.F **B.**F **C.**T **D.**F **E.**F
More than 90% of cases of carcinoma of the larynx occur in men, with the peak incidence at 55–65 years of age. Smoking is by far the most important aetiological factor. 20% are supraglottic, 70% glottic and 10% subglottic. Lymph node metastases are rare except with supraglottic tumours, which metastasize to the cervical lymph nodes and give the worst prognosis. Hoarseness and stridor are the commonest presenting complaints. Pain and haemoptysis occur when presentation is delayed. Radiotherapy is the treatment of choice if the tumour is localized or if only palliation is possible. A laryngectomy is required if radiotherapy (DXT) fails or the tumour is extensive on presentation.

3.46 A.T **B.**T **C.**F **D.**F **E.**F
HFJV employs small tidal volumes (1–3 ml/kg) at high respiratory rates (60–250 breaths per min) with a ventilatory frequency of 1–10 Hz and a variable I : E ratio. Inspiration is active, expiration is passive. The exact mechanism by which it effects gas exchange is unknown but is thought to be due to a combination of convective flow and gas diffusion. Advantages over conventional ventilation include reduced airway pressures, greater cardiovascular stability and minimal adverse effect on renal function. It is of particular value in upper airway surgery, bronchopleural fistula and to replace IPPV when 'stiff' lungs require excessively high airway pressures to maintain oxygenation or when IPPV results in significant cardiovascular depression. HFJV can also be useful for weaning as it is well tolerated and patients require less sedation than for conventional methods. Humidification is important with HFJV as high gas flows dry the airways. As this cannot be achieved directly it is provided via a separate low-pressure circuit. HFJV should be avoided in diseases with airflow limitation (asthma, chronic obstructive pulmonary disease (COPD)) as it can cause air trapping, barotrauma and eventually cardiovascular

collapse. (See: Smith BE (1990) High frequency ventilation: past, present and future? *British Journal of Anaesthesia* **65**, 130–135.)

3.47 A.F   B.F   C.T   D.F   E.T

CF is the commonest serious autosomal recessive condition to occur in Caucasians with an incidence of approximately 1 in 2500 live births. It results in disordered ion transport in epithelial cells including increased sodium and chloride in sweat, a feature used for diagnosis. The most important clinical features are pulmonary and gastrointestinal. Bronchial secretions are thick and tenacious and together with ciliary dysfunction this leads to recurrent chest infections and the development of a vicious cycle of bacterial colonization, lung inflammation, bronchiectasis and progressive loss of lung function. 80% of patients have coexisting pancreatic disease which often leads to malabsorption and DM. Babies often first present with meconium ileus, whilst in older children it is usually with recurrent chest infections and bronchiectasis. Initial presentation with cirrhosis and portal hypertension is very rare but can occur due to inspisated biliary secretions. Treatment is essentially supportive with antibiotics, physiotherapy, pancreatic enzyme supplements and lung transplantation if needed. Life expectancy is now increasing with >50% living to over 18 years of age.

3.48 A.F   B.T   C.F   D.T   E.T

Clonidine is an imidazole compound with many actions. It is an antihypertensive agent from a combination of central and peripheral effects. Centrally it acts as an α_2 agonist to inhibit vasomotor responses in the medulla, while peripherally it is a presynaptic inhibitor of noradrenaline release. It has significant analgesic action at supraspinal and spinal sites. It has sedative and anxiolytic properties comparable to benzodiazepines, making it potentially useful for premedication. It reduces the MAC of inhalational agents by up to 50% and also decreases intraocular pressure. It is not contraindicated in pregnancy but its use as an antihypertensive has been limited by rebound sympathetic overactivity occurring with sudden withdrawal. Its use nowadays centres on its analgesic effects. Despite a lack of convincing large-scale studies it is an accepted analgesic by several routes including intravenous, intramuscular, extradural and intrathecal. It also has a significant opiate-sparing action and attenuates the symptoms of acute opioid withdrawal. In addition, compared with LAs, clonidine has little effect on sympathetic reflexes so blood pressure may be better maintained during spinal or epidural anaesthesia. Other advantages of clonidine include minimal respiratory depression and no pruritus or nausea. Hypotension and bradycardia may occur due to the reduction in catecholamine release. Postural hypotension can occur with all centrally acting antihypertensives including clonidine but is not usually a problem. Lipid-soluble and rapidly absorbed orally, its peak action occurs at 60–90 min. It has an elimination half-life of 9–12 hours with 50% hepatically metabolized to inactive metabolites and the rest excreted unchanged in the kidney. (See: Hayashi Y, Maze M (1993) Alpha$_2$ adrenoreceptors and anaesthesia. *British Journal of Anaesthesia* **71**, 108–118.)

3.49 A.F **B**.T **C**.T **D**.F **E**.F
BBB is due to an interruption in the conduction system below the atrioventricular (AV) node. This normally consists of one pathway to the right ventricle and two (anterior and posterior) to the left ventricle. In both left and right BBB the QRS duration is prolonged at >0.12 s (3 small squares).

> **RBBB** – RSR pattern V$_1$–V$_2$, large slurred S in I, V$_5$–V$_6$, ST depression V$_1$–V$_3$. Can be normal, but may be found with myocardial ischaemia, hypertension, pulmonary embolus, atrial septal defect and right ventricular hypertrophy.
>
> **LBBB** – wide notched R in I, V$_5$–V$_6$, inverted T V$_5$, V$_6$. Always pathological. Causes include ischaemia, hypertension, aortic valve disease, left ventricular hypertrophy.

Bifascicular block is RBBB plus one left bundle hemiblock. ECG changes are RBBB and left axis deviation (anterior) or RBBB and right axis deviation (posterior).

3.50 A.F **B**.T **C**.F **D**.F **E**.F
A retrobulbar block deposits 3 ml or so of LA inside the cone of muscles at the back of the orbit. A peribulbar block injects about 7–10 ml more superficially. As such, the peribulbar approach is safer but at the expense of being less reliable, particularly in achieving complete akinesia. The same range of

complications occurs with both approaches and includes retrobulbar haemorrhage and muscle palsies, particularly of the inferior rectus, as injection for both methods is through the relatively avascular inferior orbital rim. The eye should be in the primary gaze position (looking straight ahead). This displaces the optic nerve medially, protecting it from damage by the needle and also from potential injection of LA through the dural cuff to the subarachnoid space. Myopic eyes are longer, and therefore more subject to perforation; if the axial length is greater than 26 mm, alternative means of anaesthesia should be considered. Care is required with glaucoma, and a large rise in intraocular pressure should be prevented by injecting small volumes of LA incrementally. The volume of LA used in peribulbar blocks tends to cause proptosis rather than enophthalmos. Alternative local techniques are sub-Tenon's block or topical anaesthesia. The latter is more suited to co-operative patients as the iris and ciliary muscle retain their sensitivity. (See: Rubin AP (1995) Complications of local anaesthesia for ophthalmic surgery. *British Journal of Anaesthesia* **75**, 93–96. Also: Hamilton RC (1995) Techniques of orbital regional anaesthesia. *British Journal of Anaesthesia* **75**, 88–92.)

3.51 A.T **B.**F **C.**F **D.**T **E.**T

Hypothermia is defined as a core temperature <35°C and as profound when core temperature is <28°C. Respiratory rate, blood pressure and heart rate fall and oxygen delivery and demand are reduced. The oxygen dissociation curve shifts to the left. Atrial arrhythmias are found between 30 and 33°C; below 30°C pathognomonic 'J' waves (positive deflections at the end of QRS) are present, along with ventricular arrhythmias, often refractory to treatment. Glomerular filtration rate decreases but there is a paradoxical diuresis due to a reduction in tubular concentrating ability and decreased response to vosopressin (ADH). Blood glucose rises and there is a metabolic acidosis. Pupillary and tendon reflexes are lost. Initial confusion progresses to loss of consciousness at approximately 26°C. Blood viscosity and haematocrit increase, favouring thrombus formation. Other effects include elevation of serum amylase due to subclinical pancreatitis, and a rise in creatine kinase as a result of muscle damage. Shivering can increase oxygen demand by 700%, but this reflex is lost below 28°C and a spontaneous return to normal temperature is thus not possible. (See: Antretter H *et al.* (1995) Management of profound hypothermia. *British Journal of Hospital Medicine* **54**, 215–220.)

3.52 A.F B.F C.T D.T E.T
A TOF count is the number of twitches seen after four pulses have been delivered at 2 Hz for 0.5 s. The presence of 1, 2, 3 and 4 twitches suggests a residual block of 95, 90, 80 and 75%, respectively; 3–4 twitches are required before attempted reversal of neuromuscular blockade. TOF can be reliably repeated every 10–15 s. Post-tetanic stimulation is used to assess intense blockade. After a 5 s tetanus, the number of twitches produced by single pulses of 1 Hz is counted; fewer than 2 suggests a profound block. The test should not be performed more than once in 5 min. Double-burst stimulation applies two short tetanic bursts at 50 Hz, 0.75 s apart. A reduction in response (fade) between the two indicates a residual non-depolarizing block. It has been shown that when the second response is at least 60% of the first, it is no longer detectable by observation or palpation, and when compared with TOF (remember, there still can be >70% blockade with 4 twitches!) it is a much more sensitive judge of action of non-depolarizing muscle relaxants. Depolarizing neuromuscular blockers normally produce equal but reduced twitches in response to single pulses and TOF. If large amounts of suxamethonium are given, it can produce a dual (desensitization) block and act like a non-depolarizing neuromuscular blocker. Dual block may be reversed by neostigmine although the response is unpredictable. (See: Crofts SL, Hutchison GL (1992) Clinical monitoring of neuromuscular function. *British Journal of Hospital Medicine* **48**, 633–638.)

3.53 A.F B.F C.T D.T E.F
For most drugs, clearance is proportional to the GFR. As this rarely saturates the renal mechanism of elimination, drug clearance is constant and it usually follows first-order kinetics; that is, a constant *fraction* of the drug is eliminated per unit time. If saturation occurs, drug elimination undergoes zero-order kinetics in that a constant *amount* of drug is eliminated per unit time and clearance will then become variable. Lipid-soluble drugs are not readily eliminated until metabolized to more water-soluble compounds. Manipulation of pH between plasma and tubule can alter the proportion of a weak acid or

base that is non-ionized and therefore passively reabsorbed. When tubular urine is made more alkaline, weak acids are excreted more rapidly as they are more ionized and passive reabsorption is less. When the urine is made more acid, the excretion of weak acids is reduced. The opposite is true for weak bases. When renal excretion is greater than GFR, active tubular secretion has taken place. Clearance cannot exceed blood supply to the kidneys.

3.54 A.F **B.**F **C.**T **D.**F **E.**T

The Apgar score assigns a score from 0 to 10 on a newborn baby, regardless of method of delivery. It is measured initially at 1 and 5 min, and then is carried out every 5 min until a score of at least 7 has been reached. Clinical signs evaluated are:

Score:	0	1	2
Heart rate	Absent	<100/min	>100/min
Respiratory effort	Absent	Weak cry	Strong cry
Muscle tone	Limp	Some flexion	Active motion
Reflex irritability (catheter in nose)	No response	Grimace	Grimace + cough
Colour	Blue, pale	Body pink, extremities blue	Pink

The Apgar scoring system is not a particularly sensitive guide to the physiological state of a neonate. This is because the causes of a low Apgar score are many and are frequently distinct from physiological disturbances such as a metabolic acidosis. Examples include extreme prematurity, intracranial pathology and the effects of maternal anaesthesia, sedation or analgesia. Nevertheless, in terms of intervention a score of 8–10 requires routine care, 5–7 often only tactile stimulation and supplementary oxygen, 3–4 immediate ventilation and 0–2 cardiopulmonary resuscitation (CPR). The decision to resuscitate, if necessary, should not be delayed to obtain the 1 min score. The Apgar score can be used in neonates of any race. Heart rate is a better index than colour, as it is less subjective; it can be used without colour to give a maximum score of 8. Although disputed, the 5 min score is thought to be a reasonable guide to ultimate prognosis. (See: Apgar V (1966) The newborn APGAR scoring system: reflections and advice. *Pediatric Clinics of North America* **13**, 645–650.)

3.55 A.T **B**.F **C**.F **D**.F **E**.T

Transducers convert one form of energy into another, e.g. arterial pressure wave to electricity. All transducing systems are inherently damped as a compromise between speed of response and accuracy of the amplitude of a pressure trace. Overdamping results in a flat and/or distorted trace and is most often the result of either excessive frictional resistance to fluid flow or artefacts in the system. As fluid flow in the transducing system is assumed to be laminar it must follow the Hagen–Poiseuille law. Therefore resistance to flow will be directly proportional to the tube length and fluid viscosity, but inversely proportional to the fourth power of the tube radius. Therefore excessive damping can be minimized by using short and wide tubing and a low-viscosity fluid such as saline. The walls of the tubing must also be fairly rigid to prevent further dissipation of energy as a result of their compliance. Examples of artefacts include kinked tubing, blood clots and air bubbles.

3.56 A.F **B**.T **C**.F **D**.T **E**.F

Phaeochromocytoma is a rare (1 in 10 000) tumour of chromaffin tissue found in the adrenal medulla in >90% of cases. 95% secrete noradrenaline, 10% are bilateral, 10% are malignant, and metastases, if any, will commonly be to the liver. It is associated with neurofibromatosis and multiple endocrine neoplasia syndrome (MEN IIb), which includes medullary carcinoma of the thyroid and hyperparathyroidism. Clinical features include paroxysmal attacks of pallor, palpitations, sweating, headache and anxiety as well as anorexia, constipation and weight loss. Hypertension (0.1% of hypertensive patients) can be episodic or sustained. Either way it may lead to a stroke, myocardial infarction or congestive cardiac failure. Phaeochromocytoma can mimic thyrotoxicosis, DM and carcinoid syndrome. Increased vanillylmandelic acid (VMA >8 g in 24 hours), metanephrines and free catecholamines in the urine confirm the diagnosis. The tumour can be difficult to localize but is best seen with computerized tomography (CT) and scintigraphy using *m*-iodobenzyl guanidine (^{131}I-MIBG), which is selectively taken up by adrenergic cells. Surgery is the best treatment but, failing this, long-term therapy with alpha and beta blockers is a suitable alternative.

3.57 A.F **B**.F **C**.T **D**.T **E**.F

Propofol (2,6-di-isopropyl phenol) occurs as a 1% (10 mg/ml) solution in soya bean oil, egg phosphatide and glycerol. It is highly lipid-soluble and is extensively bound to plasma proteins. The normal adult induction dose is 1.5–2.5 mg/kg, with re-emergence due to rapid redistribution. It is metabolized to glucuronide conjugates in the liver and is renally excreted. It is safe to use in porphyria and with malignant hyperthermia susceptibility. Propofol reduces intraocular pressure and some studies suggest that it has intrinsic antiemetic properties. Side-effects include significant hypotension from a reduction in systemic vascular resistance – the basis for giving less, and more slowly, to the elderly. Respiratory side-effects such as cough and laryngospasm are rare. Transient pain on injection is attenuated with the addition of lignocaine (0.1 mg/kg) just prior to injection. Involuntary movements occur without EEG changes. Green urine and hair have been reported. (See: Borgeat A (1992) Subhypnotic doses of propofol possess direct antiemetic properties. *Anesthesia and Analgesia* **74**, 539.)

3.58 A.T **B**.F **C**.T **D**.F **E**.F

The liver weighs up to 1500 g and is well protected by the rib cage. It is not normally palpable except in deep inspiration. Blood supply is by the hepatic artery (40%) and portal vein (60%). Three hepatic veins deliver blood to the inferior vena cava. The liver is intimately involved in homeostasis of carbohydrate, protein and lipid. It is a store for glycogen, iron and vitamins (e.g. A, D, E, B_{12}); it detoxifies endogenous (steroid hormones) and exogenous (drugs) substances; and manufactures bile and albumin. Vitamin K is obtained by dietary means (green, leafy vegetables) as phytomenadione (vitamin K_1), and is synthesized by bacteria present in the gastrointestinal tract (vitamin K_2).

3.59 A.T **B**.F **C**.F **D**.F **E**.T

Ropivacaine is a relatively new amide LA belonging to the pipecoloxylidides group, which also contains bupivacaine and mepivacaine. The molecular weight is 274 kDa, and the pK_a is 8.1 – the same as bupivacaine. Ropivacaine is 50% less toxic than bupivacaine as regards cardiovascular depression and arrhythmogenicity, and 25% less for CNS effects. There is little difference in effect between bupivacaine and ropivacaine for infiltration, brachial plexus or peripheral nerve blocks. At an equivalent dose for extradural analgesia, the sensory block of ropivacaine is similar to bupivacaine but motor block is slower in onset, less intense and shorter in duration. These factors may be advantageous for extradural analgesia in labour but reduced motor block may render the 'test' dose invalid as intrathecal placement of the catheter could not be excluded. Ropivacaine is not currently used for spinal anaesthesia owing to insufficient motor block compared with an equivalent bupivacaine dose. (See: McClure JH (1996) Ropivacaine. *British Journal of Anaesthesia* **76**, 300–307. Also: Tanelian DL (1996) American Society of Anesthesiologists' annual refresher course lectures No. 165: The new local anesthetics, benefits, risks and use.)

3.60 A.F **B.**T **C.**T **D.**F **E.**T
The pulse oximeter works by shining two wavelengths of light (660 nm and 940 nm) through a digit, ear lobe, etc. A photocell detects and electronically processes the transmitted light to obtain an arterial saturation reading. It is programmed to respond only to pulsatile flow and to compensate for ambient light. It does not fully compensate for the presence of carboxyhaemoglobin, which can be more than 10% in heavy smokers. The readings will also be inaccurate when there is cutaneous vasoconstriction or with interference from pigments such as methylene blue, bilirubin or dark-coloured nail varnish. A transcutaneous oxygen electrode heats the skin locally to dilate capillaries so that capillary oxygen tension approximates to arterial tension. It is slow, less accurate than using arterial blood samples, is adversely affected by a fall in cardiac output and skin perfusion, and burns are a possibility. (See: Stoneham MD (1995) Uses and limitations of pulse oximetry. *British Journal of Hospital Medicine* **54**, 35–41.)

3.61 A.F **B.**F **C.**T **D.**T **E.**T
An amniotic fluid embolus can occur in any parturient but is found classically in multiparous women during or following a difficult labour. Incidence is 1 in 20 000–80 000. Mortality is up to 85%, with 25–50% dying in the first hour. The condition is responsible for 5–10% of all maternal deaths. It is thought to be caused by amniotic fluid entering the maternal circulation via endocervical and uterine tears or uterine veins in the placental bed. As it contains leukotrienes, prostaglandins and fetal debris, the amniotic fluid can cause small vessel

obstruction in the lungs, leading to pulmonary vasoconstriction and complement activation. This can result in acute respiratory distress, cardiovascular collapse (from acute pulmonary hypertension and right heart failure), a severe coagulopathy, acute renal failure, seizures and ultimately coma. Abdominal pain is not a feature. There is no specific therapy apart from immediate delivery of the fetus by Caesarean section and appropriate cardiopulmonary resuscitation. Hydrocortisone has been recommended but is not proven. Some success with continuous haemofiltration has been reported. In the few who survive, the initial hypoxia may result in permanent neurological sequelae.

3.62 A.F B.T C.F D.T E.T
Acute thrombotic occlusion of the femoral and popliteal arteries is catastrophic since there are few collateral vessels in the legs. It presents with sudden onset of intense limb pallor and severe pain with muscle spasm and paralysis. After 1–2 hours nerve ischaemia results in loss of both pain and feeling in the leg except at the border between the ischaemic and non-ischaemic areas. Within 4–8 hours the muscle spasm relaxes and the limb fills with stagnant deoxygenated blood and appears blue. Unless treatment is instituted within 24 hours irreversible damage occurs. The first step is anticoagulation to prevent proximal propagation of thrombus. Arteriography is required to distinguish a thrombus from an embolus. If a thrombus is confirmed, thrombolysis should be started immediately using either streptokinase or recombinant tissue plasminogen activator. This takes between 1 and 24 hours to dissolve the clot. If the limb is still viable angioplasty or reconstructive (femoro-popliteal or femoro-tibial bypass) surgery can be carried out. The mortality rate is 15–30% with limb loss occurring in 15–50%. (See: Beattie DK, Davies AH (1996) Management of the acutely ischaemic limb. *British Journal of Hospital Medicine* **55**, 204–208.)

3.63 A.T B.F C.F D.F E.F
The presence of soda lime to absorb carbon dioxide allows for reduction of fresh gas flow. Capnography is more important with low gas flows as the risk of rebreathing is higher. Plenum vaporizers are inaccurate at low flows (<1 l/min), therefore a vapour concentration monitor is important. Circle systems offer significant resistance to breathing (mainly due to the

presence of the two unidirectional valves). This may worsen at very low flows because the greater amounts of condensation produced cause the valves to stick.

3.64 **A**.T **B**.T **C**.T **D**.T **E**.T

Hb S accounts for between 25 and 45% of the total haemoglobin in patients with sickle cell trait. It is a benign condition with sickling crises a rarity. As such, anaemia is unusual. The most common symptom is haematuria, thought to be due to minor infarcts of the renal papillae. Hb C results from a substitution of lysine for glutamic acid in the β globin chain in the same position (6th) as the substitution in Hb S. Whereas a mild haemolytic anaemia with large numbers of target red blood cells is found in the homozygous state of Hb C, Hb C trait has a normal haemoglobin and the presence of a few target cells is often the only feature. G6PD deficiency is usually asymptomatic, causing haemolytic anaemia only in response to oxidant stress (fava beans), infection and drugs. Thalassaemia is a heterogeneous group of genetic disorders resulting from impaired synthesis of α or β chains of haemoglobin. Thalassaemia minor is normally asymptomatic with near normal haemoglobin levels but low mean corpuscular volume levels and an abnormal blood film (microcytosis, hypochromia, target cells and poikilocytosis). The anaemia of pernicious anaemia may be severe, mild or even absent, but the blood film and bone marrow appearances are always abnormal.

3.65 **A**.T **B**.F **C**.T **D**.F **E**.T

Immediate complications of a tracheostomy at the time of insertion include pneumothorax, pneumomediastinum, haemorrhage occult or otherwise, air embolism and subcutaneous emphysema, particularly if the tube is placed in pretracheal subcutaneous tissues. Apnoeic attacks are more likely to occur in an infant with pre-existing lung disease, e.g. bronchopulmonary dysplasia. Other early problems include creation of a false passage and accidental decannulation. Delayed complications include chest infections, granulomata formation, tracheal stenosis, and tracheomalacia from complete collapse of the tracheal rings. Erosion of tracheal cartilages may cause a tracheo-oesophageal fistula and mediastinitis. Erosion of the inominate (brachiocephalic) artery is very rare but can lead to fatal haemorrhage. A blocked tube is a common problem at all times after insertion. Interestingly, the long-term outcome after percutaneous dilational tracheotomy is as good as conventional tracheotomy. (See: Law RC, Carney AS, Manara AR (1997) Long-term outcome after percutaneous dilational tracheostomy. *Anaesthesia* **52**, 51–56.)

3.66 A.F **B.**F **C.**T **D.**T **E.**T

Plasma acetylcholinesterase is required to hydrolyse suxamethonium. 0.03% of the population have a genetically inherited absence of the enzyme, resulting in delayed breakdown of suxamethonium. The degree of absence of the acetylcholinesterase can be quantified by finding the dibucaine or fluoride number. Normal values are 75–85 and 60, respectively. Both are reduced with deficiency. Acquired deficiency of cholinesterase can also occur with liver failure, hypoproteinaemia, pregnancy, malnutrition or following plasmapharesis. Ecothiopate, cyclophosphamide, organophosphorus compounds (not high phosphate feeds) and edrophonium inhibit the action of cholinesterases. Physostigmine is a naturally occurring anticholinesterase used for its miotic activity in glaucoma. It very rarely causes low cholinesterase levels when given topically. Pilocarpine is a parasympathomimetic agent used as a miotic and has no anticholinesterase activity.

3.67 A.T **B.**F **C.**F **D.**T **E.**F

The membranes of all red blood cells contain antigens which determine the blood group of each individual. In Caucasians they are:

A (41%), B (10%), AB (4%), O (45%)

Antibodies against antigens are agglutinins. Thus:

Blood group A has agglutinins to B known as anti-B.
Blood group B has anti-A agglutinins.
Blood group AB has no agglutinins ('universal recipient').
Blood group O has both anti-A and anti-B agglutinins ('universal donor').

Transfusion reactions occur when a patient has agglutinins against the red cells in the transfusion. Thus, group O has anti-A and anti-B and will therefore react adversely with blood group A. Blood group antigens are found in many tissues including saliva, semen and amniotic fluid. A and B antigens are inherited as allelomorphs. Other blood groups include

Kell, Duffy and Kidd; these become important after multiple transfusions. Haemolytic disease of the newborn is a result of rhesus incompatibility, not blood group antigens.

3.68 **A.**F **B.**F **C.**T **D.**F **E.**F

Haemolytic anaemia (sickle cell, spherocytosis, etc.) causes anaemia and reticulocytosis. Aplastic anaemia is due to stem cell failure resulting in pancytopaenia with severe anaemia and inability to raise the reticulocyte count. Reticulocytosis is seen in pernicious anaemia only after treatment has commenced (peaks at 6–7 days). Acute leukaemics are anaemic with little reticulocytosis owing to marrow involvement by leukaemic cells. Anaemia and raised reticulocyte (immature red blood cells in the peripheral blood) count above the norm of 0.2–2.0% excludes polycythaemia.

3.69 **A.**T **B.**F **C.**F **D.**T **E.**T

Intrathecal opiates diffuse passively from the CSF into the spinal cord to act specifically on opiate receptors (*mu, kappa* and *delta*) in the dorsal horn (substantia gelatinosa) to inhibit release of substance P, a neurotransmitter responsible for relaying nociceptive information across synapses. Unlike bupivacaine, analgesia with opiates is without somatomotor or sympathetic block and therefore postoperative reflex responses and haemodynamic stability are maintained. Unfortunately, side-effects are similar to those from intravenous administration of opiates, if not greater. Nausea and vomiting, urinary retention and pruritus are common complaints (15–40%). Naloxone can reverse all side-effects (inconsistently with nausea and vomiting) but often only at doses which antagonize analgesic action. If respiratory depression occurs it tends to do so within 1 hour of administration. A small proportion (0.5–3%) can be delayed for 6–24 hours; this is probably due to the cephalad spread of opiates to act on the respiratory centre on the floor of the fourth ventricle. This effect is found more commonly with poorly lipid-soluble opiates such as morphine; the highly lipid-soluble opiates (e.g. fentanyl) bind more avidly to the spinal cord so that little is available to spread within the CSF. Removal of opiates is by diffusion and vascular reabsorption. Piloerection is not a recognized side-effect. (See: Cheam EWS, Morgan M (1994) Editorial: The superiority of epidural opioids for postoperative analgesia – fact or fallacy? *Anaesthesia,* **49**, 1019–1021.)

3.70 A.F **B.**F **C.**F **D.**F **E.**F

This is a difficult question to answer because the rules are continually being relaxed as the advantages of performing more operations as day cases are being increasingly recognized. Not only does day case surgery allow more efficient use of limited resources (i.e. it is about 25–75% cheaper), but patients prefer it, recovery is quicker, and it decreases demand for postoperative medications as well as the likelihood of developing hospital-acquired infections. Ex-preterm infants (postconceptual age <46 weeks) have an increased incidence of postoperative apnoeic episodes and should be admitted overnight for respiratory monitoring, otherwise young age is not a bar. Stable pre-existing conditions are not a contra-indication and neither is length of procedure, as long as it does not involve large fluid shifts and is not too painful to be managed at home. The use of intubation and ventilation is increasing and spinal anaesthesia is quite commonplace. (See: Hitchcock M, Ogg TW (1995) Anaesthesia for day case surgery. *British Journal of Hospital Medicine* **54**, 202–206.)

3.71 A.T **B.**T **C.**T **D.**T **E.**T

Absolute humidity in g/m^3 or g/l is the mass of water vapour present in a given volume of air. Relative humidity is absolute humidity divided by the amount present when the gas is fully saturated at the same temperature. Humidity can be measured by: *Wet and dry bulb thermometer:* two mercury thermometers are placed side by side. The bulb of one is open to the air, whilst the other is surrounded by a wick which dips into a water reservoir. The temperature of the wet bulb depends on the rate of evaporation and hence the humidity of the surrounding air, and is therefore lower than the temperature of the dry bulb. The relative humidity can be determined from tables which relate the dry and wet bulb temperature to humidity. The *whirling hygrometer* works on an identical principle. *Hair hygrometer:* human hair increases in length as humidity is increased. This can be calibrated but it is not particularly accurate and the range is limited to a humidity of between 15% and 85%. *Mass spectrometer:* measures water vapour pressure and is sufficiently rapid to measure breath-by-breath changes. Its expense precludes general use. *Dew point hygrometer:* a silver tube is cooled gradually by evaporation of liquid ether. When the tube cools to the dew point of the surrounding air (i.e. the point at which the air becomes fully saturated), small droplets condense on the outside of the silver tube. If the temperature of the ether is measured, the absolute humidity can be read from a graph. *Humidity transducer*: utilizes change in resistance or capacitance which occurs in a substance, e.g. silica gel, when it absorbs water. It is usually extremely sensitive.

3.72 **A.**T **B.**T **C.**T **D.**F **E.**F

Kussmaul breathing is an increase in both respiratory rate and tidal volume. Although classically associated with diabetic ketoacidosis, it is due to stimulation of central chemoreceptors by hydrogen ions and can occur in severe metabolic acidosis of any cause, including renal failure from acute tubular necrosis. Cheyne–Stokes respiration is a regular cycle of gradual deepening of breathing followed, after a period of very deep rapid breaths, by a phase of slowly decreasing respiratory excursion which may cease for several seconds before the cycle is repeated. It occurs most commonly with increased intracranial pressure, e.g. after a head injury or stroke, but it also occurs with cardiac and renal failure, severe pneumonia and narcotic drug poisoning. Tidal volume is reduced in emphysema from loss of lung tissue and in ankylosing spondylitis from restriction of chest wall movement.

3.73 **A.**F **B.**F **C.**T **D.**F **E.**T

The oculocardiac reflex was first described in 1908. It results in bradycardia which may be severe enough to lead to asystole and other dysrhythmias after traction on the extraocular muscles (particularly the medial rectus) or pressure on the globe. The afferent pathway of the reflex is mediated through the ophthalmic division of the trigeminal nerve while the efferent pathway is via the vagus. It occurs after both LA and general anaesthesia, but is more likely during 'light' anaesthesia. The presence of hypoxaemia and hypercarbia increases incidence and severity. It is more common in children as they have a higher vagal tone. There are numerous techniques to obtund the response but few are consistently effective. Prophylactic atropine at normal doses is ineffective and can be associated with severe ventricular dysrhythmias in older patients. The use of retrobulbar block is controversial as although it may obtund the oculocardiac reflex in some patients it can actually worsen it in others, and performing the block is associated with potentially serious complications. Atropine given at induction is useful but the best treatment is to ask the surgeon to stop and if necessary give intravenous atropine or glycopyrrolate.

3.74 A.T **B.**T **C.**T **D.**F **E.**T

At birth haemoglobin is mainly fetal (Hb F). This has a higher affinity for oxygen than adult haemoglobin (Hb A), which results in a decrease in oxygen release from haemoglobin at the tissue level compared with that of Hb A. This is compensated to some extent by a high haemoglobin at birth. Hb F is replaced by Hb A within the first 2–3 months of life to produce physiological anaemia in the order of 10–12 g/dl. Tidal volume at birth is in the order of 17 ml/kg at a respiratory rate of 30–40 breaths per min. The average cardiac output is 350–500 ml/kg/min. This falls steadily through the neonatal period to about 150 ml/kg/min. The postnatal blood pressure gradually rises in the same period from an initial 70/40. Blood volume in a neonate is 80–85 ml/kg. It is increased in premature neonates to about 90–100 ml/kg whilst in adults it is in the order of 60–70 ml/kg. The spinal cord assumes its permanent position at L1 by 1 year of age.

3.75 A.T **B.**T **C.**T **D.**T **E.**T

All the possibilities are true for the following reasons. Marfan's syndrome, an autosomal dominant connective tissue disease, often has a high arched palate and kyphoscoliosis. Cleft lip and palate can lead to problems in placing the laryngoscope. Treacher Collins syndrome is associated with choanal atresia, mandibular hypoplasia and micrognathia. The larynx is often anterior and there may be little room for the tongue. Ludwig's angina is cellulitis with massive swelling of the floor of the mouth and the submandibular region, which can lead to laryngeal obstruction. Acromegaly due to a pituitary adenoma producing excess growth hormone leads to an enlarged jaw, tongue and larynx, and a widespread increase in soft tissue.

3.76 A.F **B.**F **C.**F **D.**F **E.**T

APKD is an autosomal dominant condition due to a defective gene on the short arm of chromosome 16. The incidence is 1 in 1000; males and females are equally affected. From infancy, small cysts begin to enlarge and gradually compress normal renal tissue resulting in progressive loss of function. Often asymptomatic until middle age, the earliest sign is hypertension. Other features include loin pain due to the expanding kidney, haematuria and urinary tract infections. Over 50% of patients ultimately require dialysis and transplantation. 30% have coexisting hepatic cysts, although hepatic dysfunction is rare. 10–20% have berry aneurysms of cerebral vessels which may bleed, resulting in subarachnoid haemorrhage. Juvenile APKD is a rare autosomal recessive condition, usually fatal in the first year of life.

3.77 A.F **B.**F **C.**F **D.**F **E.**T
Haemorrhoids are dilatations of the venous plexuses at the lower ends of the anal mucosal columns. They are normally located in the 3, 7, 11 o'clock positions when viewed in the lithotomy position. Haemorrhoids are produced by venous congestion secondary to raised intra-abdominal pressure, commonly brought about by chronic constipation. They are divided into three groups: first degree are small and do not prolapse; second degree prolapse during defaecation but return; and third degree remain prolapsed. They are considered internal when covered by mucosa, and external when covered by squamous epithelium of the anal margin. Symptoms are intermittent and include perianal irritation and itching due to perianal leakage of mucus, rectal bleeding and prolapse. Pain usually occurs only when haemorrhoids are thrombosed or strangulated. Diagnosis is by proctoscopy as they collapse on digital examination. Treatment ranges from dietary change (to high fibre) to injection with phenol, elastic band ligation and infrared coagulation. Surgical excision is a last resort if all other treatments have failed. Malaena is altered blood found in the faeces due to bleeding from the upper part of the intestinal tract. (See: Pfenninger JL (1997) Modern treatment for internal haemorrhoids. *British Medical Journal* **314**, 1211–1212.)

3.78 A.T **B.**F **C.**F **D.**F **E.**T
N_2O is a colourless, odourless gas. It has both advantages and disadvantages, the balance of which has led to some controversy over its continued use.

Advantages	Disadvantages
Fast onset, fast offset	Low potency (MAC 105)
Analgesic action	Pressure and volume effects in gas-filled cavities
Minimal airway irritation	Toxicity (patients, staff, pollution)
Not metabolized	Emetic effects (?)
Safe (no mortality)	Cardiodepressive
Cheap	Requires scavenging
Non-flammable	Supports combustion

Its insolubility (blood:gas partition coefficient 0.5) leads to rapid induction and recovery but diffusion hypoxia is possible. It rapidly enters and increases air-containing spaces (e.g. intestine, middle ear and tracheal tube cuffs), which may cause pressure-related problems. Some studies suggest that N_2O is best avoided with intracranial pathology as it increases cerebral blood flow. Although minor, it is also a contributing factor in stimulating postoperative nausea and vomiting. Mild cardiovascular depression is partially compensated by centrally mediated sympathetic stimulation but N_2O does not sensitize the myocardium to catecholamines. N_2O inhibits vitamin B_{12} acting as a cofactor with methionine synthetase in the production of methionine and thymidine important for DNA synthesis. Megaloblastic changes occur in bone marrow after several hours' exposure with agranulocytosis after prolonged use (5–6 days). These effects are accompanied by a rise in serum folate and a decrease in serum methionine. Marrow recovers within 1 week but recovery can be accelerated by folinic acid, which restores normal thymidine synthesis. (See: Raeder JC (1996) Nitrous oxide: still a role in anaesthesia? *Current Opinion in Anaesthesia* **9**, 279–284.)

3.79 A.F **B**.T **C**.F **D**.T **E**.F

Ankylosing spondylitis is a progressive spinal arthropathy with a male-to-female ratio of 4:1. HLA-B27 antigen is implicated in more than 90% of cases. The onset is insidious with recurrent episodes of low back pain and early morning stiffness. Other effects include chest pain due to involvement of the costovertebral joints, plantar fasciitis, anterior uveitis, iritis, aortic incompetence and cardiac conduction defects. Peripheral joints are affected in about 10% of cases. Radiological signs include sacroiliitis and 'bamboo' spine due to ossification of the spinal ligaments. Treatment is with analgesia and regular exercise to maintain function. Non-specific urethritis, conjunctivitis and arthritis occurring together are known as Reiter's disease, which may follow bacterial dysentery or exposure to sexually transmitted infection. Most cases of Reiter's disease are self-limiting although about 10% become chronic.

3.80 A.F **B**.T **C**.F **D**.T **E**.F

Fulminant hepatic (also known as 'hyperacute') failure is defined as severe liver failure with encephalopathy developing in less than 8 weeks in a patient with a previously normal liver. The commonest causes in the UK are viral hepatitis and paracetamol poisoning. The encephalopathy varies from slight confusion and disorientation (grades I and II) to unresponsive coma with convulsions (grade IV). Foetor hepaticus is common but signs of chronic liver disease, such as ascites and splenomegaly, are rare. The liver is usually small. Fever, vomiting, hypertension and hyperglycaemia frequently occur. The prothrombin time is the most useful index of severity and when very high (more than three times normal) indicates a poor outcome. Other important prognostic indicators include the aetiology (worse if hepatitis C), age (under 10 years, over 40 years), the serum bilirubin (if it is in excess of 300 μmol/l) and serum pH (Less than 7.3 in paracetamol poisoning). Treatment is supportive with liver transplantation a last resort. Cerebral oedema is the major cause of death and is found at postmortem in 80% of patients. (See: Gimson AES (1996) Fulminant and late onset hepatic failure. *British Journal of Anaesthesia* **77**, 90–98.)

3.81 A.F B.T C.T D.F E.T
Amyotrophic lateral sclerosis is a mode of presentation of motor neurone disease, in which anterior horn cells are destroyed leading to motor weakness, wasting and fasciculation but not sensory loss. Friedrich's ataxia is due to spinocerebellar, corticospinal and dorsal column degeneration. Sensory impairment is usually seen over time. Syringomyelia causes 'dissociated' sensory loss with spinothalamic loss and dorsal column preservation. Paterson–Brown–Kelly syndrome is a premalignant condition causing dysphagia secondary to a postcricoid web. Vitamin B_1 (thiamine) deficiency is beriberi. There are two forms: *wet*, causing high output cardiac failure; and *dry*, resulting in a peripheral neuropathy with loss of sensory, motor and reflex function.

3.82 A.T B.T C.F D.F E.F
The reduction in the proportion of total body water and relative increase in body fat in the elderly means that the volume of distribution of water-soluble drugs is reduced. Thus plasma and tissue concentrations are effectively increased. A decrease in hepatic blood flow, microsomal enzyme system activity and GFR, results in increased sensitivity to many drugs including opiates. The MAC values of all inhalational agents

progressively decline with advancing age. The ageing process also leads to an increase in lung compliance, residual volume and FRC with a decrease in vital capacity. The ventilatory response to hypoxia and hypercapnia is also reduced. The autonomic nervous system becomes less sensitive as demonstrated by increased incidence of postural hypotension and a reduced ability to maintain body temperature.

3.83 A.T **B.**T **C.**T **D.**F **E.**F
Modern criteria for the initiation of dialysis in the ICU include:

1. Oliguria: urine output of <5 ml/kg day or anuria.
2. Plasma urea concentration >30 mmol/l.
3. Serum creatinine >600 μmol/l.
4. Hyperkalaemia >6.5 mmol/l.
5. Pulmonary oedema unresponsive to diuretics.
6. Metabolic acidosis <7.2.
7. Uraemic encephalopathy, pericarditis or neuropathy.

The presence of one of the above is sufficient to justify dialysis; two or more strongly indicate the need for dialysis. Anaemia and hypoproteinaemia are a consequence of chronic renal failure and are not corrected by dialysis.

3.84 A.T **B.**F **C.**T **D.**F **E.**T
TEC6 vaporizers have been specifically designed for use with desflurane. The boiling point of desflurane is 23.5°C, and therefore it will not remain a liquid in the reservoir chamber of a conventional vaporizer at room temperature. To compensate, the TEC6 vaporizer contains two thermostatically controlled electrical heating elements which raise the temperature of the desflurane to 39°C. When vapour is required, a shut-off valve is closed and pure vapour is released. This is passed through a pressure regulator to reduce the pressure to the level of that of a normal vaporizer (1–2.5 kPa) and the vapour is then calibrated prior to being added to the fresh gas flow. An increase in the fresh gas flow is detected by two independent pressure regulators which act to increase desflurane flow and thus maintain the set vapour concentration. Calibration (0–18% on the dial) is accurate to more than 10 l of fresh gas flow. The vaporizer requires an electrical supply and a 5–10 min warm-up period before use. There are additional heaters to prevent vapour condensation inside the vaporizer. The

machine switches off automatically if there is more than a 15° tilt from the vertical axis and it can be refilled when in use via a dedicated filler nozzle which is already attached to the desflurane bottle. Like the other current inhalational agents, sevoflurane can be used with any conventional vaporizer, including the TEC4 and the TEC5, but not the TEC6. (See: Graham S (1994) The desflurane TEC6 vaporizer. *British Journal of Anaesthesia* **72**, 470–473.)

3.85 A.T **B.**T **C.**T **D.**F **E.**T

Hyponatraemia (serum sodium <135 mmol/l) is a common finding. It can be dilutional due to volume overload – as seen with cardiac, hepatic and renal failure, nephrotic syndrome and syndrome of inappropriate antidiuretic hormone (SIADH) – or the result of genuine salt loss with chronic vomiting and diarrhoea. Other causes include oat cell carcinoma of the lung, which can induce hyponatraemia due to adrenocorticotrophic hormone (ACTH) or ADH. Hyponatraemia becomes symptomatic below 120 mmol/l as the fall in extracellular osmolality pushes water into brain cells leading to confusion, convulsions and coma. Treatment involves correcting the underlying cause and fluid restriction. Hypertonic saline is restricted to patients with acute retention and neurological signs. This must be given slowly as a rapid increase in extracellular osmolality can rapidly shrink brain cells to cause central pontine myelinosis. Conn's syndrome is primary hyperaldosteronism arising from an adrenal adenoma. Hypokalaemia, metabolic alkalosis and hypertension are usually found, with normal serum sodium.

3.86 A.F **B.**T **C.**F **D.**T **E.**T

TMJD and maxillary sinusitis are frequent causes of bilateral facial pain. Guillain–Barré syndrome is an acute inflammatory demyelinating polyradiculoneuropathy causing gradual ascending weakness. Pain can be a feature and is seen in the face with bilateral involvement of the facial nerves. MS arises from demyelinating plaques within the CNS, the size and number of which are unrelated to physical symptoms. Facial pain in MS tends to be unilateral, with retrobulbar neuritis, trigeminal neuralgia or complex disturbances of sensation including bursts of pain, sensory distortion and itching. Open-angle glaucoma is insidious progressive painless loss of vision due to increased intraocular pressure. Closed-angle glaucoma is characterized by sudden onset of severe blurring, excruciating pain and nausea and vomiting. Although the pain normally affects only one eye at a time, the other eye must always be examined and often requires prophylactic treatment.

3.87 A.F   B.F   C.F   D.T   E.F

A bronchopleural fistula most commonly occurs after a pneumonectomy, although it may also follow thoracic trauma, chronic infection or erosion by lung tumour. Reducing minute volume or respiratory rate will not substantially reduce the leak but decreasing inflation pressure, flow rate and PEEP will. If conventional IPPV fails to maintain an adequate minute ventilation, transferring to high-frequency ventilation with small tidal volumes, high respiratory rates and low airway pressures may be essential. Management of a ventilated patient with a bronchopleural fistula is difficult as it is often not possible to wean him/her from the ventilator. The mortality rate is 60–70%.

3.88 A.F   B.F   C.F   D.T   E.F

The aim in hypothermia is to restore body temperature without complications. Slow rewarming of up to 1°C/hour is preferable as rapid rewarming may lead to hypotension and arrhythmias. It is best reserved for younger patients who have suffered a rapid fall in temperature. Gentle handling is also required to prevent arrhythmias. Supplementary oxygen is beneficial but intubation and ventilation are usually reserved for lower core temperatures. ECG monitoring is essential and arrhythmias should be appropriately treated as they arise. Warmed intravenous fluids are useful but gastric and colonic lavage, warm peritoneal dialysis and cardiac bypass are required only when hypothermia is profound (<28°C). Antibiotics should be reserved for established infections; steroids are of no value. Severe complications include pancreatitis, bronchopneumonia and circulatory arrest. Underlying causes include hypothyroidism, drug overdose and poor socioeconomic conditions. The outcome is favourable if spontaneous rewarming occurs at about 0.5°C/hour without adverse sequelae.

3.89 A.F   B.F   C.F   D.T   E.T

Sickle cell trait is the heterozygote form of the homozygous condition sickle cell anaemia. Unlike sickle cell anaemia, sickle cell trait has minimal effects on normal growth and development and is symptomatic only if a severe hypoxic event occurs.

The combination of other structural globin abnormalities (Hb C, Hb D) with sickle cell disease is possible and a mixture of β thalassaemia trait and sickle cell trait clinically resembles sickle cell anaemia. Exposing red cells to sodium metabisulphite is the basis of the sickling test and is useful in the emergency surgical situation. However, it does not differentiate the heterozygous from the homozygous state and it is open to observer error. Definitive diagnosis requires haemoglobin electrophoresis. The use of a tourniquet is controversial and the traditional answer is to avoid it in the presence of sickle cell trait. Nevertheless, evidence in the literature increasingly suggests that the worry is unfounded, particularly if the proportion of Hb A present is greater than 25%.

3.90 A.F B.T C.T D.F E.T
The ESR is obtained by measuring the distance from the surface meniscus to the upper limit of the red cell layer in a column of blood left standing for 60 min. Although there has been no satisfactory explanation, it is often higher in women than in men, with an upper limit of 15 mm and 10 mm, respectively. The ESR is widely used as a non-specific index of organic disease. It is often elevated to 100 mm or so in temporal arteritis and polymyalgia rheumatica, where serial measurements can be used to assess the efficacy of steroids in the management of these conditions. ESR is also elevated in anaemia, acute and chronic infections, neoplastic diseases, collagen diseases, renal failure and any disorder associated with an increase in plasma proteins. It rises during pregnancy and with increasing age, and an elevated ESR is often found over the age of 60 years without cause.

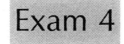

Exam 4

Questions

4.1 **Enteral feeding in the critically ill in the intensive care unit (ICU):**
A. can frequently achieve a positive protein balance.
B. is usually preferable to total parenteral nutrition (TPN).
C. reduces the incidence of septic complications.
D. is as expensive as total parenteral nutrition.
E. may result in *Clostridium difficile* diarrhoea.

4.2 **The coeliac plexus (CP):**
A. lies posterior to the inferior vena cava.
B. lies at the level of the second lumbar vertebra.
C. lies posterior to the pancreas.
D. is situated posterior to the crura of the diaphragm.
E. is in direct communication with the cervical sympathetic chain.

4.3 **Coarctation of the aorta is associated with:**
A. intracranial aneurysms.
B. most commonly a preductal position.
C. upper limb hypertension.
D. Turner's syndrome.
E. a bicuspid aortic valve.

4.4 **Hartmann's solution contains:**
A. sodium   – 112 mmol/l.
B. chloride   – 131 mmol/l.
C. bicarbonate   – 29 mmol/l.
D. calcium   – 2.0 mmol/l.
E. potassium   – 5.0 mmol/l.

4.5 **Core temperature may be reliably measured in the:**
A. external auditory canal.
B. axilla.
C. lower third of the oesophagus.
D. nasopharynx.
E. rectum.

4.6   A potassium of 2.5 mmol/l and bicarbonate of 15 mmol/l are compatible with:
   A.   diabetic ketoacidosis.
   B.   Addison's disease.
   C.   acute renal failure.
   D.   pyloric stenosis.
   E.   milk alkali syndrome.

4.7   Thermoregulation:
   A.   is centrally controlled in the hypothalamus.
   B.   is stimulated by endogenous noradrenaline.
   C.   is dependent on the temperature of blood perfusing the carotid bodies.
   D.   is stimulated by afferents from piloerector muscles.
   E.   is obtunded by inhalational agents.

4.8   Human immunodeficiency virus (HIV):
   A.   is a retrovirus.
   B.   is incorporated into host ribonucleic acid (RNA).
   C.   can be transmitted via breast milk.
   D.   sufferers commonly develop *Pneumocystis carinii* pneumonia (PCP).
   E.   should be treated as a first line with protease inhibitors.

4.9   Colorectal carcinoma:
   A.   commonly arises in the rectum.
   B.   commonly develops from a single polyp.
   C.   can have a 'signet ring' appearance.
   D.   can be amenable to chemotherapy alone.
   E.   metastasizes to liver before lymph nodes.

4.10 Glutamine is:
   A.   an essential amino acid.
   B.   stable in solution.
   C.   a substrate for polymorphonuclear leukocytes (PMNLs).
   D.   a substrate for enterocytes.
   E.   important for glutathione synthesis.

4.11 **A well-controlled, non-insulin dependent diabetic on glibenclamide is to have major surgery. The following statements are correct:**

   A. the patient should be stabilized on short-acting insulin preoperatively.
   B. increasing the dose of glibenclamide is sufficient to cover surgery.
   C. glucose infusion is essential intraoperatively.
   D. glucose and insulin should not be given together.
   E. patients with coexisting hypertension are at increased risk of having autonomic neuropathy.

4.12 **Hypoglycaemia is found with:**

   A. excessive alcohol intake.
   B. leprosy
   C. panhypopituitarism.
   D. petit mal epilepsy.
   E. phaeochromocytoma.

4.13 **The following drugs undergo considerable first-pass metabolism:**

   A. warfarin.
   B. diazepam.
   C. chlorpromazine.
   D. benzylpenicillin.
   E. phenytoin.

4.14 **The following can occur in diabetic coma:**

   A. lactic acidosis.
   B. metabolic acidosis.
   C. hypomagnesaemia.
   D. hypoviscosity.
   E. hyperlipidaemia.

4.15 **Pulmonary fibrosis is associated with:**

   A. bleomycin.
   B. bretylium.
   C. cortisone succinate.
   D. paraquat.
   E. 90% oxygen.

4.16 The probability of microshock occurring increases with:
- A. a saline-filled central venous catheter.
- B. high leakage currents.
- C. multiple earth connections.
- D. isolated circuits.
- E. use of an oesophageal temperature probe.

4.17 Neurofibromatosis is associated with:
- A. increased sensitivity to non-depolarizing neuromuscular blockers.
- B. airway obstruction.
- C. interstitial lung disease.
- D. phaeochromocytoma.
- E. prolonged action of local anaesthetics (LAs).

4.18 A blood urea of 12 mmol/l would be consistent with:
- A. gastrointestinal (GI) haemorrhage.
- B. cardiac failure.
- C. liver failure.
- D. pyloric stenosis in a neonate.
- E. acute renal failure.

4.19 Legionnaires' disease is commonly associated with:
- A. pneumonia.
- B. leucopenia.
- C. encephalopathy.
- D. cavitating lung lesions.
- E. myalgia.

4.20 The complement system plays an important role in the following:
- A. drug hypersensitivity reactions.
- B. virus inactivation.
- C. phagocytosis by macrophages.
- D. mast cell degranulation.
- E. neutrophil chemotaxis.

4.21 **Following administration of ergometrine, a previously undiagnosed twin was discovered. The following may be useful in relaxing the uterus to aid delivery:**
  A. prostaglandins.
  B. thiopentone.
  C. halothane.
  D. suxamethonium.
  E. salbutamol.

4.22 **Adrenocortical insufficiency:**
  A. may be due to pituitary dysfunction.
  B. occurs with chronic steroid therapy.
  C. is excluded by a normal response to administered adrenocorticotrophic hormone (ACTH).
  D. may present with hypoglycaemia.
  E. responds poorly to a fluid load.

4.23 **The following can be employed in the measurement of carbon dioxide (CO_2):**
  A. thermal conductivity.
  B. metacresol purple.
  C. potassium hydroxide.
  D. polarography.
  E. Severinghaus electrode.

4.24 **Late complications of a partial gastrectomy include:**
  A. anaemia.
  B. steatorrhoea.
  C. osteomalacia.
  D. weight loss.
  E. renal calculi.

4.25 **A patient taking monoamine oxidase inhibitors (MAOIs) was given ephedrine. Blood pressure rose to 300/170 mmHg. Acceptable treatment includes:**
  A. propranolol.
  B. sodium nitroprusside.
  C. labetolol.
  D. diazoxide.
  E. phentolamine.

4.26 Patients with acute intermittent porphyria should not be given:
   A. paracetamol.
   B. barbiturates.
   C. sulphonamides.
   D. propofol.
   E. pethidine.

4.27 The Valsalva manoeuvre:
   A. assesses baroreceptor reflexes.
   B. involves inspiration against a closed glottis.
   C. results in an initial fall in heart rate.
   D. blood pressure (BP) initially decreases.
   E. is abnormal in patients with raised central venous pressure (CVP).

4.28 Nephrotic syndrome is associated with:
   A. minimal change glomerulonephritis.
   B. SLE.
   C. hepatitis B.
   D. subacute bacterial endocarditis (SBE).
   E. hypercholesterolaemia.

4.29 Glycine irrigation during prolonged transurethral resection of the prostate (TURP) may cause:
   A. metabolic acidosis.
   B. hypocalcaemia.
   C. irreversible visual disturbances.
   D. bradycardia.
   E. hypokalaemia.

4.30 Appropriate management of diabetes insipidus (DI) includes:
   A. fluid restriction.
   B. hypertonic saline.
   C. intravenous vasopressin (ADH).
   D. 5% dextrose infusion.
   E. thiazide diuretics.

4.31 Transcutaneous electrical nerve stimulation (TENS):
   A. stimulates A nerve fibres.
   B. is useful for thalamic pain.
   C. uses frequencies of 30–100 Hz.
   D. uses voltage of 1–50 V.
   E. is useful for the management of peripheral nerve injury.

4.32 The following visual deficits may be caused by:
   A. blindness in one eye: retinal artery occlusion.
   B. homonymous hemianopia: lesion in occipital cortex.
   C. bitemporal hemianopia: chiasmal compression.
   D. constriction of visual fields: hysteria.
   E. tunnel vision: glaucoma.

4.33 Surfactant:
   A. consists mainly of lipoprotein.
   B. increases surface tension in the lungs.
   C. prevents alveolar collapse at low lung volumes.
   D. is found in amniotic fluid at 30 weeks.
   E. alters capillary permeability.

4.34 Secondary brain damage after head injury can be exacerbated by:
   A. hypoxia.
   B. hypotension.
   C. a decrease in serum osmolality.
   D. hyperglycaemia.
   E. raised intracranial pressure (ICP).

4.35 Likely findings with a ruptured abdominal aortic aneurysm include:
   A. raised jugular venous pressure.
   B. anuria.
   C. absent femoral pulses.
   D. bruising on the flanks.
   E. continuous abdominal pain.

4.36 Ulna nerve block at the elbow reduces the power of:
   A. finger adduction.
   B. finger abduction.
   C. thumb abduction.
   D. thumb apposition.
   E. flexion of the interphalangeal joints.

4.37 Carbon monoxide (CO) poisoning is associated with:
   A. cutaneous bullae.
   B. atrial fibrillation.
   C. cyanosis.
   D. hyperventilation.
   E. hyperpyrexia.

4.38 Ritodrine can cause:
A. vasoconstriction.
B. tachycardia.
C. pulmonary oedema.
D. hypokalaemia.
E. augmentation of uterine contraction.

4.39 In the management of oesophageal varices:
A. propranolol effectively decreases portal hypertension.
B. a Minnesota tube may be useful.
C. ADH can lead to myocardial ischaemia.
D. sclerotherapy reduces the frequency of an acute bleed.
E. successful liver transplanation leads to their regression.

4.40 Contraindications to elective major surgery include:
A. sickle cell anaemia.
B. polio immunization 10 days previously.
C. susceptibility to malignant hyperthermia.
D. acute febrile upper respiratory tract infection (URTI) in a child.
E. myasthenia gravis.

4.41 Post-herpetic neuralgia (PHN):
A. is more painful in the elderly.
B. incidence decreases with age.
C. can be effectively treated by capsaicin.
D. can be prevented by antiviral agents, e.g. acyclovir.
E. can be effectively treated by opiates.

4.42 The following features may be associated with rheumatoid arthritis (RA):
A. Heberden's nodes.
B. early involvement of the lumbar spine.
C. psoriasis.
D. early morning stiffness.
E. splenomegaly.

4.43 Regarding an exponential function:
   A. it is an example of zero-order kinetics.
   B. after three time constants, the event is 95% complete.
   C. after one time constant, 37% of the event is complete.
   D. half-life is the time taken for 50% decay.
   E. there is a constant proportional rate of change.

4.44 An infusion of albumin:
   A. carries a risk of viral transmission.
   B. commonly causes anaphylactoid reactions.
   C. can be derived from bovine or human plasma.
   D. is suitable for a volume expander.
   E. is a useful source of protein for malnourished patients.

4.45 Complications of postoperative hypoxaemia include:
   A. subarachnoid haemorrhage.
   B. silent myocardial ischaemia.
   C. basal atelectasis.
   D. decrease in cardiac output.
   E. cognitive dysfunction.

4.46 Flumazenil:
   A. has anticonvulsant properties.
   B. antagonizes the action of midazolam.
   C. is structurally similar to benzodiazepines.
   D. is indicated for all benzodiazepine overdoses.
   E. may need repeat dosage.

4.47 Gout:
   A. has a genetic predisposition.
   B. results in deposition of urates in the kidney.
   C. can cause lytic lesions in the bones.
   D. can be precipitated by surgery.
   E. should be treated acutely with allopurinol.

4.48 The pudendal nerve:
   A. passes through the lesser sciatic foramen.
   B. provides sensation to the perineum.
   C. provides motor supply to the uterus.
   D. block is useful for the first stage of labour.
   E. block has a high success rate.

4.49 Indications for immediate surgery after a head injury include:
A. unilateral pupillary dilatation.
B. decreasing level of consciousness.
C. status epilepticus.
D. cerebrospinal fluid (CSF) rhinorrhoea.
E. headache with neck stiffness.

4.50 Applied Physiology and Chronic Health Evaluation Score (APACHE) III measurements include:
A. serum glucose.
B. serum potassium.
C. a numerical score of 0–299.
D. the best physiological variables in the first 24 h.
E. a modified version of the Glasgow Coma Scale (GCS).

4.51 Post dural puncture headache (PDPH):
A. is more common with pencil-point needles.
B. may be associated with cranial nerve lesions.
C. may be associated with auditory hallucinations.
D. commonly resolves without an extradural blood patch.
E. is often successfully treated with caffeine.

4.52 Acute extracellular fluid (ECF) depletion causes:
A. increased blood urea.
B. increased sodium loss in the urine.
C. raised haematocrit.
D. raised urine osmolality.
E. reduced skin turgor.

4.53 A 45-year-old man develops a transient left hemiparesis and impaired vision in his right eye. His BP is 190/115 mmHg at rest. The following are true:
A. immediate treatment of his BP is required.
B. angiography must be performed to confirm a diagnosis.
C. if the lesion is inaccessible to surgery, anticoagulation is indicated.
D. the site of the lesion is probably in the internal capsule.
E. he may have an aneurysm of the circle of Willis.

4.54 Indications for insertion of a temporary preoperative pacing wire include:
A. asymptomatic congenital complete heart block.
B. Mobitz type II second-degree heart block.
C. Wenckebach type I second-degree heart block.
D. sick sinus syndrome.
E. Wolff–Parkinson–White (WPW) syndrome.

4.55 Hypotension during spinal anaesthesia may be due to:
A. preganglionic sympathetic blockade.
B. venoconstriction.
C. block of the dorsal root ganglion.
D. administration of low-dose adrenaline.
E. hypovolaemia.

4.56 Coeliac plexus block (CPB):
A. causes constriction of the sphincter of Oddi.
B. may cause diarrhoea.
C. may cause postural hypotension.
D. commonly causes impotence.
E. can be of value in treating pain from an abdominal malignancy.

4.57 Weakness, spasticity and impaired sensation may be associated with:
A. spinal cord compression.
B. polymyositis.
C. multiple sclerosis.
D. motor neurone disease.
E. poliomyelitis.

4.58 As regards an EMLA:
A. eutectic means that the melting point of each individual LA is increased in the presence of the other.
B. it is a combination of 2.5% prilocaine and 5% lignocaine.
C. methaemoglobinaemia is a known complication.
D. it can cause vasoconstriction.
E. local skin reactions are uncommon.

4.59 A patient breathing room air with a haemoglobin of 7.5 g/dl may:
   A. have a P_aO_2 of 13 kPa (100 mmHg).
   B. have a P_aCO_2 of 5.6 kPa (40 mmHg).
   C. have a haemoglobin oxygen saturation of 97%.
   D. have an arterial oxygen (O_2) content of 19.5 ml/dl.
   E. be cyanosed.

4.60 With a pulmonary artery (PA) flotation catheter:
   A. the thermistor is situated at 20 cm from the balloon.
   B. the pulmonary artery pressure (PAP) waveform must be displayed continuously.
   C. cardiac output can be derived from pressure measurements.
   D. readings are more accurate if it is inserted through a jugular vein.
   E. the proximal lumen is used for measuring CVP.

4.61 Carcinoma of the lung:
   A. may cause Cushing's syndrome.
   B. may present with peripheral neuropathy.
   C. can produce Horner's syndrome.
   D. can cause cerebellar degeneration without posterior fossa metastases.
   E. occurs ten times more frequently in men than women.

4.62 Heparin:
   A. is very acidic.
   B. can be given orally.
   C. abolishes the risk of deep vein thrombosis (DVT) after hip replacement.
   D. is antagonized by aprotinin.
   E. has the same mode of action as prostacyclin.

4.63 The anion gap:
   A. is usually between 8 and 12 mmol/l.
   B. is increased by alkalosis.
   C. utilizes hydrogen ion concentration.
   D. increases with renal tubular acidosis.
   E. increases with diabetic ketoacidosis.

4.64 The renal threshold for glucose:
  A. is approximately 6.5 mmol/l.
  B. is higher in women than men.
  C. is elevated in diabetics.
  D. falls in pregnancy.
  E. varies in the same person from day to day.

4.65 Pressor response to intubation can be effectively attenuated by:
  A. oral esmolol.
  B. deep inhalational anaesthesia.
  C. intravenous fentanyl.
  D. topical lignocaine.
  E. sublingual enalapril.

4.66 Which of the following are suggestive of severe aortic stenosis (AS)?
  A. angina.
  B. effort syncope.
  C. cardiomegaly.
  D. apex pulsation in 6th intercostal space in the anterior displaced apex beat.
  E. collapsing pulse.

4.67 Paracetamol:
  A. is a phenacetin derivative.
  B. is highly protein-bound.
  C. has a peripheral anti-inflammatory effect.
  D. is excreted unchanged in the urine.
  E. is safe to use in small children.

4.68 In an adult the lung function tests below are compatible with the following conditions:

FEV$_1$	1.8 l	$P_a O_2$	8.5 kPa		
FVC	2.2 l	$P_a Co_2$	4.5 kPa	TLC	3.5 l

  A. chronic obstructive pulmonary disease (COPD).
  B. respiratory acidosis.
  C. asthma.
  D. cryptogenic pulmonary fibrosis.
  E. pulmonary embolism (PE).

4.69 In established congestive cardiac failure:
- **A.** glomerular filtration rate (GFR) is reduced more than renal blood flow.
- **B.** diuretics are an important first line of treatment.
- **C.** digoxin decreases myocardial tension.
- **D.** aldosterone secretion is high.
- **E.** ACE inhibitors are contraindicated.

4.70 The following drugs can be given via the trachea:
- **A.** calcium chloride.
- **B.** naloxone.
- **C.** sodium bicarbonate.
- **D.** lignocaine.
- **E.** atropine.

4.71 Helium:
- **A.** has a low viscosity.
- **B.** has a narcotic action.
- **C.** is stored as a liquid.
- **D.** is more dense than nitrogen.
- **E.** supports combustion.

4.72 Regarding oral hypoglycaemic agents:
- **A.** metformin increases insulin release from pancreas.
- **B.** chlorpropamide can cause intrahepatic cholestasis.
- **C.** metformin can cause metabolic acidosis.
- **D.** glibenclamide is longer acting than tolbutamide.
- **E.** they can be effective in IDD.

4.73 Urinary bilirubin is increased in jaundice due to:
- **A.** acute hepatitis.
- **B.** chloropromazine therapy.
- **C.** haemolysis.
- **D.** primary biliary cirrhosis (PBC).
- **E.** sickle cell crisis.

4.74 Magnesium sulphate:
- **A.** decreases uterine contractility.
- **B.** potentiates non-depolarizing muscle relaxants.
- **C.** potentiates depolarizing muscle relaxants.
- **D.** causes epileptiform convulsions.
- **E.** increases the bleeding time.

4.75 Characteristics of type I chronic regional pain syndrome (CRPS) include:
- A. cyanosis.
- B. pain.
- C. osteoporosis.
- D. leukocytosis.
- E. occurrence in athletes.

4.76 The following contribute to the silhouette of the left heart border on a PA chest radiograph:
- A. right ventricle.
- B. left pulmonary artery.
- C. left atrial appendage.
- D. left main bronchus.
- E. aortic arch.

4.77 Pain perception and transmission occurs in:
- A. free nerve endings.
- B. A delta nerve fibres.
- C. the thalamus.
- D. C nerve fibres.
- E. dorsal columns.

4.78 Tetany may be associated with:
- A. persistent vomiting.
- B. coeliac disease.
- C. metabolic acidosis.
- D. hypokalaemia.
- E. Trousseau's sign.

4.79 Respiratory distress syndrome (RDS) in the newborn:
- A. is more likely in infants delivered by Caesarean section.
- B. is associated with meconium aspiration.
- C. occurs almost exclusively within 12 h of birth.
- D. can be effectively treated with continuous positive airway pressure (CPAP).
- E. can be effectively treated with extracorporeal membrane oxygenation (ECMO).

4.80 The following changes in an ECG may contribute to a diagnosis of right ventricular hypertrophy:
  A. tall R wave in lead I.
  B. deep S wave in leads V_5 and V_6.
  C. inverted T waves in leads V_1 to V_3.
  D. wide QRS complexes.
  E. dominant R wave in lead V_1.

4.81 The Bain breathing system:
  A. is suitable for use in small children.
  B. has an expiratory valve near the patient connection.
  C. passes the fresh gas flow (FGF) down the outer limb.
  D. increases dead space if the inner tube detaches.
  E. can be classified as both Mapleson B and D.

4.82 Penicillins:
  A. are bacteriostatic.
  B. are more active against rapidly dividing bacteria.
  C. are all degraded by penicillinases.
  D. are active only against Gram-positive organisms.
  E. affect bacterial cell wall synthesis.

4.83 Acute hyperkalaemia of 7.0 mmol/l can be satisfactorily treated by:
  A. intravenous glucose and insulin.
  B. ion exchange resins.
  C. sodium bicarbonate.
  D. glucagon.
  E. calcium chloride.

4.84 The Wright respirometer:
  A. is unidirectional.
  B. underestimates when the vanes are wet.
  C. overestimates with low fresh gas flows.
  D. underestimates at high tidal volumes.
  E. can be used with children.

4.85 The following features are consistent with end-stage hepatic cirrhosis:
 A. parotid enlargement.
 B. palmar erythema.
 C. finger clubbing.
 D. testicular hypertrophy.
 E. raised globulin level.

4.86 Peripheral nerve injuries are a well-recognized complication of:
 A. fracture of the ulna and radius.
 B. fractured shaft of tibia.
 C. fractured shaft of humerus.
 D. dislocated shoulder.
 E. fractured shaft of femur.

4.87 Sodium dantrolene:
 A. inhibits calcium ion uptake by the sarcoplasmic reticulum.
 B. can be given orally.
 C. is useful in treating neuroleptic malignant syndrome (NMS).
 D. is hepatotoxic.
 E. initial dose for treatment of malignant hyperthermia (MH) is 10 mg/kg.

4.88 An FEV_1/FVC ratio of 0.6 is consistent with:
 A. obstructive lung disease.
 B. restrictive lung disease.
 C. myasthenia gravis.
 D. the elderly.
 E. pulmonary embolus.

4.89 As regards fat embolus syndrome:
 A. petechiae are required to confirm the diagnosis.
 B. the absence of fat globules in the urine excludes the diagnosis.
 C. cerebral signs are mainly due to hypoxia.
 D. it increases serum triglyceride level.
 E. it may be associated with unilateral tremor of the hand.

4.90 Cholestatic jaundice is associated with:
  A.   increased urinary urobilinogen.
  B.   increased unconjugated serum bilirubin.
  C.   steatorrhoea.
  D.   sclerosing cholangitis.
  E.   raised alkaline phosphatase.

Answers

4.1 A.F B.T C.T D.F E.F

If possible, enteral feeding is preferred over TPN. Not only is it cheaper, but nitrogen retention and weight gain have been found to be greater together with a reduced incidence of epigastric and intestinal bleeding. In addition, it enhances blood flow to the gut, thus preserving the structure, integrity and function of gut mucosa. This also promotes the release of gut trophic hormones which helps limit bacterial translocation and potential complications of endotoxaemia. Indeed, compared with TPN the incidence of septic complications is halved. It is suggested that enteral feeding should be commenced as soon as possible, even in the absence of bowel sounds. There are several commercial preparations specifically intended for certain conditions (Traumacal, Pulmocare) but their use has not been associated with sufficient benefit to justify their extra cost. Nutritional support improves nitrogen retention but fails to prevent protein catabolism and a positive protein balance is rarely, if ever, achievable. Intolerance of feeds can be a problem and feeding should start with low volumes. The addition of cisapride may improve gastric emptying. The most common problem is diarrhoea (32–68%). Loperamide may be useful as long as both overflow leakage from faecal impaction and infective diarrhoea resulting from antibiotic use have been excluded. Infection with *C. difficile*, which can cause pseudo-membranous colitis, is particularly important to consider. (See: McMahon MM *et al.* (1993) Nutritional support of the critically ill. *Mayo Clinic Proceedings* **68**, 911–920.)

4.2 A.T B.F C.T D.F E.F

The CP lies anterolateral to the vertebral bodies of T12–L1. The two interconnected ganglia lie anterior to the diaphragmatic crura at the origin of the coeliac artery and posterior to the stomach, pancreas and left renal vein. Preganglionic sympathetic fibres, carried in the greater, lesser and least splanchnic nerves, relay within the ganglia, which also have parasympathetic (coeliac branch of right vagus) innervation. Postganglionic fibres form a network anterior to the aorta. Innervation is generally segmental and, although not in direct communication, preganglionic fibres pass through the ganglia to synapse distally, e.g. to the cervical sympathetic chain.

4.3   A.T   B.F   C.T   D.T   E.T
Coarctation of the aorta accounts for 8% of all congenital heart disease. The incidence is 1 in 10 000 and is higher in males than in females (1.7:1). Extracardiac malformations are seen in 7%, the most frequent association being Turner's syndrome (gonadal dysgenesis, webbed neck), hypospadias and ocular defects. Intracranial aneurysms are present in 8–10% of patients. The narrowing of the descending aorta is postductal (i.e. after the ductus arteriosus) in more than 95% of cases. Symptoms are dependent on the degree of narrowing. Near total obstruction of the left ventricular outflow will normally present in the first week of life with left ventricular failure. Systemic flow will thus be dependent on left-to-right shunting at atrial level and with passage through the still patent ductus arteriosus. In older children with less severe narrowing, presentation can be with upper extremity hypertension, intermittent claudication of the lower limbs (femoral pulses weak and delayed compared with radial), a cerebrovascular accident (CVA) or bacterial endocarditis involving the aortic valve, which is commonly bicuspid. Other features include a systolic heart murmur, left ventricular hypertrophy, and the characteristic chest radiograph findings of a double aortic notch, small descending aorta and rib notching (Dock's sign) from enlarged collateral vessels.

4.4   A.F   B.F   C.F   D.T   E.T
Hartmann's solution (Ringer's lactate, compound sodium lactate) has a pH of 5.7 and contains:

sodium	– 131 mmol/l
chloride	– 112 mmol/l
lactate	– 29 mmol/l
calcium	– 2 mmol/l
potassium	– 5 mmol/l

It is commonly used for perioperative maintenance and resuscitation. Ringer was the first person to devise a fluid containing the electrolytes that are essential for tissue function. At a later date (1930s), Hartmann adapted the solution by adding lactate and used it to treat acidosis in children. The lactate in solution is metabolized mainly in the liver by either gluconeogenesis (70%) or oxidation (30%). These two processes consume H^+ ions to produce a relative excess of bicarbonate ions. As this process takes about an hour to complete, a steady stream of bicarbonate is generated which can be used to reduce acidosis in a controlled fashion. If there is no acidosis, the bicarbonate is promptly excreted from the kidney and the mild alkalosis is transient. The gluconeogenesis may also result in a transient rise in blood glucose. In certain circumstances, Hartmann's solution should be used with care: e.g. in diabetics, and in some critically ill patients who are obligate excretors of acidic urine, as the added bicarbonate load cannot be excreted. This can make the patient more alkalotic whilst enhancing potassium loss. Hartmann's solution is often avoided in patients with renal failure because of the risks of hyperkalaemia, and in sick patients or those with hepatic failure because of the risk of lactic acidosis. A recent paper revealed that few of the candidates at a final FRCA examination knew the contents and purpose of Hartmann's solution, which is both unfortunate and inexcusable since it is so commonly used. (See: White SA, Goldhill DR (1997) Is Hartmann's the solution? *Anaesthesia* **52**, 422–427.)

4.5 A.F B.F C.T D.T E.F
Probes in the external auditory canal are unreliable but measurements at the tympanic membrane correlate closely with core temperature; however, perforation is a risk. The lower third of the oesophagus is accurate as it lies below the carina and is unaffected by the temperature of inspired gases. The nasopharynx is suitable for an intubated patient if the probe is correctly placed posterior to the soft palate. Rectal measurement is controversial. It is probably accurate but the probe is not close to metabolically active tissues, response is slow – particularly if inserted into faeces – and pelvic or abdominal surgery can expose the probe to cold air. Axillary measurements are unreliable due to frequent malpositioning. Skin/core temperature difference can be useful, particularly in children, as a means of assessing peripheral perfusion. Pulmonary artery catheters with thermistors provide accurate measurement of temperature. (See: Ilsey H *et al.* (1983) An evaluation of body temperature measurement. *Anesthesia in Intensive Care* **11**, 31–39.)

4.6 A.F B.F C.F D.F E.F
These figures show a metabolic acidosis and hypokalaemia. Diabetic ketoacidosis, Addison's disease and acute renal failure are associated with hyperkalaemia. Pyloric stenosis produces a hypokalaemic, hypochloraemic alkalosis with a paradoxically

acid urine. Milk alkali syndrome is an uncommon condition that results from a high intake of calcium and alkali as found in antacids. Hypercalcaemia, alkalosis and renal failure result. A probable diagnosis is primary hyperaldosteronism (Conn's syndrome).

4.7   A.T   B.T   C.F   D.F   E.T
Thermoregulation is controlled by the hypothalamus but temperature-sensitive cells are also found in brainstem, spinal cord, skin and skeletal muscle. Peripheral afferents to the hypothalamus are from A δ and C fibres, while efferents run via the sympathetic nervous system to blood vessels, piloerector muscles and sweat glands. Heat loss can be minimized by means such as curling into a ball to reduce surface area, cutaneous vasoconstriction and piloerection, while heat production is maximized by shivering, metabolizing food, activity and increasing catecholamine release. The carotid bodies are not involved in thermoregulation. During surgery, heat loss occurs by radiation, convection, evaporation (from lung and open body cavities) and conduction and cannot be corrected by the normal physiological mechanisms of conservation and production. Hypothermia increases oxygen demand postoperatively and may compromise recovery. Both regional and general anaesthesia impair central and peripheral temperature-regulating mechanisms. Inhalational agents, in particular, decrease the threshold temperature at which the body responds to hypothermia by about 2.5°C.

4.8   A.T   B.F   C.T   D.T   E.T
Acquired immune deficiency syndrome (AIDS) develops from HIV-1 and -2. They are retroviruses of the lentivirus group which invade immune cells via CD4, Fc and complement cell surface receptors. Once inside, the viral RNA converts to deoxyrubonucleic acid (DNA) by a reverse transcriptase enzyme which is then incorporated into host DNA as proviral DNA. The proviral DNA remains there until the cell is activated and new HIVs are produced under the control of viral proteases. Acute HIV infection is associated with a seroconversion illness similar to infectious mononucleosis in 50–70% of patients. The associated viraemia is controlled by cellular and antibody-mediated responses which result in resolution of symptoms. Although the majority become asymptomatic, HIV replication continues to take place until the immune system is eventually overwhelmed

and immunodeficiency develops with depletion of $CD4^+$ T cells. The median time to develop AIDS from HIV infection is 9 years. Diagnosis is by detecting the presence of anti-HIV antibodies by enzyme-linked immunosorbent assay (ELISA) or Western blot analysis. HIV is transmitted by sexual contact, contaminated blood and needles, and mother to child either *in utero*, perinatally or by breast milk (14% of babies become infected by HIV-positive mothers). The result of the progressive immunodeficiency is neoplasia and opportunistic infections with bacteria, viruses and fungi leading to dysfunction of all the major systems, particularly neurological and respiratory. PCP represents 80% of admissions into ICU of HIV-positive patients and is treated with co-trimoxazole and nebulized pentamidine. Many studies now suggest that antiviral treatment should be commenced as soon as possible after diagnosis to control HIV replication in lymphoid tissue. Combination therapy is recommended to prevent resistance, and includes reverse transcriptase inhibitors (zidovudine, didanosine) and protease inhibitors (saquinavir, ritonavir). As more than 90% of HIV-positive patients live in developing countries, few have either the funding or the access to this level of treatment.

4.9   A.T   B.T   C.T   D.F   E.F
Colorectal carcinoma is common, with an equal sex incidence. Of the 40% found in the rectum, 75% are within reach of a flexible sigmoidoscope. The condition is influenced by genetic factors, inflammatory bowel disease, excess bile salts and a low-fibre, high-fat diet. The majority develop from polyps which eventually ulcerate to encircle and constrict the bowel in a signet ring shape. The carcinoma metastasizes first to lymph nodes before entering the bloodstream to the liver. Treatment is by surgical resection and survival is related to the spread as determined by Dukes' classification. If the tumour is limited to the mucosa of the bowel (Dukes' A) the 5-year survival is 90%; with lymph node involvement (Dukes' C2) it is around 30%. Radiotherapy and chemotherapy (5-fluorouracil, levamisole) have an adjuvant role with Dukes' C tumours and above.

4.10   A.F   B.F   C.T   D.T   E.T
Glutamine is the most abundant amino acid in plasma and intracellular fluid, comprising 50% of free amino acids in the body. Glutamine has many functions. It is the major carrier of nitrogen, particularly between the organs of synthesis (e.g.

muscle, liver) and of utilization (e.g. gut, lung). It also has a key role in the production of nucleotides (DNA and RNA precursors), skeletal muscle synthesis and breakdown, ammoniagenesis in the kidney, glutathione synthesis and gluconeogenesis. It is involved in the maintenance of immune function as it optimizes both the growth and the function of lymphocytes and macrophages, whilst a lack of glutamine suppresses T cells and interleukin 2. It is also a metabolic fuel for enterocytes of the gut mucosa, PMNLs and lymphocytes. In addition, it is thought to help preserve the gut mucosal barrier and limit bacterial translocation. Nevertheless, as it can be readily synthesized in many tissues it is regarded as a conditionally essential amino acid only in catabolic states, i.e. when demand exceeds synthesis. As this occurs in surgery, trauma and sepsis, glutamine deficiency is thought to be one of the mechanisms for impaired immune function after these events. Glutamine supplements in nutrient (enteral and parenteral) feeds of the critically ill have therefore been proposed. This requires further validation. Although glutamine is unstable in solution (it decomposes to form ammonia and pyroglutamic acid), stable preparations are now commercially available in the form of glutamine precursors (e.g. α-ketoglutarate) and dipeptides such as alanine–glutamine. (See: Hall JC *et al.* (1996) Glutamine. *British Journal of Surgery* **83**, 305–312. Also: Organ CH (1996) Glutamine, cancer and its therapy. *American Journal of Surgery* **172**, 418–429.)

4.11 A.T   B.F   C.T   D.F   E.T
More than 90% of diabetics undergoing surgery will be non-insulin dependent. The incidence of perioperative problems is directly related to the severity of end-organ disease such as ischaemic heart disease, renal insufficiency and neuropathy. 50% of patients with coexisting hypertension also have an autonomic neuropathy which is associated with an increase in perioperative morbidity and mortality. Routine 'tight' glycaemic control has been shown to prevent, retard or even reverse some chronic complications in the long term but its effect in the perioperative period is less well proven. Some studies have shown an improvement in wound healing and a decrease in wound infection. This is important as more than 60% of postoperative problems and 20% of perioperative deaths in diabetics are attributable to infections (due to excess glucose adversely interfering with leukocyte function and impairing

phagocytic activity of granulocytes). Thus, stabilizing a patient on insulin perioperatively is appropriate. Increasing the dose of oral hypoglycaemics is not. Insulin always requires an infusion of glucose, which can be done separately with a sliding scale and 5% dextrose infusion or together as with the Alberti regimen. Although hypoglycaemia is unusual, the complications are severe and it must be avoided by regular checks on intraoperative glucose level.

4.12 A.T B.F C.T D.F E.F

Hypoglycaemia rarely produces symptoms until the glucose level falls to 2–3 mmol/l. Alcohol-induced hypoglycaemia is due to suppression of gluconeogenesis during metabolism of alcohol. It is found most frequently in chronic alcoholics when starvation or malnutrition is present (as gluconeogenesis is the main source of glucose) but may occur in young drinkers after the first exposure. Panhypopituitarism occurs from destruction of the pituitary by a primary or metastatic tumour, infarction (Sheehan's syndrome), postsurgery or irradiation. Hypoglycaemia is due to glucocorticoid and growth hormone deficiency causing a marked increase in sensitivity to insulin. Other causes of hypoglycaemia include drugs (salicylates increase insulin secretion, non-selective beta blockers decrease hepatic glucose efflux, pentamidine induces beta cell death and subsequent release of insulin), pregnancy, end-stage renal failure using glucose-containing intraperitoneal dialysis (stimulates insulin release), heart failure and liver failure. Leprosy and petit mal epilepsy have no association with hypoglycaemia. Phaeochromocytoma can be associated with hyperglycaemia and glucose is found in the urine of upwards of 30% of patients during paroxysmal release of the catecholamines.

4.13 A.F B.F C.T D.T E.F

First-pass metabolism is related to the amount of drug, given orally, which undergoes metabolism either in the gut wall or in the liver before gaining access to the systemic circulation and site of action. Other drugs with a high first-pass metabolism include dopamine, isoprenaline, heparin, pethidine, lignocaine and propranolol.

4.14 A.T B.T C.F D.F E.T

A diabetic coma is a consequence of either diabetic ketoacidosis (DKA) in insulin-dependent diabetes mellitus (IDDM) or non-ketotic hyperosmolar hyperglycaemia in non-insulin-diabetes mellitus (NIDDM). In DKA, the lack of insulin prevents the uptake and therefore the utilization of glucose by the tissues, as well as stimulating hepatic gluconeogenesis and glycogenolysis. This results in a high blood glucose but a low intracellular glucose. To compensate, peripheral lipolysis occurs, producing free fatty acids (FFAs) which are taken up by the liver to use as an energy substrate. Unfortunately, the amount of FFAs produced often exceeds the capacity of the Kreb's cycle to oxidize them and they are converted into ketone bodies, two of which (acetoacetate and β-hydroxybutyrate but not acetone) cause a metabolic acidosis. In NIDDM there is sufficient endogenous insulin to prevent hepatic ketogenesis, but glucose production is uncontrolled. This leads to higher blood glucose levels than in IDDM, greater hyperosmolality and thus hyperviscosity. Lactic acidosis is more commonly a feature of a diabetic coma from NIDDM, particularly if septic or with biguanides (metformin) and after excessive alcohol intake. It can be suspected if there is a large anion gap (> 40 mmol/l). Hyperlipidaemia frequently coexists with both types of diabetes mellitus (DM). Magnesium tends to move out of cells with potassium and in DKA with a high plasma potassium, magnesium will also be elevated. The commonest cause of hypomagnesaemia is through loss from prolonged diarrhoea.

4.15 A.T B.F C.F D.T E.T
The cytotoxic drug bleomycin can cause dose-related pulmonary infiltrates with fibrosis. Some cases regress with cessation of the drug. Survivors of paraquat ingestion commonly develop fibrosis. Oxygen toxicity is a well-recognized problem in premature neonates and adults alike. It is related to the duration of exposure and the inspired concentration: an inspired concentration greater than 80% can cause a deleterious effect in the lungs within hours. This ultimately results in pulmonary endothelial necrosis and hyaline membrane formation before diffuse fibrosis, and permanent structural and functional damage. Drugs such as amiodarone, busulphan, melphalan, chlorambucil, nitrofurantoin and hydrochlorothiazide have also been implicated. Bretylium can cause nausea and vomiting. The complications of steroids are many but do not include pulmonary fibrosis.

4.16 A.T **B.**T **C.**F **D.**F **E.**T

Microshock occurs when a minute amount of current (50 µA) is applied directly to the ventricular myocardium (atria need much higher current) and results in ventricular fibrillation. It occurs due to electrical contact across a small surface area in or close to the myocardium and has been reported with pacemaker wires, saline-filled central venous catheters, or cardiac catheters with a terminal electrode or filled with conductive radio-opaque dye. It is also a potential problem with oesophageal temperature probes which are positioned close to the heart. The risk of microshock is minimized by limiting leakage (< 10 µA) from all electrical equipment, using resistive material to limit earth pathways produced by hand-to-hand contacts, isolating all electrical circuits that make contact with the patient and using battery-operated equipment fully isolated from earth. Using earth-free mains supplies reduces but does not abolish leakage current and thus increases the safety margin.

4.17 A.T **B.**T **C.**T **D.**T **E.**F

Neurofibromatosis, or von Recklinghausen's disease, is an autosomal dominant condition isolated to a defective gene on chromosome 17. The incidence is 1 in 3000 and the condition is characterized by multiple cutaneous neurofibromas and café au lait pigmentation. Associated abnormalities that may give rise to anaesthetic difficulties include scoliosis, multiple endocrine adenomatosis, renal artery stenosis, phaeochromocytoma (1%), pulmonary fibrosis (20%) and obstructive cardiomyopathy. Other potential anaesthetic problems also arise from the distribution of the neurofibromata and respiratory obstruction and difficult intubation have both been recorded. Increased sensitivity to non-depolarizing neuromuscular blockers has been found in some cases; prolonged action of LAs has not.

4.18 A.T **B.**T **C.**F **D.**T **E.**T

Normal blood urea is 3–7 mmol/l. It is produced by the urea cycle from breakdown of amino acids in the liver. It is freely filtered at the glomerulus and approximately 50% is reabsorbed in the proximal tubule; it represents about 90% of daily nitrogen excretion. Urea levels can be increased as a result of increased intake or catabolism (GI haemorrhage), dehydration (neonatal pyloric stenosis) or an inability to excrete due to poor renal perfusion (cardiac failure) or intrinsic renal damage (acute renal failure). Liver failure commonly results in a decrease in serum urea.

4.19 A.T **B.**F **C.**T **D.**F **E.**T

Legionnaires' disease is caused by a Gram-negative bacillus (*Legionella pneumophilia*) spread by aerosol from infected stagnant water found in cisterns, air-conditioning systems, humidifiers and showerheads. The bacillus can cause epidemics in both immuncompromised and previously fit individuals, and particularly in institutions such as hotels and hospitals. It infects men twice as often as women. Clinical features include myalgia, headache, high fever with rigors, nausea, vomiting and diarrhoea. Seizures, confusion and cerebellar ataxia also occur. Respiratory signs include tachypnoea, dry cough and pneumonia with a chest radiography showing multilobar shadowing. Cavitating lung lesions are rare. Diagnosis is by culturing organisms and demonstrating a rising antibody titre. There is lympho penia with leukocytosis. Treatment is with erythromycin in combination with rifampicin or tetracycline. Mortality is greater than 30% in the elderly but most other patients make a full recovery.

4.20 A.T **B.**F **C.**T **D.**T **E.**T

'Complement' is the name given to a group of proteins which, when activated, form part of a cascade reaction (with amplification of effect) resulting in immunological and inflammatory reactions and the lysis of target cells. The cascade consists of a series of hepatically synthesized glycoproteins identified as C1–9, which can be activated by either the classical or the alternative pathway. The *classical* pathway was discovered first: C1 (consisting of three subunits C1q, C1r, C1s) binds to IgG Ag/Ab complexes or IgM to trigger production of complement components in sequence leading to destruction of antibody-coated microorganisms or cells. The *alternative* pathway can be stimulated either spontaneously or by aggregated IgA and infections. In this, C3 and C5 each produce C3a and C5a fragments which release histamine from mast cells, granulocytes and platelets to effect destruction. C5a and a complex of C5b, C6 and C7 are chemotactic, attract neutrophils and aid phagocytosis by macrophages. Complement, binding to IgM and IgG, is involved in hypersensitivity reactions such as adverse drug reactions. The action of complement on viruses is variable but not very important. Some viruses can activate the classical pathway without antibody involvement, others (e.g. herpes simplex virus 1 and 2 (HSV-1 and -2)) mimic the structure of some subunits to inactivate complement. Overall, the most important factors in viral inactivation are circulating antibodies and cytotoxic T cells. Deficiency of individual complement components can result in increased susceptibility to pyogenic infections, immune complex disease (systemic lupus erythematosis (SLE), coeliac disease and autoimmune endocrine disease. Conversely, deficiency of complement regulators can cause disease, e.g. C1 esterase deficiency produces hereditary angioneurotic oedema.

4.21 A.F B.F C.T D.F E.T
Tocolytic agents are used to inhibit uterine contraction. The most commonly used drugs are β_2 adrenoceptor agonists which include salbutamol, terbutaline and ritodrine. They act by increasing intracellular cAMP which increases sarcoplasmic reticular binding of calcium, inhibiting muscular activity. Ritodrine has some β_1 activity which can cause tachycardia, arrhythmias, hypokalaemia, hyperglycaemia and a metabolic acidosis. Halothane, enflurane and isoflurane are all equipotent in producing uterine relaxation at >1 minimum alveolar concentration (MAC). None of the muscle relaxants, depolarizing or otherwise, relaxes uterine muscle. Thiopentone reduces uteroplacental perfusion but has little effect on uterine tone. Prostaglandins stimulate contraction.

4.22 A.T B.T C.F D.T E.F
Primary adrenocortical insufficiency with destruction of the adrenal cortex is commonly due to autoantibodies and is known as Addison's disease. It results in reduced production of glucocorticoids, mineralocorticoids and sex hormones. Secondary adrenocortical insufficiency can also occur with chronic steroid therapy or pituitary disease. Failure to produce cortisol from a short ACTH stimulation test is diagnostically of value but a normal response does not exclude the condition as 'normal' is difficult to define individually. A long 'Synacthen' test differentiates between primary and secondary forms. The condition has an insidious onset with non-specific symptoms including weakness, weight loss, fever, depression, confusion, postural hypotension and hypoglycaemia. Abnormal pigmentation, especially buccal, is also found with primary hypoadren-

alism due to excessive ACTH stimulating melanin production. Electrolyte values can be normal but classically include hyponatraemia, hyperkalaemia, mild metabolic acidosis and raised serum urea. Patients respond poorly to stress and a 'crisis' (hypotension and acute circulatory failure) can occur with an intercurrent infection or surgery. It is important to prevent this with adequate correction of the relative hypovolaemia (responds well to a fluid load) and electrolyte abnormalities. Treatment of the primary disease requires a glucocorticoid, normally hydrocortisone, to which a mineralocorticoid (normally fludrocortisone) can be added, depending on the response of electrolyte and renin levels. In pituitary disease, mineralocorticoid secretion remains largely intact as it is predominantly stimulated by angiotensin II.

4.23 A.T B.T C.T D.F E.T
Thermal conductivity measures the degree of cooling of CO_2 (or helium) passed over a heated wire. The temperature drop can then be quantified and displayed on a meter. CO_2 concentration in gas mixtures can be determined by measuring the reduction in volume after absorption of the gas in a 10–20% potassium hydroxide solution. The Severinghaus electrode measures hydrogen ion concentration, which is directly related to CO_2 concentration as it reversibly reacts with water to produce carbonic acid before dissociating to hydrogen and bicarbonate ions. Other methods include infrared analysers found in capnographs, mass spectrometry, gas chromatography and the dye metacresol purple found in soda lime. In polarography, the basis of Clarke's electrode, current flowing between two electrodes in a buffered electrolyte solution with a potential of 0.6 V between them is proportional to the oxygen concentration in solution.

4.24 A.T B.T C.T D.T E.F
Partial gastrectomy is associated with less severe nutritional problems than a total gastrectomy. The commonest problem is weight loss due to malabsorption. This is most likely due to a faster gastric emptying and intestinal transit time. The same mechanism underlies 'dumping syndrome', characterized by weakness, fainting, tachycardia, abdominal cramps, bloating and urgent diarrhoea. The somatostatin analogue, octreotide, may be a useful treatment. Stasis in the afferent loop with bacterial overgrowth from a combination of poor mixing of

food with pancreatic enzymes and bile salts can lead to protein and fat malabsorption, resulting in steatorrhoea. Upwards of 30% develop anaemia within 15 years of surgery from a mixture of iron and folate but rarely vitamin -B_{12} malabsorption. Osteomalacia occurs in up to 33% after 10–20 years from vitamin D and calcium malabsorption. There is a slight increased risk of developing carcinoma in the gastric remnant. Renal calculi do not appear to be a problem.

4.25 A.F   B.T   C.T   D.T   E.T

A rapid rise in blood pressure requires a rapid fall back to normal (the opposite is true for chronic hypertension due to resetting of the autoregulatory parameters). Ephedrine increases blood pressure by stimulating α and β adrenergic receptors, releasing noradrenaline from nerve endings and inhibiting MAO, which is important for metabolism and inactivation of active amines including catecholamines. Thus, control of blood pressure can occur only with drugs that have a direct vasodilatory action on blood vessels or combined α and β blockade. This would include sodium nitroprusside as it causes arteriolar and venular dilatation by a direct action on the blood vessels. Moreover, it is extremely potent, has a rapid onset and short duration of action, and is therefore ideal as blood pressure can be tightly controlled by titrating the infusion. It must always be covered when used as it forms toxic cyanide ions when exposed to light. Diazoxide is structurally similar to thiazide diuretics (paradoxically, it has sodium-retaining effects) and acts by relaxation of arteriolar smooth muscle. It reduces blood pressure quickly in a hypertensive crisis but, by antagonizing the effects of insulin, has diabetogenic properties. Labetolol combines selective α and non-selective β adrenergic receptor activity in a ratio of 3:1 or 5:1 (different sources!). It is quick acting and has a short half-life of 4 hours which makes it effective. Phentolamine is an α adrenergic blocker with an additional direct relaxant effect on vascular smooth muscle. It works within 2 min for about 15 min and is effective in controlling hypertensive episodes. Propranolol is ineffective as it has no α adrenergic blocking action. Although this scenario is uncommon, it may become more frequent as a result of a new generation of effective short-acting MAOIs being introduced for a wide spectrum of psychiatric illnesses. (See: McFarlane HJ (1994) Anaesthesia and the new generation monoamine oxidase inhibitors. *Anaesthesia* **49**, 597–599.)

4.26 A.F   B.T   C.T   D.F   E.F
Barbiturates, phenytoin and sulphonamides must be avoided. Etomidate, lignocaine and chlordiazepoxide have been implicated in laboratory and animal studies but not in humans. Diazepam, halothane, steroids, pancuronium, ketamine and propofol have been subjected to conflicting reports but many have been given without problems. Drugs considered safe include opiates (except pentazocine and maybe alfentanil), nitrous oxide, suxamethonium, vecuronium, atropine, neostigmine, bupivacaine, prilocaine, propranolol, droperidol, aspirin, paracetamol and insulin. (See: Jensen NF *et al.* (1995) Anesthetic considerations in porphyrias. *Anesthesia and Analgesia* **80**, 591–599.)

4.27 A.T   B.F   C.F   D.F   E.T
The Valsalva manoeuvre assesses the integrity of baroreceptor reflexes, which are important in maintaining postural changes in heart rate and blood pressure. It involves forced expiration against a closed glottis at 40 mmHg for 10 s. Initially, BP increases due to an increase in intrathoracic pressure but then falls due to compression of the intrathoracic veins, which decreases venous return and cardiac output. This inhibits the baroreceptors, causing tachycardia and a rise in peripheral resistance. When intrathoracic pressure returns to normal, cardiac output is restored but peripheral resistance is still high causing the BP to rise above normal, which stimulates the baroreceptors causing bradycardia and a drop in BP to normal. There is an abnormal response with cardiac failure, constrictive pericarditis, tamponade and with high CVP. The response is lost with autonomic neuropathy (diabetes mellitus, primary hyperaldosteronism), when BP falls and remains low until intrathoracic pressure returns to normal.

4.28 A.T   B.T   C.T   D.T   E.T
Nephrotic syndrome results from structural damage to the glomerular basement membrane. It is characterized by heavy proteinuria, hypoproteinaemia and oedema. Hypercholesterolaemia is almost always present. The prognosis reflects the underlying disorder which can be:

renal	– all types of glomerulonephritis
systemic	– SLE, polyarteritis nodosa, DM, amyloidosis

infective   – SBE, malaria, hepatitis B, syphilis
malignant   – carcinomatosis, Hodgkin's disease
drug-induced   – penicillamine, captopril, gold

Basic management includes low-salt diet (a high-protein diet is now considered ineffective), diuretics and, occasionally, salt-poor albumin to initiate a diuresis. Treating the underlying cause is important (usually with steroids and immunosuppressive agents), as is preventing the potential complications including: sepsis; venous thrombosis, from the hypovolaemia and hypercoagulable state; and oliguric renal failure, as a result of acute tubular necrosis from a combination of low blood volume and hypotension.

4.29 **A**.T **B**.T **C**.F **D**.T **E**.F

TURP syndrome occurs in up to 10% of cases. It is due to absorption of irrigating fluid, normally 1.5% hypotonic glycine, through open prostatic vessels. Incidence is related to the hydrostatic pressure of the irrigation fluid, duration of surgery and experience of the surgeon. Signs and symptoms result from a combination of volume overload, dilutional hyponatraemia with intracellular oedema and the direct toxic effects of glycine and its by-product, ammonia. The effects are mainly cardiovascular and cerebral and include hypotension, dyspnoea, angina, reversible visual and mental changes, seizures and coma. Metabolic acidosis and hypocalcaemia also occur. Serum potassium increases by about 0.5 mmol/l, thought to be due to hypotonic glycine causing mild haemolysis and interference with transmembrane electrolyte exchange. Treatment requires early recognition. In this respect regional block is superior to general anaesthesia as mental changes can be detected much earlier. Treatment is aimed at correcting both the fluid overload and the hyponatraemia. Diuresis is usually brisk as the result of the absorbed fluid but can be further encouraged by diuretics. Correction of the hyponatraemia must not be too rapid as there is a possible risk of intracranial and central demyelinating lesions such as pontine myelinosis. TURP syndrome is largely avoidable if resection time is limited to 1 hour and hydrostatic pressure of the irrigation fluid to less than 6.9 kPa (70 cm H_2O). (See: Jensen V (1990) The TURP syndrome. *Canadian Journal of Anaesthesia* **38**, 90–97.)

4.30 A.F B.F C.F D.T E.T

DI results from a deficiency of ADH. The most common causes include pituitary surgery, head injuries and other intracranial events (infection, radiotherapy, vascular event, etc.). DI can vary in severity from minor to complete deficiency of ADH. The symptoms are polyuria, nocturia and compensatory polydipsia. Lethargy, confusion and coma are possible but convulsions are uncommon. Daily urine output may be as much as 10–15 l daily and the urine is often very hypotonic (sp. gr. 1.002–1.005). Biochemically serum sodium is high, as is the plasma osmolality. Definitive diagnosis relies on the measurement of a low plasma ADH, failure to concentrate urine with fluid restriction, and restoration of urine-concentrating ability following administration of ADH or its analogue. The priority of treatment is to restore haemodynamic stability by rehydration. Water loss is far in excess of electrolyte loss so intravenous fluid replacement with 5% dextrose is satisfactory, although large volumes may lead to hyperglycaemia and further exacerbation of polyuria. It is best not to use hypertonic saline as large sodium loads are unnecessary and may confuse the diagnosis. Potassium requirements are usually small. Definitive treatment is with synthetic ADH. Although rarely used, thiazide diuretics, carbamazepine and chlorpropamide are alternative agents in mild DI. They probably work by sensitizing renal tubules to endogenous vasopressin. DI must not be confused with psychogenic polydipsia. Nephrogenic diabetes insipidus is another condition where renal tubules are resistant to normal or high levels of vasopressin. It may be inherited as a sex-linked recessive disorder or acquired as a result of renal disease, drugs (lithium, glibenclamide) and chromic hypercalcaemia or hypokalaemia.

4.31 A.T B.F C.T D.T E.T

TENS attempts to stimulate preferentially large A nerve fibres to block transmission of nociceptive impulses carried by A δ and C fibres according to Melzack's gate theory of pain. Using skin electrodes, a pulse generator delivers impulses for 0.1–0.5 ms in the frequency range 30–100 Hz. A voltage of up to 50 V is needed as much of the current is lost in the tissues. It is useful when pain originates peripherally. It is safe, cheap, portable and non-addictive. The main side-effect is a reaction to the electrode gel used to decrease impedance. TENS is best avoided in patients with implanted cardiac pacemakers (particularly unipolar pacemakers) as it may inhibit or alter their function as a result of mechanical interference from production of skeletal myopotentials.

4.32 A.T B.T C.T D.F E.F
Retinal artery occlusion leads to optic nerve destruction and complete blindness. Homonymous hemianopia is blindness affecting either the right or left half of the visual field. Tumours and vascular events in the contralateral optic tract and optic radiation (post-chiasmal) are the main causes. Unilateral posterior cerebral artery infarction of the occipital cortex can also cause homonymous hemianopia, often with macular sparing as there is a dual blood supply to the occipital region from the middle and posterior cerebral arteries. Bitemporal hemianopia is blindness in the outer half of each visual field from chiasmal lesions compressing the decussating nerve fibres from the nasal half of each eye. Glaucoma leads to visual field constriction. Tunnel vision is seen with retinitis pigmentosa.

4.33 A.F B.F C.T D.T E.T
Surfactant is a mixture of lipoprotein (10%) and phospholipid (90%) produced from type II alveolar cells (pneumocytes). It is present in amniotic fluid from 28 weeks. According to Laplace, surface tension in small spheres is higher than in larger ones. If spheres are interconnecting, as in alveoli, the higher pressure would empty the smaller spheres into the larger ones. This is prevented by surfactant, which lowers surface tension by aligning its hydrophilic ends on the alveolar surface to increase repulsion by adjacent molecules when the alveoli are small. Thus, the alveoli do not collapse and stability is maintained. Surfactant reduces transepithelial protein leakage to maintain alveolar fluid homeostasis, and also has a role in host defence by increasing the phagocytosis of alveolar macrophages. Immaturity at birth leads to hyaline membrane disease (atelectasis, low lung compliance) which can be treated with human, bovine or synthetic surfactant to reduce both morbidity and mortality.

4.34 A.T B.T C.T D.T E.T
Brain damage at the time of injury (i.e. primary) is usually irreversible. Thus, management must be directed at maintaining oxygenation and cerebral perfusion whilst limiting factors that lead to secondary brain damage. These include raised ICP,

hypoxia, hypercarbia, hypotension and decreased serum osmolality. Accurate monitoring is essential. Suitable interventions include intubation, sustaining systolic BP >90 mmHg, fluid restriction, reducing ICP by moderate hyperventilation, mannitol, and adequate sedation and analgesia to reduce cerebral metabolism. Hyperglycaemia is increasingly recognized as causing a worse outcome after head injury. This is probably due to glucose-induced intracellular lactic acidosis with the excess hydrogen ions damaging neurones. Normoglycaemia is recommended by restricting glucose-containing fluids and judicious use of insulin. (See: Wass CT, Lanier WL (1996) Glucose modulation of ischaemic brain injury: review and clinical recommendations. *Mayo Clinic Proceedings,* **71**, 801–812.)

4.35 A.F B.F C.T D.T E.F
A ruptured aortic aneurysm causes sudden severe back pain, diminished or absent femoral pulses, a pulsatile abdominal mass and signs of hypovolaemic shock. CVP will be low. 20% rupture anteriorly into the peritoneal cavity and are associated with a much higher mortality than the 80% which rupture posteriorly into the retroperitoneal space, as the tissues temporarily tamponade the bleeding (and also result in blood staining the flanks). Urine output will be reduced due to hypovolaemia but anuria is rare and occurs only if there is mechanical obstruction. 95% of aortic aneurysms occur below the renal arteries. An asymptomatic aneurysm found incidentally needs repair if over 5 cm in diameter. The annual incidence of rupture rises from 5% at 5 cm to 75% at 7 cm. Mortality is 2–5% for elective repair, but approaching 50% following rupture.

4.36 A.T B.T C.F D.F E.T
At the elbow the ulnar nerve (C6, C7, C8, T1) supplies an articular branch to the elbow joint, muscular branches to the flexor carpi ulnaris and the ulnar half of the flexor digitorum profundus, as well as a cutaneous branch to the skin covering the hypothenar eminence and the palmar and dorsal aspect of the lateral 1½–2 fingers. In the hand it also supplies the hypothenar muscles, the interossei, third and fourth lumbricals and adductor pollicis. The ulnar nerve can be blocked where it passes near the medial epicondyle. This will result in inability to flex and adduct the hand at the wrist joint (flexor carpi

ulnaris), abduct and adduct the fingers (interossei) and adduct the thumb (adductor pollicis). Thumb abduction and apposition is by the median nerve. Flexion of the interphalangeal joints is mainly by the flexor digitorum superficialis supplied by the median nerve but the flexor digitorum profundus, as well as flexing the distal phalanx of the fingers, also contributes to flexion of the middle and proximal phalanges. Thus ulnar nerve block will cause some weakness. In practice the ulnar nerve is rarely blocked at the elbow due to an unacceptably high incidence of complications.

4.37 A.T **B.**T **C.**F **D.**T **E.**T

Toxicity from CO poisoning arises from the fact that the affinity of haemoglobin for CO is 240 times greater than for oxygen. This leads to reduced oxygen-carrying capacity and a left shift of the oxyhaemoglobin dissociation curve, i.e. more avid binding of oxygen and reduced unloading of oxygen resulting in tissue hypoxia. Oximeter readings remain normal as carboxyhaemoglobin (COHb) cannot be distinguished from oxyhaemoglobin. Features of CO poisoning include headache, agitation, confusion, nausea and vomiting, hyperventilation, bullous lesions, hyperpyrexia, cardiac arrhythmias, acute renal failure and muscle necrosis. Neurological sequelae include peripheral neuropathies, hemiplegia, cerebral and cerebellar damage. Cyanosis is absent because the presence of carboxyhaemoglobin reduces the amount of reduced haemoglobin seen. Treatment is supplementary oxygen, preferably hyperbaric oxygen.

4.38 A.F **B.**T **C.**T **D.**T **E.**F

Ritodrine is a β_2 adrenoceptor agonist used to relax uterine smooth muscle to delay delivery in premature labour. It can also cause hypokalaemia as a result of intracellular shift of potassium by action on the Na^+/K^+ pump (although as total body stores are maintained, replacement therapy of potassium is unnecessary) and increases insulin secretion secondary to glycogenolysis. β_2 stimulation results in systemic vasodilatation and hypotension, which is partially compensated for by a tachycardia and fluid retention. Reports of pulmonary oedema are probably due partly to these physiological changes and to fluid overload from the relatively large volumes often infused with ritodrine. As the dose of ritodrine is increased adverse β_1 effects begin to appear, including myocardial ischaemia and cardiac arrhythmias. General anaesthesia is contraindicated in the presence of ritodrine. This is not a great problem as its half-life is 6–9 min. Although ritodrine delays the onset of labour its benefits are unproven as regards improved perinatal survival or ability to prolong labour to term. In addition, its value has been brought to question as there are significant maternal risks associated with its use. Incompletely but rapidly absorbed, most is excreted in the urine as inactive conjugates. (See: Rodgers SJ, Morgan M (1994) Tocolysis, β_2 agonists and anaesthesia. *Anaesthesia* **49**, 185–187.)

4.39 A.T **B.**T **C.**T **D.**T **E.**T
Initial treatment of bleeding oesophageal varices is resuscitation with blood and intravenous fluids to achieve haemodynamic stability. Vasopressin, somatostatin and octreotide all reduce portal pressure but are a stopgap measure to help control bleeding before definitive treatment can be instituted. ADH can worsen any coagulopathy by stimulating release of plasminogen activator and causes myocardial ischaemia in about 10% of cases. Endoscopic injection sclerotherapy or variceal ligation with rubber bands controls 80–90% of acute bleeding episodes as well as reducing incidence of rebleeding when performed regularly (although whether overall survival is greater is controversial). Balloon tamponade with a four lumen Minnesota tube (replacement for Sengstaken–Blakemore) is useful but limited to 24 hours to prevent tissue necrosis. A transjugular intrahepatic portosystemic shunt (TIPS) places a stent between the hepatic vein and a branch of the portal vein. It effectively reduces portal pressure in more than 90% of cases and thus potential bleeding from varices. Surgery should be considered only when bleeding continues or frequently recurs. Survival is not much improved and hepatic encephalopathy is a a major complication (as with TIPS). Propranolol in a dose sufficient to reduce resting pulse by 25% decreases portal pressure. This is probably as good as sclerotherapy at reducing rebleeding in patients with well-compensated liver disease. Liver transplantation is a potentially curative procedure for patients with portal hypertension and end-stage liver disease. It is effective for the acute situation when all other methods have failed to stop the bleeding. (See: Parks RW, Diamond T (1995) Emergency and long term management of bleeding oesophageal varices. *British Journal of Hospital Medicine* **54**, 161–168.)

4.40 A.F B.F C.F D.T E.F

A common problem with URTIs in children is distinguishing them from a non-infective chronic purulent nasal discharge. However, if one or more of the following features are present – pyrexia, general malaise, sore throat and productive cough – elective cases should be cancelled for at least 2–3 weeks as there is an increased incidence of bronchospasm, hypoxaemia and critical incidents. As long as suitable precautions are taken and the patient is maximally prepared, elective surgery is not contraindicated in the other conditions listed. However, what constitutes maximal preparation is always subject to controversy. This includes the preoperative role of blood transfusion with sickle cell anaemia and whether drug therapy should be discontinued prior to surgery in patients with myasthenia gravis. There is no contraindication to surgery after any type of immunization.

4.41 A.T B.F C.T D.F E.F

PHN occurs in 10% of all shingles sufferers. With age, there is a preferential loss of large nerve fibres which impairs pain-modulating systems and therefore allows increased transmission of nociceptive information through the dorsal horns to the CNS. Thus PHN is more common and more severe in the elderly, occurring in over 50% at 60 years and over 75% at 70 years. PHN is rarely severe or persistent under 40 years of age. There is little consensus to treatment. Topical anaesthetic cream (e.g. eutectic mixture of local anaesthetics (EMLA)) or capsaicin (depletes substance P and causes degeneration of C fibres) has been shown to ameliorate and reduce the incidence of pain, but some find it messy and painful to apply. Antiviral agents (e.g. acyclovir) reduce the duration but not the incidence of pain. Although often reserved for those who are immunocompromised, some believe antiviral agents should be routinely given during an acute attack in an attempt to ameliorate symptoms. Antidepressants, anticonvulsants, simple analgesics, nerve blocks, transcutaneous nerve stimulation, acupuncture and cold packs are some of the many other treatment options. Some of these help for part of the time and are probably worth trying in patients who have not responded to better-validated therapies. Neuroablative procedures (dorsal root entry destruction, cordotomy) and strong opioids are of no value. Prompt initiation of treatment, and the personality and psychological profile of the sufferer, has the most profound effect on outcome. (See: Lee JJ, Gauci CAG (1994) Postherpetic neuralgia: current concepts and management. *British Journal of Hospital Medicine* **52**, 565–570.)

4.42 A.F B.F C.F D.T E.T

RA is a symmetrical chronic arthritis. The synovium becomes infiltrated by inflammatory cells (lymphocytes, plasma cells and macrophages) to form a pannus which destroys cartilage by spreading over and under it. Typical presentation is morning stiffness with pain and swelling of small joints of the hands and feet, which can lead to swan-neck or boutonniere deformities. This ultimately results in joint subluxation and instability. The lumbar spine is often spared. Extra-articular involvement is common and includes pulmonary (pleural effusion, rheumatoid nodules), cardiac (pericardial effusion, pericarditis) and neurological (atlantoaxial subluxation, sensory neuropathy) conditions. 80% of patients have positive rheumatoid factor, 30% have antinuclear factor. The condition must be distinguished from psoriatic seronegative arthropathy. Felty's syndrome is RA with splenomegaly and neutropaenia. First-line drug treatment of symptoms is with non-steroidal anti-inflammatory drugs (NSAIDs). Second-line treatment, to halt progression, includes gold, penicillamine, methotrexate, chloroquine and steroids. The outcome is variable. After 10 years, 10% are severely crippled, 25% have minimal symptoms. Heberden's nodes are bony outgrowths of the terminal interphalangeal joints found in osteoarthritis.

4.43 A.F B.T C.F D.T E.T

An exponential function is where the rate of change of a variable is proportional to the said variable. It is found in first-order kinetics such as the one-compartment model of drug distribution. The half-life is the time taken for 50% decay to occur. The time constant relates to the progress of the exponential function if the initial rate of change had continued. Thus, after one time constant 63% of the event will be complete, after two 86.5% and after three 95%. When plotted on semilogarithmic paper, the exponential processes become straight lines.

4.44 A.F B.F C.F D.T E.F

Albumin is prepared from human plasma as a 4.5% or 20% solution. It is heat-treated and so is the only blood product which does not carry the risk of virus transmission. It can be used as a volume expander and approximately increases circulating volume by the amount infused. However, it is expensive and there is little evidence that it is significantly more effective than cheaper solutions (gelofusine, dextrans) in terms of survival, length of stay in intensive care or reduction in incidence of renal failure or pulmonary oedema. Fewer than 1% of patients develop anaphylactoid reactions such as flushing, urticaria, fever and, rarely, hypotension. It should not be used to treat patients with hypoalbuminaemia from malnutrition, chronic renal failure or liver disease. (See: Stockwell MA *et al.* (1992) Colloid solutions in the critically ill. *Anaesthesia* **47**, 3–9.)

4.45 **A**.F **B**.T **C**.F **D**.T **E**.T
Postoperative hypoxaemia is a common problem and may last for several days. It arises from a mixture of airway obstruction, basal atelectasis, reduction in functional residual capacity and hypoventilation as a result of anaesthetic-induced respiratory depression, pain and inability to cough. The extent of the deleterious effects depends on the condition of the patient and nature of the operation, being more common in the elderly, the obese, those with pre-existing respiratory disease, and after thoracic and upper abdominal procedures. Hypoxaemia has been associated with myocardial ischaemia, arrhythmias and a decrease in cardiac output. Adverse neurological effects depend on the degree of hypoxaemia. Minor falls in satura-tions to about 80% are associated with mild but usually reversible cognitive dysfunction. Severe hypoxaemia of less than 65% results in unconsciousness. However, the evidence for permanent neurological sequelae with episodic hypoxae-mia is scanty. Current recommendations for postoperative care include oximetry until patients are able to maintain saturations of more than 93% in air. Supplementary oxygen is required for 'at risk' groups. The percentage of patients who rely on hypoxic drive for ventilation is overrated and as graded amounts of oxygen can be given safely it should never be withheld. Subarachnoid haemorrhages are more likely to arise from a berry aneurysm or an arteriovenous malformation. (See: Powell JF *et al.* (1996) The effects of hypoxaemia and recommendations for postoperative anaesthetic therapy. *Anaes-thesia* **51**, 769–772.)

4.46 **A**.T **B**.T **C**.T **D**.F **E**.T

Flumazenil is an imidazobenzodiazepine which rapidly and effectively terminates the action of benzodiazepines by competitive antagonism at their receptor sites in the CNS. Despite its association with convulsions, flumazenil has intrinsic anticonvulsant activity. It is useful for elucidation of undiagnosed comas but not for all benzodiazepine overdoses. It has a rapid onset but relatively short half-life (0.8–1.2 hours), which means repeat dosage or infusion may be required to prevent resedation. It is eliminated almost entirely by hepatic metabolism to inactive products. Side-effects include nausea and vomiting, flushing, anxiety and agitation. An initial dose of 0.2 mg should be given, with 0.1 mg increments until recovery is complete.

4.47 **A**.T **B**.T **C**.T **D**.T **E**.F

The features of gout are a result of hyperuricaemia. Deposition of sodium urate crystals may occur in joints causing arthritis, in soft tissues producing tophi, and in the renal tract forming urate stones and ultimately renal failure. It is commoner in men (10:1) and is usually due to a genetically determined inadequacy of uric acid excretion after a purine load; the remainder generally result from increased production of uric acid (e.g. Lesch–Nyhan syndrome). Diagnosis is mainly clinical as serum urate is often normal and, paradoxically, asymptomatic hyperuricaemia is common. Isolation of needle-shaped crystals in joint synovial fluid may be useful and radiographs may show punched out bone erosions below soft tissue tophi. Gout can be precipitated by surgery, starvation, excess alcohol, and thiazide diuretics. The first-line treatment of an acute attack is analgesia with NSAIDs or colchicine. Long-term treatment is with allopurinol as it lowers serum urate by inhibiting xanthine oxidase. As it can precipitate an acute attack, it should be given only once an attack has subsided.

4.48 **A**.T **B**.T **C**.F **D**.F **E**.F

The pudendal nerve (S2, S3, S4) passes through the greater and lesser sciatic foramen to the ischiorectal fossa. There it divides into the perineal nerve, the dorsal nerve to the clitoris/ penis, and the inferior haemorrhoidal nerve to supply the perineum and pelvic floor. A pudendal block provides analgesia for the second stage of labour (after full cervical dilatation), episiotomies, low forceps deliveries and repair of perineal lacerations. As the pain of the first stage of labour is a result of uterine distension and cervical dilatation and is transmitted by sympathetic fibres, pudendal nerve block (PNB) is ineffective. In reality PNB is no longer recommended in any stage of labour as LA deposited near the uterine artery may cause vasoconstriction with a reduction of uterine blood flow, leading to fetal bradycardia and cardiac depression. In addition, the block has been estimated to be effective in less than 50% of cases.

4.49 A.T B.T C.F D.F E.F
The classic clinical picture of an extradural haematoma is loss of consciousness with or without an initial lucid interval, severe headache, rapid development of a fixed dilated pupil on the side of the injury and a contralateral hemiparesis. It occurs in approximately 10% of severe head injuries, most often within 24 hours of the traumatic event, and is due to rupture of the middle meningeal artery secondary to (but not always) a temporal skull fracture. Immediate surgery is required for evacuation as rapid accumulation of blood between the vault and the dura compresses the underlying brain and increases intracranial pressure. CSF rhinorrhoea occurs with a base-of-skull fracture and surgery may be required if it does not stop spontaneously. Status epilepticus can occur after a severe head injury and it may be an indication for elective intubation and ventilation, but not surgery. Headache and neck stiffness, again, could be the result of trauma or meningitis secondary to skull fracture.

4.50 A.T B.F C.T D.F E.T
The APACHE I, II and III scoring systems were devised to enable comparisons to be made as to the effect of different treatment strategies and survival rates between ICUs by allowing accurate matching of patients with similar expectation of survival. They are not individually predictive. APACHE III (1991) is analogous to APACHE II (1985) in that it produces a score that reflects the weight given to three principal groups: physiological measurements, chronic health status and age. APACHE III adds five physiological variables not found in APACHE II: albumin, urea, bilirubin, glucose and urine output; and omits two: potassium and bicarbonate. A modified version of the GCS is used in which verbal

response is excluded. The chronic health component has also been modified from that in APACHE II and is now based on seven variables referring to presence/absence of lymphoma, haematological malignancies, HIV, metastatic cancer, immune suppression, hepatic failure and cirrhosis. APACHE II included only emergency or elective procedures, or if there was any major organ insufficiency, or whether patients were immunocompromised. APACHE III also takes into account the patient's treatment location prior to admission to the ICU. The worst physiological score is measured in the first 24 hours except for neurological assessment which may be altered by sedation. Studies suggest that there are only small differences between APACHE II and III. Both tend to underestimate death and in one study APACHE III appeared to have a better discriminating ability but at the expense of increased complexity of data collection and cost of installing a new computer program. (See: Knaus WA *et al.* (1991) The APACHE III prognostic syndrome: risk prediction of hospital mortality for critically ill hospitalised patients. *Chest* **100**, 1619–1639. Also: Beck DH *et al.* (1997) Prediction of outcome from intensive care: a prospective cohort study comparing APACHE II and III prognostic systems in a UK intensive care unit. *Critical Care Medicine* **25**, 9–15.)

4.51 A.F B.T C.T D.T E.F
PDPH is characterized by a severe pounding headache, typically beginning in the occiput before spreading to the frontal area. It is worse on standing and relieved by lying down. Neck stiffness, photophobia, auditory hallucinations, nausea and vomiting, and VIth cranial nerve involvement can accompany the headache. It is thought to be due to loss of CSF (a loss of only 20 ml is needed) through the dural tear. The incidence has reduced with the introduction of smaller-gauge and pencil-point (i.e. blunt) needles where the LA is ejected through a hole in the side of the needle (Sprötte, Whitacre) as opposed to the tip (Quincke). The blunt needle is thought to pass between the dural fibres without cutting them, enabling the dura to seal more quickly after removal. The incidence of PDPH with 25 g Whitacre needles is less than 1%. Most cases of PDPH resolve with bedrest, NSAIDs and good hydration with a fluid intake of at least 3 l daily. An extradural blood patch is reserved for patients with severe or disabling symptoms, neurological sequelae or if headache persists for more than

48 hours. Although these are the definitive treatment of choice, success is not guaranteed (70–90%) and, as they are not without their problems (radicular pain, backpain), they should not be used indiscriminately. Caffeine is thought to improve headache by inducing cerebral vessel constriction but studies suggest that it is not of much value as the action is transient. Theophylline may last longer. (See: Morgan P (1995) Spinal anesthesia in obstetrics. *Canadian Journal of Anaesthesia* **42**, 1145–1163.)

4.52 A.T **B.**F **C.**T **D.**T **E.**T

As water is lost from the body, ECF becomes hypertonic. Plasma sodium and urea rise, as do haemoglobin and the haematocrit. Compensatory mechanisms include stimulation of aldosterone secretion. This reduces water loss by promoting sodium and chloride reabsorption from the kidney. As such, urinary sodium will be reduced. Oliguria occurs, causing a rise in urine osmolality. Water migrates from cells in an attempt to re-establish osmotic equilibrium. Intracellular dehydration develops when more than 8% of body water is lost. By then, skin turgor will be substantially reduced.

4.53 A.F **B.**F **C.**F **D.**T **E.**F

This clinical picture suggests a transient ischaemic attack (TIA) with amaurosis fugax, most probably from an embolus from internal carotid artery atheroma. The hemiparesis suggests damage at a site where the pyramidal (motor) fibres are closely compacted, which is likely to be the internal capsule. Lesions of the cerebral cortex tend to be more discrete, i.e. one limb or part of it. TIAs often proceed to a stroke or myocardial infarction and, particularly in view of his age, warrant full investigation and treatment. This should be carried out initially by non-invasive means. The preferred method is duplex Doppler scanning which simultaneously images the carotid arteries as well as measuring velocity of blood flow. Angiography and a computerized tomography (CT) brain scan are useful for management but need not be performed to confirm the diagnosis. Hypertension immediately following a TIA is possible and treatment should be delayed until it is known to be chronic. Initial treatment is with antiplatelet agents (e.g. aspirin) despite lack of effect seen in randomized clinical trials. Anticoagulation is indicated for cardiac thromboemboli from atrial fibrillation. Carotid endarterectomy is increasingly being performed as it reduces the incidence of TIAs and strokes when the carotid artery is more than 70% occluded. Blood supply to the brain arises from four main arteries (left and right carotid and vertebral arteries), which link together in the base of the brain to form the circle of Willis. This provides a collateral channel for blood to the brain if one of the main extracranial channels is occluded. An aneurysm of the circle of Willis results in a subarachnoid haemorrhage which classically presents with a severe headache, often occipital, vomiting and loss of consciousness. Neck stiffness is common. It must be differentiated from severe migraine or meningitis.

4.54 A.F   B.T   C.F   D.T   E.F

Sick sinus syndrome is due to impaired sinoatrial node activity or conduction leading to alternating periods of profound bradycardia and sinus arrest with supraventricular tachycardia or atrial fibrillation (brady-tachy syndrome). As with complete heart block, it tends to occur in elderly patients with ischaemic heart disease and as such preoperative pacing is required. Second-degree heart block is either Wenckebach type I or Mobitz type II. Wenkebach is characterized by atrioventricular (AV) delay with gradual lengthening of PR interval until AV block occurs, i.e. a P wave is not followed by a QRS complex. Mobitz type II is when AV block occurs intermittently. Whereas there is little doubt that Mobitz type II requires preoperative pacing, the situation for Wenckebach is undecided. The British Pacing and Electrophysiological group say pacing is required. The American College of Cardiology and American Heart Association disagree. Take your pick! Congenital heart block, unless symptomatic, does not require pacing. WPW syndrome is characterized by a short PR interval and a wide QRS complex as a result of an accessory AV pathway: the bundle of Kent. It predisposes to paroxysmal tachycardia. Pacing is not required.

4.55 A.T   B.F   C.F   D.T   E.T

Hypotension following spinal anaesthesia is primarily mediated through preganglionic sympathetic blockade. The reduction in sympathetic tone below the block produces hypotension by two mechanisms: firstly, and more importantly, from a reduction in arterial systemic vascular resistance, and secondly from a fall in cardiac output due to a fall in preload and stroke volume as a result of venous pooling. In practice the heart compensates for the latter by increasing its contractility and rate unless the decrease in preload is substantial. In addition the sympathetic cardio-acceleratory fibres (T1–T4) may be affected by the spinal block, causing bradycardia and further decreases in cardiac output. Any coexisting hypovolaemia will exacerbate these effects and is therefore a contraindication to spinal anaesthesia. As long as hypotension is treated promptly, there is no evidence that its brief appearance is harmful to the patient (unfortunately this cannot be assumed in the case of the unborn fetus). Administration of low-dose adrenaline may contribute to hypotension by β_2 adrenoceptor-mediated vasodilatation. Prevention of hypotension by preoperative volume loading has not been found to be effective and treatment is currently thought to be best with vasopressors. Choice is between a mixed α and β adrenoceptor agonist such as ephedrine or an α agonist such as metaraminol or phenylephrine. There are arguments for using either but as a simple guide alpha blockers are probably best if there is a coexisting tachycardia and ephedrine if heart rate is normal. A poor response should lead to a reassessment of other causes, particularly exclusion of blood loss. The dorsal root ganglion contains cell bodies of afferent neurones conveying heat, pain and light touch sensations. (See: Critchley LAH (1996) Hypotension, subarachnoid block and the elderly patient. *Anaesthesia* **51**, 1139–1143. Also: McCrac AF, Wildsmith JA (1993) Prevention and treatment of hypotension during central neural blockade. *British Journal of Anaesthesia* **70**, 672–680.)

4.56 A.F B.T C.T D.F E.T
CPB inhibits nociceptive pathways to upper abdominal viscera. It is useful for chronic pancreatitis, abdominal malignancy and, more recently, hepatic artery embolization. The block is usually performed initially with LAs to confirm its effect before performing the definitive block. The commonest complication is postural hypotension (20%) due to extensive vasomotor block. Pleural puncture and a chylothorax have also been reported. A permanent neurolytic block can, rarely, result in impotence due to involvement of the hypogastric plexus. The sphincter of Oddi will relax and transient diarrhoea can occur due to unopposed parasympathetic action. It has been suggested that splanchnic nerve blocks are equally effective and have fewer complications.

4.57 A.T B.F C.T D.F E.F

It is easy to answer this question by exclusion. Poliomyelitis is due to infection by RNA enteroviruses which specifically destroy anterior horn cells. This results in a lower motor neurone lesion (flaccid weakness) but normal sensation as spinothalamic tracts remain unaffected. Motor neurone disease is due to progressive degeneration of motor neurones in the spinal cord. This can present either as a spastic paresis (amyotrophic lateral sclerosis) or as flaccid weakness with progressive muscular atrophy or progressive bulbar palsy. The sensory system is not involved. Polymyositis presents with proximal muscle weakness and wasting due to muscle fibre inflammation and necrosis. Sensation is normal. Treatment is high-dose corticosteroids and physiotherapy. Multiple sclerosis arises as a result of demyelinating plaques within the brain and spinal cord. Signs and symptoms are variable and are related to position of the plaques but all of the above are possible; similarly with spinal cord compression.

4.58 A.F B.F C.T D.T E.F

EMLA cream is a mixture of 2.5% prilocaine and 2.5% lignocaine. 'Eutectic' means a mixture whose melting point is lower than that of either of its individual constituents. In this case prilocaine and lignocaine melt to form an oil at temperatures greater than 16°C. This increases the concentration of LAs in the oil phase to over 80%, despite an initial anaesthetic concentration of 5%. This is sufficient for the LAs to diffuse through the intact skin to block neuronal transmission and produce topical anaesthesia. It takes 60 min to work and is primarily used for paediatric intravenous cannulation, although it is also of value in skin graft harvesting and cautery of warts. Vasoconstriction and local skin reactions such as erythema, oedema, itching and rash are common but generally mild and transient. EMLA is not recommended for skin wounds because of the increased risk of wound infection, nor for use on mucous membranes due to increased absorption. Methaemoglobinaemia has been reported in neonates and use should be limited to once daily. Amethocaine and iontopheric lignocaine are suitable alternatives. (See: Garjraj NM *et al.* (1994) Eutectic mixture of local anesthetics (EMLA) cream. *Anesthesia and Analgesia* **78**, 574–583.)

4.59 A.T **B.**T **C.**T **D.**F **E.**F

A + B: P_aO_2 and P_aCO_2 are unaffected by anaemia.

C: Hb saturation = oxygen content of Hb/oxygen capacity of Hb, therefore saturation is unchanged.

D: Oxygen content = $1.31 \times Hb \times sat. + 0.002$. Therefore normal haemoglobin is 19.5 g/dl; this is reduced in anaemia.

E: Cyanosis requires at least 5 g/dl of reduced Hb and is therefore difficult to detect in anaemia.

4.60 A.F **B.**T **C.**F **D.**F **E.**T

The PA flotation catheter was introduced by Swan and Ganz in 1970. Most have at least three lumens; a distal lumen for PAP and mixed venous blood samples; a proximal lumen (about 25 cm from the tip) in the right atrium or superior vena cava for CVP measurement and infusions; and a third lumen for inflation of the balloon. Most are inserted via the right internal jugular vein as this is technically easier, but this route is no more accurate than any other. Continuous monitoring of PAP waveform is required to prevent continuous wedging causing infarction of lung tissue. Cardiac output measurements are based on the Fick principle and thermodilution is the most commonly employed technique. Cold injectate is injected through the proximal lumen and a thermistor registers temperature change at the tip of the catheter. Relative contraindications to the use of a PA catheter include prosthetic tricuspid and pulmonary valves, left bundle branch block and coagulopathy. Complications are similar to central venous catheterization but include intracardiac problems such as ventricular arrhythmias, subacute bacterial endocarditis, pulmonary artery rupture, pulmonary infarction and emboli. It is best left in place for only the shortest possible time, i.e. 2–3 days. There is huge controversy over its value as there is no conclusive evidence that it leads to a decreased mortality. (See: Soni N (1996) Editorial: Swansong for Swan–Ganz catheter. *British Medical Journal* **313**, 763–764.)

4.61 A.T **B.**T **C.**T **D.**T **E.**F

Lung cancer is responsible for 8% of all deaths in men. The male-to-female ratio is 2–3 : 1. Cigarette smoking is the most important cause. Apart from finger clubbing, non-metastatic manifestations are relatively rare. They include cerebellar degeneration, polyneuropathies and myasthenic syndrome (Eaton–Lambert syndrome), along with hypertrophic pulmonary osteoarthropathy and thrombophlebitis migrans. Small cell carcinomas of the lung arise from endocrine cells and secrete polypeptide hormones including ADH (hyponatraemia), adrenocorticotrophic hormone (Cushing's syndrome) and parathyroid hormone (hypercalcaemia). Apical lung cancer (Pancoast's tumour) can disrupt the sympathetic supply to the eye to cause a Horner's syndrome. Surgery is the only viable option for non-small cell tumours. Of the 20% suitable for resection, the 5-year survival is 25–30%.

4.62 **A**.T **B**.F **C**.F **D**.F **E**.F

Heparin is a naturally occurring mucopolysaccharide found in the liver and in lung mast cells. Its physiological function is unknown. Clinically it acts via a cofactor, antithrombin III, to inactivate thrombin and inhibit factor Xa-mediated conversion of prothrombin to thrombin. Higher doses neutralize clotting factors IXa, XIa, XIIa to suppress thrombin-induced platelet aggregation. Heparin is ineffective orally due to its polarity and size (MW 16 000). Equally it does not easily traverse the placenta or blood–brain barrier. Its half-life is 60 min. It is metabolized by liver heparinase and renally excreted. In low doses it is used to reduce the incidence (but does not completely abolish the risk) of DVT. High doses are required for the management of DVT, pulmonary emboli and in cardiac surgery. Its use is relatively contraindicated in hypertensives (diastolic >110 mmHg), peptic ulceration and after ophthalmic or neurosurgical procedures. Reversible thrombocytopaenia occurs in 1–5% of patients after commencing both low- and high-dose therapy. *Protamine* is the low molecular-weight, highly alkaline antagonist of heparin. Approximately 1 mg is needed to reverse each 100 units of heparin. *Aprotinin* is a proteolytic enzyme inhibitor which exerts antiplasmin activity causing reduced fibrinolysis and reduced platelet aggregation. It has been used to reduce postoperative blood loss, particularly after cardiac surgery and in hyperfibrinolytic states. It will oppose the actions of heparin but is not a direct antagonist. *Prostacyclin* acts differently from heparin by strongly inhibiting platelet aggregation by increasing cAMP levels.

4.63 **A**.T **B**.F **C**.F **D**.F **E**.T

The anion gap is the sum of the sodium and potassium concentrations minus the sum of the serum chloride and bicarbonate concentrations:

$([Na^+] + [K^+] - [Cl^-] + [HCO_3^-])$

The normal range is 8–12 mmol/l, due to non-buffered anions such as sulphate, phosphate and lactate. Acidosis due to loss of bicarbonate or an increase in hydrogen ions has no effect on the anion gap (e.g. renal tubular acidosis, diarrhoea, ureteral diversions) but will increase when non-bufferable acids are added to plasma either exogenously (salicylate and methanol overdose) or by disorded metabolism (diabetic ketoacidosis, uraemia, lactic acidosis). Occasionally, elevation can be seen with raised bicarbonate in mixed acid–base disorders. A low anion gap can be seen with multiple myeloma, lithium poisoning and severe hypercalcaemia and hypermagnesaemia.

4.64 A.F **B.**F **C.**F **D.**T **E.**F
Glucose is freely filtered by the glomerulus and is completely absorbed from the proximal convoluted tubule. The threshold is constant and is approximately 10 mmol/l in men, slightly lower in women. A small proportion of the population have glycosuria without diabetes owing to a genetic defect of absorption. The renal threshold does not change in diabetics with otherwise normal renal function. The presence of glycosuria implies poor glycaemic control resulting in hyper-glycaemia. Upwards of 60% of pregnant women develop glycosuria, mainly in the second and third trimester, without diabetes; this normally resolves within 1 week of delivery. (See: Butterfield WJH *et al.* (1967) Renal glucose threshold variations with age. *British Medical Journal* **4**, 505–507.)

4.65 A.F **B.**T **C.**T **D.**F **E.**F
Intubation and extubation stimulate the sympathetic nervous system to increase heart rate, blood pressure and intracranial pressure. As this can be up to 20–70% above normal, it is undesirable in patients with ischaemic heart disease, hyperten-sion, head injury, etc. Of all the agents tried, none is completely satisfactory. Esmolol is a relatively new intravenous cardioselective β adrenoceptor antagonist with a rapid onset but short duration of action from esterase-mediated metabo-lism (half-life of 9 min). When used as an i.v. bolus or infusion, it significantly reduces the pressor response. Topical lignocaine is ineffective as the pressor response is stimulated by laryngo-scopy but intravenous lignocaine 1–2 mg/kg 1–2 min prior to induction is of value, as is i.v. fentanyl. Deep inhalational

anaesthesia and the calcium channel antagonists verapamil and diltiazem are also useful. Hydralazine, GTN and sodium nitroprusside have all been used with some success. A number of angiotensin-converting enzyme (ACE) inhibitors (e.g. enalapril) have been given as oral, sublingual and intravenous preparations in an attempt to attenuate the response. As regards enalapril, it is ineffective unless given intravenously, when there is a potential problem with excessive hypotension and bradycardias. (See: Vucevic M *et al.* (1992) Esmolol hydrochloride for management of the cardiovascular stress responses to laryngoscopy and tracheal intubation. *British Journal of Anaesthesia* **68**, 529–530. Also: Miller KA, Harkin CP, Bailey PL (1995) Postoperative tracheal extubation. *Anesthesia and Analgesia* **80**, 149–172.)

4.66 A.T B.T C.F D.F E.F
AS may be due to calcification of a congenital bicuspid valve, rheumatic heart disease or degenerative changes. Angina, dyspnoea and effort syncope are the main symptoms and occur only with severe stenosis. Signs include a slow rising pulse, a non-displaced apex beat and a harsh ejection systolic murmur in the aortic area radiating to the carotids. Left ventricular enlargement may be seen on chest radiographs but heart size is frequently normal. ECG changes include left atrial and ventricular hypertrophy with left bundle branch block (LBBB) but may also be normal in the elderly despite severe stenosis. The diagnosis can be confirmed by echocardiography and Doppler cardiography to calculate the systolic gradient across the aortic valve. Valve replacement is required if symptomatic and/or the gradient is more than 50 mmHg.

4.67 A.T B.F C.F D.F E.T
Paracetamol is an effective analgesic and antipyretic agent derived from acetanilid and phenacetin. It inhibits central prostaglandin synthesis to produce a centrally mediated antipyretic action but has no effect on peripheral prostaglandin synthesis and therefore has minimal anti-inflammatory action. Paracetamol is well absorbed throughout the gastro-intestinal tract and it does not cause gastric irritation or bleeding. It is not significantly bound to plasma proteins. It is metabolized by the liver and is principally excreted by the kidney as glucuronide, sulphate and cysteine residues. Its half-life is about 2 hours but its effects are longer-lasting. Side-

effects are minimal (rash). Although phenacetin has been implicated in causing a nephropathy, paracetamol is safe in renal impairment. Rectal absorption is often delayed and adequate plasma concentrations are not reached with conventional oral doses. As such, doses of between 25 and 45 mg/kg 6-hourly have been suggested as necessary to provide analgesia. It is safe to use in children of any age. (See: Montgomery CJ *et al.* (1995) Plasma concentration of high dose acetaminophen in children. *Canadian Journal of Anaesthesia* **42**, 982–986.)

4.68 A.F B.F C.F D.T E.F
These results show a small total lung capacity (TLC), reduced forced expiratory volume (FEV_1) and forced vital capacity (FVC) but a normal ratio (>75%), hypoxia and a low to normal CO_2 concentration. COPD and asthma are excluded as the FEV_i/FVC ratio for these should be less than 75%. Respiratory acidosis would have an increase in P_aCO_2. Lung volumes should be normal with a PE. This leaves pulmonary fibrosis, a diagnosis which fits all the above values.

4.69 A.F B.T C.F D.T E.F
Congestive cardiac failure is biventricular and occurs when the heart is unable to maintain a sufficient cardiac output (CO) to meet the metabolic demands of the body. Main causes are hypertension, coronary artery disease and valvular disease. Cardiac function is initially improved by compensatory mechanisms but these ultimately contribute to worsening heart failure. For example low CO stimulates the sympathetic nervous system to increase peripheral vascular resistance and redirect blood flow to essential organs. However, the increased afterload imposes a further burden on the heart, impairing CO further. As heart failure progresses renal blood flow falls (GFR will be preserved for a time), stimulating renin and aldosterone secretion which leads to salt and water retention. This further increases preload (atrial pressures), resulting in pulmonary and hepatic congestion, ascites and pleural effusion. Treatment includes bedrest to decrease the work of the heart and diuretics to promote sodium and therefore water excretion. This in turn decreases preload, relieving pulmonary and hepatic congestion. Vasodilators such as ACE inhibitors improve survival by further enhancing salt and water excretion, decreasing afterload and improving myocardial contractility. Digoxin improves

myocardial wall tension but nowadays is more often reserved for heart failure complicating atrial fibrillation because of its narrow therapeutic index. (See: Doughty RN, Sharpe N (1996) Current management of congestive cardiac failure. *British Journal of Hospital Medicine* **55**, 539–544.)

4.70 A.F   B.T   C.F   D.T   E.T
Drugs given via the trachea potentially have a rapid onset of action since there is an extensive epithelial surface available for absorption. Unfortunately neither the optimal dose of drug required nor significant advantages of this route have been established and it must be reserved for when the intravenous route is unavailable. Nevertheless, as a guide the minimum required should be taken as the intravenous dose, although it may be 2–3 times higher. Adrenaline can also be given. The drug has to pass beyond the endotracheal tube (ETT) and this is best achieved either by diluting the drug or instilling it via a catheter that has been inserted beyond the ETT. A saline flush can be given followed by several positive pressure ventilations. The intraosseous route is an often forgotten mode of administration that is of particular value in babies and children under 6 years of age. Complications are rare and include fat and bone marrow emboli, tibial fracture, compartment syndrome, skin necrosis and osteomyelitis. It should also be regarded as a temporary measure until vein cannulation is possible.

4.71 A.F   B.F   C.F   D.F   E.F
Helium is an inert gas present to a small extent in air. It can be used to make breathing easier in cases of upper airway obstruction (stridor) because during turbulent flow density is the factor determining gas flow, and helium is less dense than nitrogen. It is not useful in asthma because lower airway flow is laminar and flow is thus dependent on viscosity, which is actually greater with helium than nitrogen. Helium is supplied in cylinders with brown shoulders and body as a compressed gas at 137 bar. Unlike nitrogen it has no narcotic effect and is combined with oxygen and used extensively by deep-sea divers. Helium has been successfully used as a replacement for CO_2 in laparoscopic procedures as it is very insoluble (which limits absorption from peritoneal cavity), is metabolically inactive (unlike CO_2), neither flammable nor explosive, and is safe with diathermy and lasers.

4.72 A.F B.T C.T D.F E.F
Tolbutamide, glibenclamide and chlorpropamide are sulphonylureas with half-lives of 5, 6 and 36 hours, respectively. Glycaemic control is achieved by promoting release of insulin and reducing glucagon secretion from the pancreas. This requires functioning islet cells; sulphonylureas are therefore unsuitable for IDD. Side-effects include skin reactions, alcohol intolerance and blood dyscrasias. All are metabolized except for chlorpropamide, which is eliminated unchanged in urine (can be associated with profound hypoglycaemia in renal impairment and in the elderly). Metformin is a biguanide which is used exclusively in NIDDM. Its exact mechanism of action is unknown but it probably decreases carbohydrate absorption from the small intestine increasing peripheral uptake and metabolism of glucose. Lactic acidosis is its most serious side-effect.

4.73 A.T B.T C.F D.T E.F
Jaundice is due to raised serum bilirubin. Unconjugated bilirubin (non-water-soluble) is derived from breakdown of haemoglobin in the spleen. Bound to albumin, it is transferred to the liver where it is conjugated by glucuronyl transferase to bilirubin glucuronide (water-soluble), excreted into the gut, converted to urobilinogen, and excreted in the faeces (as stercobilinogen) or reabsorbed and disposed off by the kidneys. Thus, bilirubin in the urine can be found only after glucuronidation, which excludes haemolysis and sickle cell anaemia. Acute hepatitis causes cholestatic jaundice, as does chloropromazine (allergic) and PBC (progressive destruction of intrahepatic bile ducts, leading ultimately to cirrhosis).

4.74 A.T B.T C.T D.F E.T
Magnesium sulphate has increasingly become the drug of choice for the management of pre-eclampsia. As an anticonvulsant it is superior to phenytoin and diazepam in the prophylaxis and treatment of eclamptic convulsions. It reduces blood pressure by vasodilatation and acts as a tocolytic agent to inhibit uterine contraction. Magnesium acts peripherally at the neuromuscular junction both to decrease release of acetylcholine and to reduce endplate sensitivity to acetylcholine as well as having a central action resulting in cortical depression. Other potential uses include bronchodilation (although it has no effect on airway reactivity) in asthma, as

an alternative to nitric oxide to relieve pulmonary hypertension, and as an adjuvant to postoperative analgesia. Side-effects may be significant. They include cardiac conduction defects, drowsiness, muscle weakness, decreased reflexes, hypoventilation and potentiation of non-depolarizing and depolarizing neuromuscular blockers. It crosses the placenta to cause neonatal hypotonia and inhibits platelet activity to increase the bleeding time. It can be given intravenously or intramuscularly at an empirical dose between 2 and 4 g followed by 1–2 g/hour. Therapeutic plasma levels are 2.0–3.5 mmol/l. Side-effects emerge at serum levels in excess of 4–5 mmol/l. Cardiac arrest will occur at more than 12 mmol/l. Treat excess with intravenous calcium. (See: James MFM (1992) Clinical use of magnesium infusions in anesthesia. *Anesthesia and Analgesia* **74**, 129–136. Also: Tramer MR *et al.* (1996) Role of magnesium sulfate in postoperative analgesia. *Anesthesiology* **84**, 340–347.)

4.75 A.T **B.**T **C.**T **D.**F **E.**F

Type I CRPS replaces the term 'reflex sympathetic dystrophy'. It is characterized by a burning pain, trophic and pseudomotor changes with loss of function in a limb. The underlying cause is often obscure but can include trauma, surgery (e.g. arthroscopies) or inflammatory conditions. The acute stage is associated with burning pain, hyperalgesia and warm (or cyanotic) skin in the affected area. This is followed by a dystrophic stage: the skin is cold and cyanotic with oedema and muscle wasting. The final, atrophic stage is associated with smooth, waxy skin subject to ulceration, flexor tendon contractions and osteoporosis. There are no pathognomonic blood tests. Prompt diagnosis and treatment are required to halt progression. Psychological support, pain relief and physiotherapy are important. Using a tourniquet, intravenous sympathetic block with guanethidine (20–30 mg) and prilocaine (40–60 ml 0.5%) can give pain relief for several weeks. Up to 40% of patients have features of CRPS type I at 10 years. I have found no studies that suggest athletes are more susceptible. Causalgia has been redefined as type II CRPS. It is a burning pain often associated with a partially damaged nerve, commonly median, ulnar or sciatic. This tends to occur shortly after injury (1–2 months) and may radiate beyond the nerve's cutaneous distribution. Features are similar to type I CRPS and the spectrum of treatment is the same.

4.76 A.F **B.**F **C.**T **D.**F **E.**T

From top to bottom, the structures visualized are: the aortic knuckle (posterior part of the aortic arch), the pulmonary trunk, left atrial appendage and the left ventricle. Pulmonary arteries are not visible until they emerge from the pericardium and are surrounded by aerated lung. The left hilum is 2.5 cm higher than the right. The right heart border consists of the superior vena cava, right atrium and inferior vena cava.

4.77 A.T **B.**T **C.**T **D.**T **E.**F

The sense organs for pain – nociceptors – are free nerve endings found in almost every tissue of the body. There are two broad types: *thermomechanoreceptors* respond to pinprick and sudden changes in temperature and are responsible for rapid pain sensation; *polymodal* receptors respond to general tissue damage from pressure, heat, histamine and other chemical substances, and are responsible for slow pain sensation and immobilization of the affected part. The former tend to travel to the spinal cord by A delta myelinated fibres which conduct at rates of 12–30 m/s; the latter pass via unmyelinated C fibres at a slower rate of 0.5–2 m/s. Integration of the fibres occurs in the substantia gelatinosa of the dorsal horn. This is an important site for modification of the quality and intensity of the pain. It is also influenced by larger A fibres which ascend in the dorsal columns, and by descending tracts from the reticular activating system. Second-order neurones relay in the dorsal horn and decussate before ascending in the contralateral spinothalamic tract and the more diffuse spinoreticular pathways to terminate in the thalamus. This is probably the main region responsible for appreciation of pain but projections pass to the postcentral gyrus of the cerebral cortex, which is associated with the localization of pain. Although there are no pain fibres in the dorsal columns, transection may render painful stimuli more severe and unpleasant.

4.78 A.T **B.**T **C.**F **D.**T **E.**T

Tetany is increased neural excitability presenting as peripheral muscle spasm. It occurs with hypocalcaemia, alkalosis, hypokalaemia and magnesium deficiency. The alkalosis can be from either excessive bicarbonate therapy, as with treatment for chronic renal failure, or loss of acid from excessive vomiting. Alkalotic tetany can be diagnosed by an increase in plasma bicarbonate and an alkaline urine. Hyperventilation alters the protein binding of calcium such that the ionized fraction falls and may therefore cause hypocalcaemic tetany despite a normal plasma calcium. Other causes of hypocalcaemia include acute pancreatitis, low plasma albumin, hypoparathyroidism, vitamin D deficiency or resistance, drugs (calcitonin) and citrated blood in massive transfusion. Coeliac disease is an allergy to gluten leading to loss of intestinal villi. Severe malnutrition can occur and tetany is a well-recognized if rare complication. Clinical features of hypocalcaemia include numbness around the mouth and in the extremities followed by cramps, tetany, convulsions and death if untreated. Chvostek's sign shows twitching of facial muscle when tapping over the facial nerve, and Trousseau's sign is carpopedal spasm when the brachial artery is occluded. Immediate treatment is with 10 ml of 10% calcium gluconate intravenously, repeated as necessary as an infusion.

4.79 A.T B.T C.T D.T E.T
Hyaline membrane disease is the commonest cause of RDS and respiratory failure during the first few days of life. It is commonly due to prematurity, as before 34–36 weeks' gestation there is both insufficient alveolar development and a lack of surfactant. Without surfactant surface tension is high and atelectasis results from inability to maintain alveolar expansion. This increases both intrapulmonary shunting and V/Q mismatch, resulting in hypoxaemia. When combined with the limited respiratory capacity of a neonate compensatory mechanisms are poor and respiratory failure with tachypnoea, grunting, chest recession and cyanosis can occur soon after birth. Pneumothorax, pulmonary hypertension and persistent fetal circulation may be added complications. Apart from prematurity, predisposing factors include being male, Caucasian, delivered by Caesarean section (particularly prior to labour) and the child of a diabetic mother. Meconium aspiration causes a chemical pneumonitis and airway obstruction to produce atelectasis. Prompt recognition and suctioning of the airway may prevent progression to RDS. Most cases of RDS are self-limiting, resolving in 4–5 days with endogenous surfactant production. Any treatment intervention reflects the clinical state of the neonate. If supplementary oxygen is insufficient the addition of CPAP is very useful. It improves oxygenation and pattern and regularity of respiration whilst retarding the progression of disease and reducing morbidity.

Instillation of surfactant (either bovine or synthetic) into the trachea improves oxygenation and lung compliance to reduce incidence of pneumothorax, intracranial haemorrhage, morbidity and mortality. Severely affected neonates require conventional ventilation, which may be difficult because of the high pressures required. If so, both ECMO and nitric oxide individually have been shown to be promising in carefully selected individuals. 80–90% of infants with RDS survive: most have normal lungs by 1 month of age but between 15 and 40% develop bronchopulmonary dysplasia requiring increased oxygen concentration for many weeks, although eventually lung function becomes normal.

4.80 A.F **B.**T **C.**T **D.**F **E.**T
Right ventricular hypertrophy is associated with a tall R wave in AVR and V_1, right axis deviation, deep S waves in V_5 and V_6, and inverted T waves in V_1 to V_3. Possible causes include chronic lung disease with or without cor pulmonale, massive or multiple pulmonary emboli and pulmonary stenosis. Wide QRS complexes suggest a bundle branch block. *Left ventricular hypertrophy* produces tall R waves in V_5 and V_6, deep S waves in V_1 to V_3, ST depression and T inversion in I, AVL, and V_4 to V_6. In contrast, left axis deviation is not a feature.

4.81 A.F **B.**F **C.**F **D.**T **E.**F
The Bain breathing system is classified as a Mapleson D, not B. It is a coaxial tube with FGF through the inner tube and waste gases through the outer tube. The reservoir bag and expiratory valve are at the machine end. It is inefficient for spontaneous breathing as waste gases enter the reservoir bag and a high FGF (2–3 times minute ventilation) is necessary to prevent rebreathing by purging exhaled gases out through the expiratory valve. It is more efficient for controlled ventilation as exhaled anatomical dead space gas passes into the reservoir bag first to mix with the fresh gas which fills the bag during expiration. The bag is full by the time alveolar expired gas reaches it so the latter is voided through the expiratory valve. The relatively high resistance to breathing limits its use in small children. The dead space will increase with inner tube detachment, resulting in hypoxaemia and hypercapnia.

4.82 A.F   **B.**T   **C.**F   **D.**F   **E.**T

Penicillins consist of a thiazolidine ring and a β-lactam ring attached to a side chain. The nucleus confers biological activity while the side chain determines the characteristics of the penicillin. All are bactericidal as they interfere with cell wall synthesis and are therefore more active against rapidly dividing bacteria. Resistance develops in some bacteria producing β-lactamase and penicillinase which destroy the β-lactam ring of some penicillins (e.g. benzylpenicillin, amoxycillin and ampicillin), but not flucloxacillin as its structure prevents access to the β-lactam ring. The addition of clavulanic acid to amoxycillin (co-amoxyclav) also confers resistance. Gram-negative bacteria possess an outer phospholipid membrane which inhibits access to the bacterial wall. Amoxycillin and ampicillin are moderately hydrophobic and can pass through the membrane to destroy some Gram-negative bacteria (*Haemophilus influenzae, Escherichia coli*). (See: Ellis R, Pillay D (1996) Antimicrobial therapy: towards the future. *British Journal of Hospital Medicine* **56**, 145–150.)

4.83 A.T   **B.**F   **C.**T   **D.**F   **E.**F

Hyperkalaemia exceeding 7.0 mmol/l requires immediate treatment to avert a cardiac arrest. Intravenous glucose and insulin which rapidly drive potassium is the initial treatment of choice. Alkalinization with sodium bicarbonate has the same effect and is useful when acidosis is a feature, although it must be avoided in patients who are unable to cope with the high sodium load (i.e. renal failure). As both methods only buy time, they must be followed by definitive treatment such as haemodialysis. Whether ion exchange resins such as sodium or calcium resonium should be used to treat acute hyperkalaemia is a tricky one to answer as they do remove potassium but can take up to an hour to exert any effect, and so cannot be recommended as first-line treatment. Calcium chloride or gluconate may be used to stabilize the myocardium against the effects of hyperkalaemia but has no effect on potassium levels. Glucagon is used in diabetics to raise low blood glucose resulting from insulin-induced hypoglycaemia.

4.84 A.T   **B.**T   **C.**F   **D.**F   **E.**T

The Wright respirometer consists of a light mica vane within a cylinder perforated with tangential slits which allow the vane to rotate unidirectionally with expiration. The vane is either attached to a gear chain which drives a pointer around a dial or linked electronically to give a measurement of tidal volume. It is accurate at normal tidal volumes and respiratory rates. It overestimates at high tidal volumes and underestimates at low tidal volumes due to its inertia. Fresh gas flows and oxygen concentration are unimportant. Condensation increases the inertia, thus decreasing accuracy. A paediatric version is available.

4.85 A.T B.T C.T D.F E.T
Cirrhosis is the end result of a diffuse, progressive necrosis of liver cells followed by fibrosis and nodule formation. There are many causes, with alcohol being the most common in developed countries and viral hepatitis (mainly hepatitis B) commonest worldwide. Jaundice, ascites (secondary hyperaldosteronism from reduced albumin), splenomegaly (portal hypertension) and a small liver (continuing hepatocyte destruction) are commonly found. Cutaneous manifestations are considerable and include xanthelasma, spider telangiectasia (>2), clubbing, purpura, oedema and scratch marks from bilirubin-induced pruritus. Palmar erythema is a consequence of an increase in peripheral blood circulation. Endocrine changes include gynaecomastia and testicular atrophy. Parotid enlargement is not uncommon. Hyperglobulinaemia is invariable and, once established, tends to persist. This is probably due to an increase in immunoglobulins or as a response to low colloid oncotic pressure from the coexisting hypoalbuminaemia.

4.86 A.F B.F C.T D.T E.F
Fractured shaft of humerus can cause a radial nerve injury resulting in wrist drop and sensory loss over the thumb. Anterior dislocation of the shoulder, commonly associated with fracture of the proximal humerus, can cause axillary nerve damage. This is usually temporary. Nerve injury is uncommon after fractures of the ulna, radius, and shafts of femur and tibia.

4.87 A.F B.T C.T D.T E.F
Dantrolene is a highly lipid-soluble furhydantoin, initially used for control of severe muscle spasms but now chiefly used for treatment of MH. It acts by blocking calcium efflux from sarcoplasmic reticulum into T tubules, thus preventing neuromuscular excitation–contraction coupling. It has no

effect on the neuromuscular junction, EMG, T tubule or calcium re-uptake by sarcoplasmic reticulum. The initial dose is 1 mg/kg i.v., increasing to 10 mg/kg. Its half-life is 9–12 hours and it is broken down in the liver and renally excreted. The intravenous preparation contains mannitol and sodium hydroxide, which results in a pH of 9.5. It is difficult to dissolve. Dantrolene can be used orally to relieve spasticity but side-effects are common including hepatitis, sedation, weakness and diarrhoea. NMS is a disorder of central dopamine transmission found mainly in patients treated with neuroleptic agents such as sulpiride, haloperidol, fluphenazine and the antiemetics prochlorperazine and metoclopramide. Characteristic features are muscle rigidity, pyrexia, cardiovascular disturbances and depressed level of consciousness. These can be fatal and the use of dantrolene is generally recommended on empirical grounds. (See: Bristow MF, Kohen D (1996) Neuroleptic malignant syndrome. *British Journal of Hospital Medicine* **55**, 517–520.)

4.88 A.T B.F C.F D.F E.F
FEV_1 and FVC are measured by spirometry. The patient exhales as fast and as long as possible after full inspiration. The normal FEV_1/FVC ratio is about 75%; a low ratio is typical of obstructive lung disease (COPD, asthma). Restrictive lung disease (pulmonary fibrosis) can have a normal or increased ratio. Old age and myasthenia gravis both give rise to reduced FEV_1 and FVC, leaving the ratio unchanged. Pulmonary emboli do not affect ventilation and should theoretically have no effect on the FEV_1/FVC ratio.

4.89 A.F B.F C.F D.F E.T
Fat embolism is the release of fat droplets into the circulation. Typically, this occurs after major trauma with long bone fractures liberating fatty bone marrow into the blood vessels. It can also occur after prosthetic joint replacements, pancreatitis and parenteral nutrition. Further progression to fat embolism syndrome is, fortunately, rare. The syndrome tends to present 1–3 days after the precipitating event and its features are related both to blood vessel obstruction and to the toxic effect of free lipids. The classic triad of respiratory insufficiency, encephalopathy and petechial rash is found in fewer than 5% of cases. The fat liberated from exposed marrow or adipose tissue obstructs pulmonary capillaries stimulating

production of inflammatory mediators and resulting in an adult respiratory distress syndrome (ARDS)-type picture, i.e. bronchospasm, dyspnoea, tachypnoea, hypoxaemia and cor pulmonale. 40–50% of patients develop a petechial rash in non-dependent areas, e.g. chest, axillae and conjunctiva. Cerebral signs of headache, irritability, coma and fits are thought to be due to fat emboli passing to the systemic circulation as a result of increased raised atrial pressure inducing foramen ovale patency. Odd focal neurological signs are also possible, together with retinal changes (haemorrhages, oedema), pyrexia, hypotension and renal and hepatic impairment. Urine examination is neither specific nor sensitive enough to aid diagnosis. Serum triglyceride and lipid concentrations do not reflect severity. The disease is mostly self-limiting and treatment is essentially supportive with oxygen and ventilation if necessary. Recovery is unrelated to severity. Heparin, steroids, aspirin and aprotinin are of uncertain, if any, value. Early fixation of fractures decreases the incidence of fat embolism. (See: van Besouw JP, Hinds CJ (1989) Fat embolism syndrome. *British Journal of Hospital Medicine* **42**, 304–311.)

4.90 A.T B.F C.T D.T E.T
Cholestatic jaundice arises from obstructed bile flow and the cause may be intrahepatic, as with cirrhosis and drug allergies, or extrahepatic with sclerosing cholangitis, tumours, strictures or stones in the biliary tract. Absence of bile salts in the gut leads to steatorrhoea. The conjugated bilirubin passes back through the liver to the bloodstream and is excreted by the kidney producing dark urine from increased urobilinogen as well as being responsible for pruritus. Alkaline phosphatase rises with obstructive jaundice but does not provide information as to where the obstruction lies nor is it of any prognostic significance.

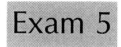

Exam 5

Questions

5.1 An overdose of tricyclic antidepressants (TCAs) can cause:
- **A.** ataxia.
- **B.** jaundice.
- **C.** hypertension.
- **D.** hypothermia.
- **E.** constricted pupils.

5.2 In severe acute pancreatitis:
- **A.** abdominal rigidity and guarding are early signs.
- **B.** serum amylase is not elevated for the first 12 hours.
- **C.** hypocalcaemia occurs within the first week of illness.
- **D.** hyperglycaemia is a common finding.
- **E.** neutropenia is a common finding.

5.3 The following can be used to estimate glomerular filtration rate (GFR):
- **A.** inulin clearance.
- **B.** serum creatinine.
- **C.** ethylenediaminetetraacetic acod (EDTA) clearance.
- **D.** urea clearance.
- **E.** *para*-aminohippuric acid (PAH).

5.4 Carcinoma of the tongue:
- **A.** generally involves the posterior third.
- **B.** is a late complication of gonorrhoea.
- **C.** can be due to dental sepsis.
- **D.** has a worse prognosis than carcinoma of the lip.
- **E.** is associated with leukoplakia.

5.5 Side-effects of amiodarone include:
- **A.** photosensitivity.
- **B.** hypothyroidism.
- **C.** pulsus bigemini.
- **D.** corneal microdeposits.
- **E.** peripheral neuropathy.

5.6　Extracorporeal membrane oxygenation (ECMO):
 A. is not suitable for use in adults.
 B. can cause systemic hypertension.
 C. is contraindicated in immunocompromised patients.
 D. is suitable for use in a neonate with a diaphragmatic hernia.
 E. requires anticoagulation.

5.7　Myocardial infarction (MI) during the perioperative period:
 A. is most likely to occur 3–5 days postoperatively.
 B. is less common with regional anaesthesia.
 C. is more common in upper abdominal surgical procedures.
 D. is more common after prolonged procedures.
 E. can be largely prevented by postoperative monitoring.

5.8　A paramagnetic analyser:
 A. detects diamagnetic gas.
 B. detects gas in a liquid.
 C. may use null deflection.
 D. detects oxygen in a gas mixture.
 E. is used to detect CO_2 .

5.9　Cryoanalgesia:
 A. cools by adiabatic expansion.
 B. uses helium (He).
 C. produces irreversible nerve lesions.
 D. cools to $-273\,K$.
 E. forms ice crystals.

5.10　A 42-year-old woman was found to be oliguric 48 hours after a cholycystectomy for gallstones. The following values were noted:
 urine osmolality　–　300 mosmol/kg
 urine sodium　　 –　180 mmol/l
 serum urea　　　–　30 mmol/l (preop. 10 mmol/l)
Possible conclusions include:
 A. she is unlikely to be dehydrated.
 B. changes are compatible with hypovolaemia.
 C. the urinary sodium is compatible with the normal stress response to surgery.
 D. the preoperative urea excludes intrinsic renal damage.
 E. a diagnosis of chronic renal failure is unlikely.

5.11 Petit mal epilepsy:
- **A.** is more common after puberty.
- **B.** has a characteristic pattern of EEG.
- **C.** can be precipitated by hyperventilation.
- **D.** is worsened by watching television.
- **E.** is normally self-limiting.

5.12 After splenectomy:
- **A.** there is thrombocytopenia.
- **B.** there is an increased tendency to thrombosis.
- **C.** antibiotic therapy is mandatory.
- **D.** serum amylase is raised.
- **E.** opsonins are depressed.

5.13 Methohexitone:
- **A.** has active metabolites.
- **B.** is reconstituted to a pH of 8.6.
- **C.** is painful on injection.
- **D.** is more potent than thiopentone.
- **E.** produces more involuntary movements than thiopentone.

5.14 Perfluorocarbons:
- **A.** can be used as a blood substitute.
- **B.** are metabolized in the liver.
- **C.** are antigenic.
- **D.** have a long elimination half-life.
- **E.** can be used for gas exchange in the lungs.

5.15 Awareness during anaesthesia:
- **A.** is always avoidable.
- **B.** may occur in the absence of pain.
- **C.** can occur in a spontaneously breathing patient.
- **D.** is most commonly found during Caesarean sections.
- **E.** can be effectively treated with benzodiazepine administration.

5.16 Surgery is the definitive treatment of choice for:
- **A.** triple vessel coronary artery disease.
- **B.** metastatic seminoma.
- **C.** stress incontinence.
- **D.** Graves' disease in a 23-year-old woman.
- **E.** chronic renal failure.

5.17 Expected findings in a healthy patient with a pneumoperitoneum include:
   A. minimal change in cardiac output.
   B. a decrease in preload.
   C. an increase in afterload.
   D. an increase in venous admixture.
   E. an increase in airway resistance.

5.18 As regards hepatitis C:
   A. it is a known cause of post-transfusion hepatitis.
   B. it frequently results in fulminant hepatic failure.
   C. vertical transmission is common.
   D. it is frequently associated with hepatitis E.
   E. it is a ribonucleic acid (RNA) virus.

5.19 Lactic acidosis can be caused by:
   A. severe anaemia.
   B. metformin.
   C. cardiac failure.
   D. pancreatitis.
   E. total parenteral nutrition.

5.20 With closed abdominal injury:
   A. all cases must be admitted for observation.
   B. a retroperitoneal haematoma alone is common.
   C. the spleen is the most vulnerable organ.
   D. there will always be guarding if visceral injury has occurred.
   E. pancreatitis is a common sequela.

5.21 The following generally hold true for normal children:
   A. a 4-year-old child requires a 5 mm internal diameter tracheal tube (TT).
   B. a 6-year-old child requires an oral tracheal tube length of 13 cm.
   C. the upper weight limit for a size 2 laryngeal mask is 10 kg.
   D. a 2-year-old child should weigh in the order of 24 kg.
   E. the blood volume of a 3.5 kg full-term neonate is in the order of 300 ml.

5.22 Reflux oesophagitis is associated with:
- **A.** pernicious anaemia.
- **B.** *Helicobacter pylori.*
- **C.** Barrett's oesophagus.
- **D.** a rolling hiatus hernia.
- **E.** angina-like pain.

5.23 Residual volume (RV) is increased in:
- **A.** asthma.
- **B.** fibrosing alveolitis.
- **C.** emphysema.
- **D.** unilateral phrenic nerve palsy.
- **E.** chronic obstructive pulmonary disease (COPD).

5.24 A chronic subdural haematoma may cause:
- **A.** ipsilateral papilloedema.
- **B.** hemiparesis.
- **C.** cerebellar dysfunction.
- **D.** fluctuating level of consciousness.
- **E.** dysphasia.

5.25 Cough:
- **A.** may be the only manifestation of asthma.
- **B.** is a side-effect of enalapril.
- **C.** can be present after brainstem death.
- **D.** can generate intrathoracic pressures greater than 100 kPa.
- **E.** is reduced by morphine administration.

5.26 Atracurium besylate:
- **A.** is stable in acid solutions.
- **B.** relies on pH-dependent metabolism.
- **C.** is not safe to use in liver failure.
- **D.** can cause a severe bradycardia.
- **E.** is contraindicated in renal failure.

5.27 Features of neuropathic pain include:
- **A.** hyperalgesia.
- **B.** allodynia.
- **C.** improvement with sodium channel blockers.
- **D.** improvements with 5-hydroxytryptamine (5-HT) antagonists
- **E.** no improvement with opiates.

5.28 Serum creatinine phosphokinase (CPK) is increased in:

A. Duchenne muscular dystrophy.

B. angina.

C. acute liver cell damage.

D. Paget's disease.

E. malignant hyperthermia (MH).

5.29 Decompression sickness:

A. can cause pruritus.

B. can cause reversible paraplegia.

C. can be treated by a helium–oxygen mixture.

D. is due to low alveolar partial pressure of oxygen.

E. is a known cause of disseminated intravascular coagulation.

5.30 High output cardiac failure can occur with:

A. an arteriovenous (AV) fistula.

B. Paget's disease.

C. aortic regurgitation.

D. acute pulmonary embolus.

E. iron deficiency anaemia.

5.31 An otherwise fit 50-year-old man presents with painless rectal bleeding. Appropriate investigations include:

A. barium meal.

B. fibreoptic colonoscopy.

C. a prothrombin time.

D. an abdominal CT scan.

E. Schilling test.

5.32 An air embolism during a neurosurgical procedure in the sitting position may be indicated by:

A. the presence of cyanosis.

B. atrial fibrillation.

C. a fall in CVP.

D. a sudden increase in heart rate.

E. a sudden increase in blood pressure (BP).

5.33 After birth:
A. The foramen ovale closes due to reversal of the pressure gradient between the right and left atria.
B. the ductus arteriosus normally closes within 24 hours.
C. lung compliance decreases.
D. umbilical artery cannulation is possible only up to 1 hour following delivery.
E. the flow in the ductus arteriosus is from aorta to pulmonary artery.

5.34 Chronic lead poisoning is associated with:
A. punctate basophilia.
B. abdominal colic.
C. diarrhoea.
D. polycythaemia.
E. encephalopathy.

5.35 Cauda equina syndrome typically causes:
A. lower limb hyperreflexia.
B. impotence.
C. persistent numbness.
D. bladder atony.
E. reduced anal tone.

5.36 In a normal distribution:
A. 68% of observations lie within 1 standard error of the mean.
B. the mean, median and mode are the same.
C. 99% of observations lie within 2 standard deviations.
D. the standard deviation is the square root of the variance.
E. calculation of the variance gives a measure of dispersion.

5.37 Acute pulmonary oedema may be a feature of:
A. left atrial myxoma.
B. a severe head injury.
C. naloxone administration.
D. constrictive pericarditis.
E. myocardial infarction.

5.38 Lasers:
A. produce ionizing radiation.
B. always require gas as a medium.
C. produce energy of variable wavelengths.
D. can be used to debulk tumours.
E. produce highly monochromatic light.

5.39 Methods of sterilization include:
A. pasteurization.
B. autoclaving.
C. ethylene oxide.
D. glutaraldehyde.
E. gamma irradiation.

5.40 Nocturia is a common feature of:
A. chronic pyelonephritis.
B. hyperglycaemia.
C. chronic glomerulonephritis.
D. acute tubular necrosis.
E. chronic prostatic obstruction.

5.41 The following suggest inadequate perfusion of vital organs in a 70 kg adult:
A. hydrogen ion concentration of 80 nmol/l.
B. arterial BP of 90/50 mmHg.
C. cardiac index of $1.5 l/min/m^2$.
D. urine output of 300 ml in 24 hours.
E. mixed venous oxygen saturation of 40%.

5.42 Reliable screening tests for MH include:
A. muscle biopsy histology.
B. genetic studies.
C. serum CPK.
D. ryanodine contracture test.
E. plasma cholinesterase.

5.43 An adverse drug reaction:
- A. can be mediated through immunoglobulin G.
- B. is more likely with amide LAs than with ester LAs.
- C. can have a genetic predisposition.
- D. is very unlikely with fentanyl.
- E. is rare without previous sensitization.

5.44 Malignant hypertension can cause:
- A. papilloedema.
- B. cerebrovascular accident (CVA).
- C. left ventricular failure.
- D. pulmonary hypertension.
- E. renal failure.

5.45 The following have significant interactions with inhalational anaesthetic agents:
- A. chlorpropamide.
- B. monoamine oxidase inhibitors (MAOIs).
- C. non-steroidal anti-inflammatory drugs (NSAIDs).
- D. warfarin.
- E. calcium channel antagonists.

5.46 Intubation is more difficult in a neonate because the:
- A. epiglottis is vestigial.
- B. head is small in relation to the body.
- C. tongue is large in relation to the size of the oral cavity.
- D. larynx is more caudal.
- E. narrowest part of the upper airway is infraglottic.

5.47 Metabolic acidosis can be associated with:
- A. hyperventilation.
- B. pancreatic fistulae.
- C. Zollinger–Ellison syndrome.
- D. chronic diarrhoea.
- E. Fanconi's syndrome.

5.48 Delayed gastric emptying occurs with:
- A. anxiety.
- B. extradural opioids.
- C. cisapride.
- D. acute renal failure.
- E. diabetic ketoacidosis.

5.49 Fluid loss in burns:
A. should be replaced by blood.
B. is maximal during the first 24 hours.
C. is a non-protein-containing fluid.
D. is partly due to increased urinary output.
E. is proportional to the size of the area burnt.

5.50 Cholelithiasis is a feature of:
A. type IV hyperlipoproteinaemia.
B. thalassaemia.
C. jejuno-ileal bypass.
D. long-term administration of the oral contraceptive pill (OCP).
E. DM.

5.51 Patients with Down's syndrome are at risk from anaesthesia because of:
A. a high incidence of atlanto-axial instability.
B. a low resistance to infection.
C. associated congenital cardiac defects.
D. increased incidence of (MH).
E. a poor airway.

5.52 Anterior uveitis is associated with:
A. toxoplasmosis.
B. ulcerative colitis.
C. sarcoidosis.
D. adult rheumatoid arthritis (RA).
E. ankylosing spondylitis.

5.53 Early signs of MH include:
A. muscle rigidity.
B. pyrexia.
C. raised end-tidal CO_2.
D. cyanosis.
E. metabolic acidosis.

5.54 ACE inhibitors:
  A. are the first-line treatment for hypertension caused by renal artery stenosis.
  B. have a diuretic action.
  C. improve survival after myocardial infarction.
  D. can be associated with loss of taste.
  E. are contraindicated in pregnancy.

5.55 Normal daily requirements for an adult male are approximately:
  A. potassium – 1 mmol/kg/day.
  B. sodium – 10 mmol/kg/day.
  C. calcium – 200 mg/day.
  D. iron – 8 mg/day.
  E. water – 10 ml/kg/day.

5.56 A transfusion of sodium chloride, adenine, glucose and mannitol (SAG-M) blood 12 days old would be expected to:
  A. contain no platelets.
  B. have no significant change in clotting factors.
  C. have a pH less than 6.0.
  D. contain no ionized calcium.
  E. contain potassium of 8 mmol/l.

5.57 Bony metastases are associated with:
  A. papillary carcinoma of the thyroid.
  B. carcinoma of the prostate.
  C. hypernephroma.
  D. bronchial carcinoid.
  E. hepatocellular carcinoma.

5.58 The laryngeal mask (LM):
  A. is safe for use in patients with latex sensitivity.
  B. is suitable for use in neonates.
  C. allows near-normal respiratory physiology with spontaneous ventilation.
  D. can be accidentally inserted into the oesophagus.
  E. can be used safely with a full stomach.

5.59 Sympathectomy is indicated in the treatment of:
  A. Raynaud's disease.
  B. intermittent claudication.
  C. diabetic neuropathy.
  D. hyperhidrosis.
  E. chronic regional pain syndrome (CRPS) type II.

5.60 On an ECG the following suggest a tachycardia to be ventricular in origin:
  A. absence of P waves.
  B. QRS duration greater than 0.14 s.
  C. left axis deviation.
  D. heart rate greater than 160 beats per minute.
  E. presence of a fusion beat.

5.61 Continuous positive airway pressure (CPAP) in an adult:
  A. requires a fresh gas flow less than maximal inspiratory gas flow.
  B. increases functional residual capacity.
  C. may increase the work of breathing.
  D. will reduce compliance if used efficiently.
  E. needs to maintain a positive pressure of at least 0.5 cm H_2O during inspiration.

5.62 The following nerves exit the skull through the routes stated:
  A. the optic nerve via the superior orbital fissure.
  B. the mandibular nerve via the foramen rotundum.
  C. the maxillary nerve via the foramen ovale.
  D. the vagus through the jugular foramen.
  E. the facial nerve through the internal auditory meatus (IAM).

5.63 Hypothyroidism (myxoedema) may present with:
  A. ataxia.
  B. hypertension.
  C. carpal tunnel syndrome.
  D. macrocytic anaemia.
  E. oligomenorrhoea.

5.64 Lasers are safe to use for an ENT procedure with:
   A. nitrogen.
   B. jet ventilation.
   C. a fleximetallic tracheal tube.
   D. a tracheal cuff filled with water.
   E. helium.

5.65 Brainstem death criteria require:
   A. $P_a\text{CO}_2$ to be greater than 6.7 kPa.
   B. 'dolls eyes' movement when rotating the head.
   C. a flat EEG.
   D. absence of spinal reflexes (e.g. knee).
   E. a core temperature in excess of 35°C.

5.66 The following occur after major surgery:
   A. natriuresis.
   B. a decrease in circulating thyroid hormone.
   C. reduced lipolysis.
   D. increased peripheral glucose uptake.
   E. potassium retention.

5.67 Pulmonary artery enlargement occurs in:
   A. Fallot's tetralogy.
   B. atrial septal defect (ASD).
   C. mitral stenosis.
   D. pulmonary stenosis.
   E. cor pulmonale.

5.68 The following are true of myotonia congenita:
   A. it is transmitted as a sex-linked recessive gene.
   B. life expectancy is 20–30 years.
   C. vecuronium should be avoided.
   D. serum potassium is usually raised.
   E. tonic spasms are usually precipitated by exercise.

5.69 Pre-eclampsia is associated with:
   A. laryngeal oedema.
   B. hyporeflexia.
   C. thrombocythaemia.
   D. hypovolaemia.
   E. proteinuria.

5.70 With surgical diathermy:
  A. direct current is required.
  B. current frequency is more than 1 kHz.
  C. heat produced is proportional to current density.
  D. bipolar diathermy is more powerful than monopolar diathermy.
  E. bipolar diathermy is contraindicated in patients with a cardiac pacemaker.

5.71 The following are useful in assessing recovery from anaesthesia:
  A. Steward score.
  B. Romberg test.
  C. p deletion test.
  D. EEG.
  E. Maddox wing test.

5.72 NSAIDs:
  A. inhibit leukotriene production.
  B. may cause respiratory depression.
  C. can cause thrombocytopenia.
  D. inhibit cyclo-oxygenase production.
  E. promote sodium retention.

5.73 Paroxysmal supraventricular tachycardia can be effectively treated by:
  A. pressure on the carotid sinus.
  B. intravenous lignocaine.
  C. verapamil.
  D. adenosine.
  E. rapid atrial pacing.

5.74 Regarding lung function:
  A. an FEV_1/FVC ratio of more than 70% is normal.
  B. carbon dioxide is used to calculate the gas transfer factor.
  C. FRC can be measured by helium dilution spirometry.
  D. closing capacity is always larger than closing volume.
  E. total lung capacity can be measured by plethysmography.

5.75 Halothane hepatotoxicity is influenced by:
- **A.** body mass index.
- **B.** duration of anaesthesia.
- **C.** perioperative hypoxia.
- **D.** age of the patient.
- **E.** sex of the patient.

5.76 Tramadol:
- **A.** suppresses monoamine reuptake activity.
- **B.** acts on kappa opioid receptors.
- **C.** is moderately addictive.
- **D.** has active metabolites.
- **E.** is potentiated by carbamazepine.

5.77 A 68-year-old man becomes unresponsive in the recovery ward after a routine hernia repair. The ECG shows ventricular fibrillation (VF). The following actions are appropriate:
- **A.** an initial precordial thump.
- **B.** an initial 1 mg dose of adrenaline.
- **C.** commence DC shock at 360 J.
- **D.** initiate a compression-to-ventilation ratio of 5 to 1.
- **E.** administer calcium chloride if all else fails.

5.78 The following are associated with chronic autoimmune thrombocytopenic purpura (AITP):
- **A.** bleeding time greater than 10 min.
- **B.** response to treatment with corticosteroids.
- **C.** splenomegaly.
- **D.** improvement within 24 hours following splenectomy.
- **E.** age less than 40 years.

5.79 Long-term administration of thiazide diuretics may result in:
- **A.** hypercalcaemia.
- **B.** hypomagnesaemia.
- **C.** hyponatraemia.
- **D.** hyperuricaemia.
- **E.** glucose intolerance.

5.80 Isoflurane is similar to enflurane as regards:
   A. structure.
   B. analgesic properties.
   C. uterine relaxation.
   D. EEG changes.
   E. metabolism.

5.81 A raised CVP in a hypotensive patient may be due to:
   A. a tension pneumothorax.
   B. a large pulmonary embolus.
   C. adrenocortical insufficiency.
   D. a venous air embolus.
   E. haemorrhage.

5.82 Immediately following complete transection of the spinal cord there will be:
   A. motor loss but retained sensation.
   B. sensory loss but retained motor function.
   C. areflexia.
   D. clonus.
   E. hypotension.

5.83 Cardiac catheterization in a 55-year-old man revealed:

Right atrial (RA) pressure	– 5 mmHg
Right ventricular (RV) pressure	– 80/30 mmHg
Pulmonary artery (PA) pressure	– 80/40 mmHg
Pulmonary capillary wedge pressure (PCWP)	– 9 mmHg
Left ventricular (LV) pressure	– 100/70 mmHg

   The values are consistent with:
   A. mitral stenosis.
   B. mitral regurgitation.
   C. primary pulmonary hypertension (PH).
   D. non-myocardial disease.
   E. pulmonary stenosis.

5.84 Hypomagnesaemia:
   A. can cause tetany.
   B. increases myocardial contractility.
   C. causes muscle weakness.
   D. causes vasodilatation.
   E. increases susceptibility to cardiac arrhythmias.

5.85 **The quality of lumbar extradural block with local anaesthetics (LAs) may be enhanced by addition of:**
   A. adrenaline.
   B. fentanyl.
   C. clonidine.
   D. dextran.
   E. hyaluronidase.

5.86 **The following indicate that oliguria is due to acute tubular necrosis (ATN):**
   A. urinary sodium   – 10 mmol/l
   B. urine osmolality   – 300 mosmol/l
   C. specific gravity of urine   – 1.025
   D. urine : plasma urea ratio   – 3 : 1
   E. urine : plasma creatinine ratio – 80 : 1

5.87 **Ranitidine:**
   A. inhibits cytochrome P-450 activity.
   B. has the same mode of action as omeprazole.
   C. neutralizes gastric acid.
   D. is more potent than cimetidine.
   E. is useful in Zollinger–Ellison syndrome.

5.88 **Minimum alveolar concentration (MAC):**
   A. increases during pregnancy.
   B. is a measure of potency.
   C. is directly related to the oil : gas partition coefficient.
   D. increases with hypothermia.
   E. remains the same throughout a particular anaesthetic.

5.89 **In a rhesus-negative mother with a rhesus-positive baby there is an association between a high level of maternal anti-D antibody and:**
   A. fetal red cells entering the maternal circulation.
   B. antigen alone crossing the placenta.
   C. neonatal anaemia.
   D. neonatal jaundice.
   E. first trimester maternal sensitization.

5.90 Myasthenic syndrome:
   A. produces marked post-tetanic facilitation.
   B. responds to anticholinesterase medication.
   C. shows sensitivity to non-depolarizing muscle relaxants.
   D. shows sensitivity to depolarizing muscle relaxants.
   E. improves with exercise.

Answers

5.1 A.T B.T C.F D.F E.F

TCAs (e.g. imipramine, amitriptylline) exert antihistamine (H_1) and anticholinergic effects, α_1 adrenergic antagonism and monoamine uptake inhibition. The consequences of overdose therefore include:

anticholinergic effects   – delayed gastric emptying, constipation, urinary retention, dry mouth, mydriasis and blurred vision

sympathetic blockade   – postural hypotension, impotence and cardiac arrhythmias

CNS effects   – tremor, sedation, convulsions, confusion, ataxia, dysarthria and muscle twitching; coma and respiratory depression are rare.

miscellaneous reactions   – skin rashes, cholestatic jaundice and pyrexia

Treatment with gastric lavage and activated charcoal is possibly useful if within 4 h of a significant overdose (more than 15 tablets). The patient should be monitored for cardiac arrhythmias but treatment is rarely needed and of limited effectiveness as the volume of distribution of TCAs is large and rapid hepatic metabolism usually results in spontaneous resolution. Correction of acidosis and hypoxia is more important and may require intubation and ventilation. Physostigmine has been used to treat all the toxic effects with variable success but it is no longer recommended as it has been associated with asystole and convulsions. More recently introduced tricyclics, e.g. lofepramine, mianserin and viloxazine, are safer in overdose as they have less antimuscarinic and cardiotoxic effects than the earlier drugs.

5.2 A.T B.F C.T D.T E.F

Gallstones and alcohol account for 80% of cases of severe acute pancreatitis. The disease usually presents with early onset of abdominal tenderness, rigidity and guarding often associated with nausea, vomiting and pyrexia. Hypovolaemic shock may occur and is proportional to the degree of pancreatic destruction and consequent fluid shift. There is an associated neutrophilia. The amylase level does not reflect severity of the attack; it peaks at 12–24 hours before falling. Serum trypsin remains elevated for longer. Up to 70% of patients develop a degree of hypocalcaemia within the first 24 hours. Hyperglycaemia is due to relative hypoinsulinaemia and hyperglucagonaemia and insulin therapy may be required. Other features include pleural effusion, jaundice and an ileus. The mortality is 30–50%.

5.3   A.T   B.F   C.T   D.F   E.F
GFR can be measured by comparing the excretion and plasma level of a substance that is freely filtered through the glomeruli but neither secreted nor reabsorbed by the tubules. Inulin, a polymer of fructose found in dahlia tubers, and EDTA are ideal examples as they are not metabolized, nor secreted or reabsorbed by the tubules. In addition more than 95% is excreted within 24 hours by glomerular filtration and they are unaffected by changes in flow rate or pH. Serum creatinine alone cannot determine GFR although creatinine clearance is useful, despite a variable amount being secreted and reabsorbed in the tubules. Urea clearance depends on dietary intake of protein and urine flow rate. PAH is freely filtered by the glomeruli and secreted by tubular cells and is used to measure effective renal plasma flow which, in turn, is used to derive renal blood flow.

5.4   A.F   B.F   C.T   D.T   E.T
75% of malignant tumours of the tongue are found in the anterior two-thirds, most commonly on the lateral margins. The majority arise from carcinomatous change of leukoplakia, a hyperkeratotic plaque which is white in colour from being kept moist by saliva. Causes include the six S's, i.e. smoking, syphilis, sepsis (i.e. dental), sharp edge of a tooth (chronic frictional irritation), spirits (alcohol) and spices (betel nut). Candidiasis is also a known cause, but not gonorrhoea. Cessation or treatment of these factors will lead, in time, to regression of the leukoplakia. Advanced cases of carcinoma of the tongue present with pain (infection or involvement of the lingual nerve), dysphagia, inability to protrude the tongue, bad breath, a lump in the neck and hoarseness as a result of metastases. After excision biopsy to confirm the diagnosis, treatment is with a combination of surgery and radiotherapy. Despite advances in treatment mortality has remained static, although the prognosis is better for women, with 50% survival

at 5 years, compared with 20% for men. A second tumour of the tongue is not unusual despite successful treatment of the first. Radiotherapy can also be used to remove the leukoplakia but there is evidence that it increases likelihood of malignant change. Carcinomas of the lip tend to occur in older men with an outdoor occupation or in smokers. As the carcinoma is easily seen it is noticed earlier and, whether treated by surgery or radiotherapy, 5-year survival is greater than 70%.

5.5 **A.**T **B.**T **C.**F **D.**T **E.**F

Amiodarone was initially developed as an anti-anginal drug but is now regarded as an antiarrhythmic agent (Vaughan-Williams class III). Amiodarone promotes electrical stability of heart by reducing sinoatrial node automaticity and prolonging the refractory period. As such it is used to treat supraventricular tachycardias and pre-excitation syndromes such as Wolff–Parkinson–White. It also raises the threshold for ventricular fibrillation and is effective for refractory ventricular tachycardia when given acutely. It also has some α and β adrenergic blocking effects but the importance of these is unclear. It is poorly absorbed orally and has a slow onset of action at 3–7 hours. The half-life with chronic therapy is also prolonged, ranging from 14 to 100 days. Long-term use is limited by side-effects, some of which are severe. These include photosensitivity, rashes, pigmentation, corneal deposits as well as 'pulmonary syndrome' with cough, dyspnoea, hypoxia and reduction in diffusion lung tests. Hyperthyroidism and hypothyroidism can also occur, although the mechanism of action is unknown. Amiodarone contains iodine, but the amount by itself should not interfere with thyroid action.

5.6 **A.**F **B.**T **C.**F **D.**T **E.**T

ECMO is a system whereby venous blood is removed from a patient by gravity and passed through a membrane oxygenator working on a countercurrent principle. Once oxygenation and removal of carbon dioxide (CO_2) have occurred the blood is warmed and returned to the arterial circulation. Although ECMO is still used in adults, results of ECMO for adult respiratory distress syndrome have been disappointing as it has not been proven to reduce either mortality or hospital stay compared with the less expensive conventional therapy such as inverse ratio ventilation. ECMO is now predominantly used in children, in whom it has been considerably more successful.

This is particularly true in neonates with severe respiratory failure from meconium aspiration, hyaline membrane disease, pulmonary hypertension or pneumonia. It can also be used for a diaphragmatic hernia but these cases have the lowest survival rate (59%). Complications are many and include hypertension with a risk of consequent intraventricular haemorrhage in neonates (58%), fluid overload, haemorrhage from the heparin required to prevent clot formation in the ECMO circuit, thrombocytopenia and permanent neurological sequelae in about 20%. IVOX (intravenous oxygenator) aims to simplify extracorporeal support by inserting a miniature 'membrane lung' composed of numerous microporous hollow fibres into the vena cavae via a femoral vein cut down. IVOX gives 20–30% gas exchange which does not allow for much decrease in ventilatory support but is a useful 'top-up' in patients already receiving maximal mechanical ventilation. (See: Levy FH *et al.* (1992) Extracorporeal membrane oxygenation. *Anesthesia and Analgesia* **75**, 1053–1062. Also: Skoiles J, Pepperman M (1993) Editorial: IVOX. *British Journal of Anaesthesia* **70**, 603–604.)

5.7   A.F   B.F   C.T   D.F   E.F
The incidence of MI after non-cardiac surgery is 0–0.7%. Most occur within 24 hours of surgery and tend to be silent non-Q wave infarcts. No study has definitively judged any anaesthetic regimen as being superior to another, provided haemodynamic variables are controlled. Intraoperative tachycardia and hypotensive episodes (more than 30% drop for longer than 10 min) are important predictors, as are both the preoperative functional state of the patient and the type of surgery being performed. Emergency, major vascular, thoracic and upper abdominal procedures give rise to increased risk of MI. There is little correlation between length of procedure and postoperative complications, once high-risk procedures have been excluded. Postoperative monitoring may marginally reduce the incidence but does not consistently prevent MI. (See: Fleisher LA, Barash PG (1992) Preoperative cardiac evaluation for noncardiac surgery. *Anesthesia and Analgesia* **74**, 586–598. Also: Goldman L (1995) Cardiac risk in noncardiac surgery – an update. *Anesthesia and Analgesia* **80**, 810–820.)

5.8   A.F   B.F   C.T   D.T   E.F
Because of their molecular structure, most gases are repelled from a magnetic field and are known as diamagnetic. Oxygen

and nitric oxide are the only two gases in clinical use that are strongly attracted by a magnetic force and can therefore be paramagnetically analysed. An analyser consists of a cell containing a magnetic field and two nitrogen-filled glass spheres connected by a short bridge to a taut wire suspension. The spheres are free to rotate, though their suspension tends to maintain them in position in the strongest part of the magnetic field. When oxygen enters the cell, the molecules are attracted to the strongest part of the magnetic field. The amount by which the spheres are displaced is proportional to the concentration of oxygen present. This can be measured by deflection of a beam of light reflected by a mirror mounted on the suspensory wire (Pauling, 1946) or by measuring the current required to prevent movement of the spheres (null deflection). Both methods are very accurate but errors can arise from the presence of water vapour or a very high concentration of diamagnetic gas, e.g. CO_2.

5.9 **A.**T **B.**F **C.**F **D.**F **E.**T
Cryoanalgesia is the interruption of peripheral nerves by extreme cold to achieve pain relief. Nitrous oxide (N_2O) or CO_2 is released at high pressure, resulting in an adiabatic expansion and cooling to $-60°C$ (Joule–Thomson effect) of the probe, which has been inserted into the target nerve. Contact for 60 s creates an iceball which destroys a 2–4 mm length of nerve. Nerve sheaths are spared, allowing nerve axons to regenerate so that loss of sensation is only temporary (up to a few months). It is useful for trigeminal neuralgia, neuromas, postherpetic neuralgia (sometimes) and self-limiting conditions such as post-thoracotomy pain and fractured ribs. (See: LLoyd JW *et al.* (1976) Cryoanalgesia, a new approach to pain relief. *Lancet* **2**, 932–934.)

5.10 **A.**T **B.**F **C.**F **D.**F **E.**F
Normal values are:

> urine osmolality – 300–1300 mosmol/l
> urine sodium – 40–210 mmol/l
> serum urea – 3–8 mmol/l

In this case the patient has a low to normal urine osmolality, a high urinary sodium and an elevated preoperative and postoperative serum urea. Plasma urea and creatinine levels begin to rise only when more than 50% of nephrons have been lost. A serum urea in excess of 13 mmol/l normally represents definite renal impairment, but in this case a serum urea of 10 mmol/l still suggests underlying intrinsic disease. This value, in combination with the low urine osmolality and high urinary sodium, confirms impaired concentrating ability associated with chronic renal failure. It is unlikely to be due to either dehydration or hypovolaemia, as both increase urine osmolality. Neither can it be the normal postoperative stress response which results in sodium conservation, leading to low levels in the urine.

5.11 A.F   **B.**T   **C.**T   **D.**F   **E.**T
Petit mal epilepsy is a generalized epilepsy, almost invariably a disorder of childhood. Most attacks commence between 5 and 10 years of age. It causes characteristic changes in the EEG and an attack is associated with a 3 Hz spike and wave discharges. Clinically, the child normally stops all activity, stares and pales slightly. The eyelids may twitch and a few jerks may occur. It commonly lasts 3–20 s. There is no residual confusion or incontinence and the child carries on as if nothing had happened. These attacks cannot be attributed to identifiable local cerebral lesions. They can be precipitated by hyperventilation, but not by watching television. Although normally self-limiting, about one-third go on to develop grand mal epilepsy in adulthood. Treatment includes sodium valproate and clonazepam.

5.12 A.F   **B.**T   **C.**T   **D.**T   **E.**T
After a splenectomy there is an immediate thrombocytosis which may be associated with an increased risk of thromboembolism in the first 2–3 weeks, particularly if there is an underlying myeloproliferative disorder. The white cell count increases but this is variable in magnitude and duration. The production of the opsonins tuftsin and properidin is depressed, which is partly responsible for an increased susceptibility to infection from encapsulated bacteria. As such, polyvalent vaccine against capsular polysaccharides from pneumococcal strains is essential and if possible should be given 2–3 weeks prior to surgery. Prophylaxis with penicillin V or erythromycin is mandatory for the first 2 years at least after excision. Atelectasis, pneumonia, left pleural effusion, acute gastric distension and gastric necrosis are all possible complications. Pancreatitis (with an increase in amylase) can arise from

iatrogenic trauma during surgery or if abdominal trauma was responsible for surgery.

5.13 A.T B.F C.T D.T E.T

Methohexitone is a methylated oxybarbiturate reconstituted as a 1% solution with a pH of 11. It is approximately three times as potent as thiopentone. Compared with thiopentone, methohexitone causes less tissue reaction after extravasation but a greater incidence of pain on injection (which can be reduced by addition of lignocaine) and more excitatory effects (involuntary muscle movements, tremor, hypertonus, etc.). Convulsions may occur in patients with underlying epilepsy. Methohexitone is broken down in the liver to hydroxymethohexitone which also has some hypnotic activity. Its half-life is 2–4 hours, making it suitable for use in day surgery and short procedures. It is often the induction agent of choice for electroconvulsive therapy.

5.14 A.T B.F C.T D.F E.T

Perfluorocarbons are biologically inert, colourless, odourless clear liquids with a high density composed of 8–10 carbon atoms. They have been used as a blood substitute because they carry oxygen in solution, the amount dissolved being proportional to arterial oxygen tension. They are insoluble in water and are administered as an emulsion, similar to intralipid. They are not metabolized but are either excreted unchanged by the lungs or following storage by the reticuloendothelial system are also eliminated through the lymphatic system. Unfortunately, they have a number of limitations which have precluded their widespread use; these include instability at room temperature, short elimination half-life and antigenic side-effects from complement activation. Because of their low surface tension and ability to dissolve oxygen and carbon dioxide, promising results have been reported with their use in partial liquid ventilation, i.e. instilling perfluorocarbons into the lungs. Clinical trials have shown improvement with respiratory distress syndrome (RDS) in both neonates and adults (particularly if requiring extracorporeal membrane oxygenation). They are also thought to improve gas exchange by increasing functional residual capacity in the most dependent areas of the lungs by opening up previously collapsed segments. However, their slow elimination and storage in the reticuloendothelial system has led to as yet unresolved concerns as to potential long-term side-effects. (See: Kelly KP (1997) Editorial: Partial liquid ventilation – turning back a PAGE on evolution. *British Journal of Anaesthesia* **78**, 1–3. Also: Hischl RB *et al.* (1995) Liquid ventilation in adults, children and full term neonates. *Lancet* **346**, 1201–1202.)

5.15 A.F **B.**T **C.**T **D.**T **E.**F
The aim of anaesthesia is to avoid awareness, but it would be impossible to say that it can always be avoided. Despite considerable research, no simple, reliable monitor of depth of anaesthesia has been developed. Thus we remain dependent on clinical signs which are not foolproof. The extent of awareness ranges from unpleasant and vivid dreams through factual recall to pain. It is more commonly associated with use of muscle relaxants but can occur in spontaneously breathing patients even in the absence of the autonomic signs of light anaesthesia (sweating, tachycardia, hypertension, mydriasis, lacrimation). Most cases of awareness occur during the first 5–10 min after induction for emergency Caesarean section under general anaesthesia. The rush to deliver the baby in conjunction with avoidance of opiates, low concentration of volatile anaesthetic agents and a high inspired oxygen concentration may prevent an adequate depth of anaesthesia being achieved. Using oxygen and N_2O without volatile agents resulted in about 25% of patients being aware. The addition of 0.5% halothane, 1.0% enflurane or 0.75% isoflurane has reduced the incidence to near zero with $50:50$ $O_2:N_2O$ mixture. Benzodiazepines cannot be guaranteed to prevent recall as they are not significantly associated with retrograde amnesia. Moreover in obstetric anaesthesia they should be avoided prior to delivery as they can cause neonatal hypotonia.

5.16 A.T **B.**F **C.**T **D.**F **E.**T
Most patients with coronary artery disease can be managed medically. Where medical management fails, coronary angioplasty provides symptomatic relief in more than 90% with lesions in one or two vessels. Re-stenosis occurs in 30% within 3–6 months and 40% of patients come to definitive surgery within 2–3 years. Prospective randomized trials have shown patients with angina and left main stem stenosis or triple vessel disease are best treated with revascularization surgery, preferably using the internal mammary artery. Orchidectomy is performed for testicular masses to allow for histological

diagnosis. It may also be the only treatment required for disease confined to the testes. Metastatic disease requires radiotherapy which cures in more than 95% of cases. In very advanced cases chemotherapy (carboplatin) is also indicated. True stress incontinence requires surgery. In the unfit or elderly, periurethral injection of collagen may cure or substantially improve symptoms. Graves' disease normally produces a diffuse, vascular toxic goitre. Therapies available include drugs (normally carbimazole, occasionally propylthiouracil), radioiodine and surgery. Patients are initially rendered euthyroid by drug therapy for 12–18 months. If patients subsequently relapse, alternative therapies including surgery may be considered. Chronic dialysis preserves life in patients with chronic renal failure but the cost in terms of quality of life is high. Renal transplantation is the only definitive treatment, even though it may not prove to be a permanent cure. Kidney survival may be as high as 90–95% in the first year but it falls by 5–10% each subsequent year.

5.17 A.T **B.**F **C.**T **D.**F **E.**T

This question refers to the potential problems associated with laparoscopic surgery. In the supine position there may be small decreases in cardiac output and mixed venous oxygen saturation and increases in central venous pressure (CVP), mean arterial pressure (MAP) and systemic vascular resistance (SVR). Venous return and hence cardiac output is thought to be maintained by increased filling pressure of the central circulation, e.g. transfer of pooled blood from compression of splanchnic vessels counterbalanced by an increase in vascular resistance. Respiratory changes include increased airways resistance and decreased compliance. Although increased intra-abdominal pressure might be expected to compress basal lung regions to cause atelectasis and increases in V/Q mismatch, oxygenation is unaffected and both oxygen consumption and venous admixture remain unchanged. One explanation for this is increased airways resistance may act as 'auto PEEP' (positive end-expiratory pressure) to compensate for any lung compression. A moderate increase in renin secretion also occurs, but is of doubtful clinical significance as it is not enough to have a pressor effect. CO_2 retention occurs during CO_2 insufflation unless adequately compensated for by increased ventilation. All these changes are more marked in the head-down position or if the patient is cardiovascularly compromised. (See: Odeberg-

Wernerman S, Sollevi A (1996) Cardiopulmonary aspects of laparoscopic surgery. *Current Opinion in Anaesthesia* **9**, 525–535.)

5.18 A.T   B.F   C.F   D.F   E.T

Hepatitis C is a single-stranded RNA virus first identified in 1988. Prior to screening, it was responsible for 70–90% of post transfusion hepatitis cases but the incidence is now considerably less. In the UK about 1 in 1800 samples of donated blood are HCV-positive. The virus is mainly transmitted by blood and blood products (76% of haemophiliacs are HCV-positive), intravenous drug abuse and sexual contact, although vertical transmission (mother-to-fetus) occurs rarely. Symptoms are non-specific in the acute phase: mainly a 'flu-like illness with a rise in liver enzymes. Fewer than 20% of patients develop jaundice, which is usually mild and self-limiting, with less than 1% proceeding to fulminant liver failure. Diagnosis is often delayed until patients present years later with chronic liver disease. This occurs in about 50%, of whom 15% will develop hepatocellular carcinoma. Diagnosis is by detecting antibodies to HCV by enzyme-linked immunosorbent assay (ELISA) and recombinant immunoblot assay. Viral RNA can also be detected by an expensive polymerase chain reaction (PCR) test. Guidelines for treatment are uncertain but interferon has been used in some acute cases. Hepatitis E is an RNA virus which causes enteral (water-borne) hepatitis. Epidemics have been seen in many developing countries but it is often self-limiting, has no carrier status and does not progress to chronic liver failure.

5.19 A.T   B.T   C.T   D.T   E.T

Lactic acidosis is a metabolic acidosis accompanied by lactate levels in excess of 5–7 mmol/l. It is classified as either *type A*, when inadequate tissue perfusion generates lactate faster than it can be removed, or *type B*, where overt tissue hypoxia does not play a major role. Examples of type A include shock, hypoxia, severe anaemia and cardiac failure. Examples of type B include hepatic failure, diabetes mellitus, pancreatitis, leukaemia, infections, lymphoma, and high levels of ethanol, salicylates and fructose and sorbitol in total parenteral nutrition (which is metabolized to lactate). Treatment is directed at correction of the underlying cause. In addition, as the severity of lactic acidosis in critically ill patients correlates with the overall oxygen debt and cardiac dysfunction is a common feature, therapy should therefore be designed to maximize oxygen delivery in order to reduce tissue hypoxia while also maintaining haemoglobin levels. The use of buffering agents, e.g. sodium bicarbonate, has not been shown to affect outcome, particularly from type A lactic acidosis. Moreover, the benefit of other therapies, e.g. peritoneal dialysis with bicarbonate-buffered solution or haemodiafiltration, to reduce the severity of lactic acidosis in the critically ill also remains unproven. Although phenformin is the main biguanide associated with lactic acidosis, it has also been reported with metformin. (See: Mizock BA, Falk JL (1992) Lactic acidosis in critical illness. *Critical Care Medicine* **20**, 80–93.)

5.20 **A.**T **B.**F **C.**T **D.**F **E.**F
The commonest causes of blunt trauma are road traffic accidents (RTAs), falls, assaults and industrial accidents. The most vulnerable organ is the spleen, followed by the liver and small bowel. Pancreatic damage is relatively uncommon (10%). A retroperitoneal haematoma is most commonly the result of pelvic fractures. Pain, tenderness and guarding, the typical signs of penetrating abdominal injury, can be absent despite significant damage. All patients should therefore be admitted to hospital and closely observed, as any serious injury will become manifest within 24 hours. Peritoneal lavage is simple, safe and cheap but has a high false positive rate (only 10 ml of blood are needed to obtain a positive tap), and should not be relied upon as the sole indicator for laparotomy unless the patient is haemodynamically unstable, despite fluid resuscitation.

5.21 **A.**T **B.**F **C.**F **D.**F **E.**T
Knowing some simple formulae for the normal child is useful as this can prevent serious mishaps with airway control, fluids and drug dosages during anaesthesia. Formulae are:

TT size	– (age/4) + 4.0 cm	
TT length (oral)	– (age/2) + 12.0 cm	
Weight at age		
1–8 years	– (2 × age) + 8 kg	
Blood volume	– premature:	90–100 ml/kg
	newborn (full-term):	80–90 ml/kg
	3–12 months:	75–80 ml/kg
	3–6 years:	70–75 ml/kg
	>6 years:	65–70 ml/kg

Fluid requirements	– 0–10 kg:	4 ml/kg/h
	11–20 kg:	2 ml/kg/h
	>20 kg:	1 ml/kg/h
Laryngeal mask	– size 1:	neonate to 6.5 kg
	size 2:	6.5–20 kg
	size 2½:	20–30 kg
	size 3:	30–50 kg
	size 4–5:	>50 kg

These are only a guide and different textbooks tend to have minor variations of the same formulae.

5.22 **A.**F   **B.**F   **C.**T   **D.**F   **E.**T

Reflux oesophagitis is due to acid, pepsin and bile salts entering the oesophagus from the stomach. Oesophagogastric sphincter incompetence is a prerequisite for reflux to occur, although poor lower oesophageal motility and epithelial resistance may also play a role. It is exacerbated by bending, lying, acid food and alcohol. Heartburn is the characteristic symptom and can be mistaken for angina. It is due to oesophageal spasm and as it is relieved by glyceryl trinitrate this can further confuse the diagnosis. A hiatus hernia is not a prerequisite for reflux but in the sliding type the lower oesophageal sphincter lies above the diaphragm, becomes defective and reflux can occur as it is no longer reinforced by intra-abdominal pressure. This is not a problem with a rolling hernia as the sphincter remains below the diaphragm while a bulge of stomach projects through the hiatus alongside the oesophagus. Strictures and formation of potentially premalignant Barrett's mucosa (epithelial changes from squamous to columnar cells) can occur with long-standing disease. Despite the Gram-negative bacterium *H. pylori* being the most important cause of gastritis, studies have failed to show that it has a significant role in the development of reflux. Pernicious anaemia produces a thin atrophic gastric mucosa with achlorhydria. As acid is required for oesophagitis the two conditions are rarely associated. The diagnosis of reflux oesophagitis is made clinically, and confirmed by barium swallow and endoscopy with biopsy. Treatment is conservative with weight reduction if necessary, smaller and more frequent meals, stopping smoking, alginates, cisapride, omeprazole and other drugs which reduce acid secretion. Surgery is best reserved for intractable symptoms. (See: Barbezat GO (1995) Reflux oesophagitis. *British Journal of Hospital Medicine* **54**, 583–586.)

5.23 A.T B.F C.T D.T E.T

RV is the air remaining in the lungs after maximal expiratory effort. It is approximately 1.2 kg in an average 70 kg man. Asthma and COPD both cause airway narrowing, thus limiting expiration and increasing RV. Emphysema results from the loss of 'elastic recoil' which normally maintains airway patency during expiration; thus there will be air flow limitation, air-trapping and an increase in RV. The phrenic nerve supplies the diaphragm and a unilateral nerve palsy is most commonly due to a bronchial carcinoma. At rest, the paralysed diaphragm assumes a resting expiratory posture. Physiological measurements show a reduction in vital capacity and maximum voluntary ventilation which results in an increase in RV. Fibrosing alveolitis is usually either a pulmonary manifestation of a connective tissue disorder (e.g. rheumatoid arthritis (RA)) or cryptogenic. It is an interstitial lung disease due to cellular infiltration and thickening of the alveolar wall leading to progressive fibrosis, lung shrinkage and a reduction in RV.

5.24 A.F B.T C.T D.T E.T

A subdural haematoma can arise from an acceleration–deceleration head injury or from a forgotten trivial injury. It is due to bleeding between the pia mater and arachnoid and thought to result from disruption of the bridging veins between the cortical surface, dura and venous sinuses. It occurs more commonly in the presence of cerebral atrophy, where the initial haematoma has space to enlarge gradually due to a combination of slow bleeding from the dural veins and fluid absorbed from cerebrospinal fluid (CSF) by osmosis. It commonly presents with increasingly severe headaches, although it is often only with the onset of drowsiness and, occasionally, a hemiparesis that hospital admission is precipitated. The diagnosis is often overlooked in the elderly and in alcoholics, particularly as it can also present with mood changes and incontinence which can be mistaken for senility. The course may be steadily downhill or interspersed with periods of improvement. A slow pulse, seizures, dysphasia, pupillary inequality, double vision, limited upward gaze, extensor plantar responses and ataxia from cerebellar dysfunction may occur but are not consistent signs. The diagnosis is suspected clinically and confirmed by computerized tomography (CT) scanning. Treatment is evacuation through burr holes.

Papilloedema can occur with a rise in intracranial pressure. It is virtually always bilateral with a chronic subdural haematoma, although it can be asymmetrical, usually greater on the side of a supratentorial lesion. It is usually unilateral with an orbital lesion.

5.25 A.T   B.T   C.F   D.F   E.T

A cough is a deep inspiration followed by a forceful expiration against a closed glottis which is then forced open to allow explosive exhalation. Intrathoracic pressures can be up to 40 kPa and the speed of exhaled air can be in the order of 900 km/hour. Although asthma commonly presents with episodic wheezing, a cough may be the only feature in children. It is a well-recognized side-effect of all angiotensin-converting enzyme (ACE) inhibitors. Cough is a result of stimulation of afferent pathways from mucosa of larynx, trachea and bronchi. As this requires integrity of the ninth and tenth cranial nerves it must be absent for a diagnosis of brainstem death. Opiates are antitussive agents.

5.26 A.T   B.T   C.F   D.F   E.F

Atracurium besylate is a non-depolarizing neuromuscular block-ing drug introduced in 1980. It is a bisquaternary nitrogenous plant derivative which is stable in acid solutions at 4°C but at normal physiological pH and temperature it is rapidly broken down to a tertiary amine – laudanosine – by a spontaneous reaction (Hoffmann elimination). Up to 50% of atracurium is also metabolized by the lung and plasma esterases to inactive metabolites. As such, accumulation is unlikely and it is often the drug of choice in liver and renal disease. Laudanosine, however, is accumulative, and as it is known to cause cerebral irritation in animals it may pose a problem with long-term use in critically ill patients. Nevertheless atracurium has a wide safety margin, is cardiostable (minimal change in heart rate) and has an elimination half-life of 20 min. It can release histamine to cause adverse reactions such as flushing. Although these reactions are rarely severe the incidence of histamine release can be reduced by using doses less than 0.5 mg/kg, slow injection and concomitant use of antihistamines.

5.27 A.T   B.T   C.T   D.F   E.F

Neuropathic pain is an abnormal perception of pain which may arise from any part of the nociceptive pathway. The possible underlying causes are numerous, and many painful conditions have a neuropathic element, e.g. trigeminal and postherpetic neuralgia, scar pain, postirradiation neuropathy and thalamic pain. The presentation is variable, but characteristic symptoms include pain from a stimulus such as light touch (allodynia), or inappropriately severe pain (hyperalgesia). The pain can be continuous, intermittent, paroxysmal or may be delayed, appearing only after repeated stimulation (hyperpathia). Theories as to the cause of neuropathic pain are many but both peripheral and central components are probably involved. Possibilities include increased sensitivity of C fibres, abnormal electrical connections (ephaptic), dorsal root hypersensitivity, abnormal central feedback loops and central chemical changes. Treatment is often ineffective but tricyclic antidepressants are used to increase brainstem 5-HT and noradrenaline as this has an inhibitory effect on pain via descending pathways. Sodium channel blockers, carbamazepine, lignocaine and mexiletine are thought to block sodium channels in A δ and C fibres to suppress spontaneous discharge. Although there is no consensus regarding the use of opiates, they may offer partial or complete relief. Other methods include capsaicin cream, topical aspirin, ketamine, clonidine and transcutaneous electrical nerve stimulation (TENS). Unsurprisingly, 5-HT antagonists have no beneficial effect on neuropathic pain. (See: McQuay HJ *et al.* (1992) Opioid sensitivity of chronic pain: a patient controlled analgesic model. *Anaesthesia* **47**, 757–767.)

5.28 A.T **B.**F **C.**F **D.**F **E.**T

As CPK is found in heart muscle, brain and skeletal muscle, damage to any of these increases levels, e.g. massive muscle necrosis with MH. Duchenne muscular dystrophy is characterized by progressive proximal limb weakness with pseudohypertrophy of the calves. Although the diagnosis is often made clinically the CPK can be 100–200 times higher than normal. CPK rises within 4–8 hours after a myocardial infarction, peaking at 1–2 days. The magnitude of the rise is a rough index of the extent of damage. A second rise suggests extension of the infarction, but levels are normal in angina. Other causes of raised CPK include physical exertion, surgery and intramuscular injections. Acute liver cell damage (hepatitis) leads to an increase in aspartate transaminase, lactate dehydrogensae and, if there is biliary obstruction, alkaline phosphatase. Paget's disease increases alkaline phosphatase but CPK is normal.

5.29 A.T B.T C.T D.F E.T
Decompression sickness results from the liberation of nitrogen (N) bubbles into the circulation on passing from a high to a low atmospheric pressure, e.g. when a diver surfaces. Apart from generalized weakness and malaise, symptoms depend on where the bubbles embolize. They include:

neurological	– ataxia ('the staggers'), visual field defects, peripheral neuropathies
musculoskeletal	– gas in muscles, joints and tendons causes pain and stiffness ('the bends')
skin	– pruritus, subcutaneous emphysema ('the creeps'), rashes
respiratory	– hyperventilation, chest pain and a cough ('the chokes')

Treatment includes immediate recompression followed by gradual decompression. Breathing a helium–oxygen mixture and hyperbaric oxygen may also be useful. Other supportive measures include supine positioning, rehydration and sedation. This usually results in a complete cure if initiated within an hour of the symptoms developing. Without adequate treatment decompression sickness may progress to acute respiratory distress syndrome (ARDS) and generalized cardiovascular shock with an associated high mortality. (See: Pennefather J, Lowry C, Edmonds C (1994) *Diving and Subaquatic Medicine*, 3rd edn. Butterworth–Heinemann, Oxford.)

5.30 A.T B.T C.T D.F E.T
High output cardiac failure is uncommon. It occurs when the heart is unable to meet the perfusion requirements of tissue metabolism despite an increased cardiac output. This is classically found in severe anaemia (loss of oxygen-carrying capacity), thyrotoxicosis (increased basal metabolic rate and therefore demand) and Paget's disease (rare, but with increased demand due to new bone formation). High output can also occur from an increase in preload as found with systemic to pulmonary shunts, AV fistulae used for haemodialysis and in aortic incompetence. Pulmonary embolus is associated with hypotension and low cardiac output.

5.31 A.F B.T C.F D.F E.F
The commonest cause of painless rectal bleeding is haemorrhoids but rectal cancer, inflammatory disease and angiodys-

plasias can occur at any age and must be excluded. Digital examination is mandatory and should be followed by sigmoidoscopy, particularly as haemorrhoids cannot be felt. Fibreoptic colonoscopy is also appropriate as it can visualize the bowel as far as the caecum. A double-contrast barium enema is the investigation of choice where change in bowel habit is the presenting symptom. A barium meal is not suitable for investigating rectal bleeding – it looks at the stomach or small bowel in cases of melaena. Prothrombin time will not isolate the cause of bleeding to the gut. CT scanning is insufficiently sensitive to pick up causes of rectal bleeding. However, it is useful in assessing local spread of malignant tumours and confirming a clinical diagnosis of acute diverticulosis. Angiodysplasia may require radioisotope scanning using the patient's own red blood cells or highly selective arteriography to localize the source of bleeding. The Schilling test is used to confirm a diagnosis of pernicious anaemia.

5.32 A.T **B.**T **C.**F **D.**T **E.**F

An air embolism occurs when venous pressure is lower than atmospheric pressure. As such it is particularly likely to occur in the sitting position with neurosurgical procedures as venous pressure in the head will be low and the dural sinuses, prevented from collapsing by their bony attachments, can allow air to be sucked in. This finds its way to the right side of the heart and, as it is compressed but not expelled by each beat, blood flow to the lungs will be impeded. This leads to a fall in end-tidal CO_2 (although this is quite insensitive, requiring 1.5–4.0 ml of air per kg), cyanosis, increases in pulmonary artery pressure (PAP) and CVP, a tachycardia, and a decreased cardiac output resulting in hypotension. The ECG may show signs of strain and atrial fibrillation or ventricular ectopics can occur. N_2O, if in use, diffuses into the air bubbles, increasing their volume to exacerbate the problem. The air can also pass into the systemic circulation through the pulmonary vasculature or from septal defects (20–30% of the population have a probe patent foramen ovale). This is catastrophic as the bubbles can obstruct the coronary or cerebral vessels. Air embolism can be detected by auscultation, listening for the characteristic tinkling sounds or a 'mill wheel' murmur. Doppler ultrasonography, transoesophageal echocardiography, a rise in end-tidal oxygen concentration and fall in dynamic lung compliance (measured by sideline spirometry) have also been found useful. Treatment is to prevent further embolism by sealing the open veins (i.e. flood wound with fluids) or by increasing venous pressure whilst attempting to remove the air via a central venous line or a special multiport retrieval catheter.

5.33 **A**.T **B**.F **C**.F **D**.F **E**.T
Prior to birth, oxygenated blood passes through the umbilical vein to the great veins and then to the right atrium. Most passes through the foramen ovale to the left atrium but some enters the right ventricle to the pulmonary artery. High pulmonary pressure forces blood through the ductus arteriosus to the aorta. Deoxygenated blood exits through the umbilical arteries which arise from the internal iliac vessels. At birth, placental blood flow stops, peripheral vascular resistance increases and the pressures in the left side of the heart increase. At the same time, lung expansion increases compliance and decreases pulmonary vascular resistance. This promotes blood flow through the lungs and the fall in right heart pressure leads to closure of the foramen ovale. The ductus arteriosus normally takes a few days to close after birth; closure is due to an increase in oxygen tension and a decrease in prostaglandins. Some situations (e.g. prematurity, acidosis, hypoxia) can lead to persistent fetal circulation with reversal of blood flow through ductus arteriosus, i.e. from aorta to lungs via pulmonary artery. Indomethacin or surgery may be required to close the duct. In some types of congenital heart disease (Fallot's, aortic coarctation), patency of the duct is vital to life. Prostaglandin E_1 may be used to buy time prior to surgery to create a temporary connection from the aorta to the pulmonary artery or curative surgery. Umbilical artery cannulation is best carried out within the first 15–30 min after birth as any delay makes it increasingly difficult. After 24 h or so cannulation requires a cut down.

5.34 **A**.T **B**.F **C**.F **D**.F **E**.T
Lead interferes with haem and globin synthesis and binds to bone. Clinical symptoms include anorexia, nausea and vomiting, a blue line on the gums, constipation often with severe abdominal colic, peripheral neuropathy and an encephalopathy. The haematological effects include a sideroblastic anaemia, mild haemolysis due to red cell membrane damage and punctuate basophilia (red cells containing aggregates of

RNA). Treatment following removal of the source is chelation of iron by sodium calcium edetate, D-penicillamine or dimercaprol.

5.35 A.F B.T C.T D.T E.T
A lesion in the spinal canal at any level below T10 can cause a cauda equina syndrome. Lumbar disc prolapse is the commonest cause, although spinal stenosis from degenerative disease (e.g. old age or ankylosing spondylitis), neurofibromas and ependymomas must be excluded. Arachnoiditis, a very rare but well-recognized complication of spinal and extradural anaesthesia, can also cause this devastating condition. Suggested aetiological factors of arachnoiditis following these anaesthetic techniques include poor asepsis technique and infection, spinal cord trauma, use of distilled water, blood, ischaemia, direct local anaesthetic (LA) toxicity plus additives such as sodium bisulphite, LA contaminants and accidental injection of neural toxins. More recently, it has been associated with use of indwelling spinal catheters (possibly due to poor mixing of hyperbaric lignocaine with CSF, leading to local toxicity), repeat attempts after 'failed spinal' and after transient radicular irritation following single-shot injection. Clinical signs can present slowly over days to weeks and are so variable that delay in diagnosis often occurs. Symptoms include a mixture of lower limb weakness, loss of reflexes, perineal numbness, loss of anal tone, bowel and bladder dysfunction and impotence. There is little effective treatment and chances of recovery are poor. (See Cheng ACK (1994) Cauda equina syndrome. *Anesthesia and Analgesia* **8**, 157–159.)

5.36 A.F B.T C.F D.T E.T
A normal, or Gaussian, distribution is graphically represented as a bell-shaped curve. It requires continuously variable data (e.g. height, weight, age) as opposed to discrete data (e.g. dead/alive, yes/no). Its importance lies in the fact that a sample population undergoing statistical analysis by parametric test is required to be 'normal' In this situation the mean (sum of the data divided by sample number), mode (most commonly occurring value) and median (value of the middle observation of a ranked sample) will be the same. The mean value and range give no information about the distribution of observations around the mean. This is achieved, instead, by calculating the *variance*. As this is often difficult to manipulate statistically,

it is more conventional to use the square root of the variance, i.e. the *standard deviation*. Thus, standard deviation expresses the variability of a sample and conventionally 1, 2 and 3 standard deviations are taken to contain 68%, 95% and 99.7% of the data, respectively. The *standard error of the mean* is different as it is an indication of how well the mean of a sample represents the true population mean. It is derived by dividing the standard deviation by the square root of the sample number. Thus the standard error of the mean is large when sample number is small, i.e. the sample mean is less likely to represent the population mean.

5.37 A.T B.T C.T D.F E.T
Pulmonary oedema results from a large increase of fluid in the alveoli and is characterized by dyspnoea, orthopnoea, wheezing and cough with production of frothy blood-stained sputum. Certain factors promote fluid transfer from the vascular compartment to the alveoli:

1. Increased pulmonary capillary (hydrostatic) pressure (e.g. left ventricular failure (LVF), mitral stenosis).
2. Decreased plasma oncotic pressure (e.g. hypoalbuminaemia).
3. Damage to alveolar–capillary membrane, i.e. increase in permeability (e.g. ARDS),
4. Acute severe subatmospheric airway pressure (e.g. large airway obstruction).

Other causes that have an uncertain aetiology, e.g. severe head injury and naloxone, are thought to cause pulmonary oedema via a neurogenic mechanism whereby sudden catecholamine release causes vasoconstriction and increases in both lung capillary pressures and capillary permeability. An atrial myxoma is a benign tumour found most often in the left atrium. It can obstruct the mitral valve to mimic the signs and symptoms of mitral stenosis including LVF and pulmonary oedema. Constrictive pericarditis prevents cardiac filling in late diastole. This results in a considerable rise in venous pressure, causing hepatomegaly, ascites and peripheral oedema. Pulmonary oedema is not a problem and chest radiographs usually show an enlarged heart due to pericardial thickening with clear lung fields.

5.38 A.F B.F C.F D.T E.T

Lasers (light amplification by stimulated emission of radiation) use non-ionizing radiation to destroy tissue by heat. This is achieved by passing a high voltage between two electrodes at each end of a long narrow tube, usually containing gas. The current produced 'excites' the atoms of the gas to a higher energy level. Light energy of a particular wavelength is given out as the excited atoms return to their original state. Mirrors are used to bounce this light back and forth through the tube, stimulating the excited atoms to give out their energy. This amplifies the light to produce the laser beam. Laser light differs from ordinary light in three ways: firstly, it is highly monochromatic light consisting of photons with a well-defined, very narrow band of wavelengths; secondly, the light is coherent, i.e. the electromagnetic fields of all photons in the laser beam oscillate synchronously; and thirdly, the light is collimated, i.e. has minimal dispersion. These characteristics allow lasers to generate intense light beams efficiently and accurately to deliver energy to small target sites. Gases used include argon (photocoagulation in ophthalmology) and carbon dioxide (ENT and neurosurgery for precise cutting and coagulation), while NdYAG (neodymium–yttrium–aluminium–garnet) for debulking tumours and prostatectomies is a solid rod in which the atoms are excited by a discharge lamp beside the rod. (See: Rampil IJ (1992) Anesthetic considerations for laser surgery. *Anesthesia and Analgesia* **74**, 424–435.)

5.39 A.F B.T C.T D.F E.T

Sterilization refers to the killing of all organisms. This can be achieved by autoclaves, ethylene oxide and gamma irradiation. Autoclaving employs steam at high pressure and temperature and is probably the most efficient, quickest, simplest and cheapest method available, but it can damage delicate equipment. Ethylene oxide provides a useful alternative but it is expensive, takes several hours, and is inflammable and toxic. In addition, to allow the gas to escape a period of 10 days must elapse before the equipment is safe to use. Gamma irradiation requires a high capital outlay and is thus not economically viable other than for large companies producing pre-packaged disposable sterile items. Not all equipment requires sterilization and there are less stringent forms of cleansing such as *decontamination* and *disinfection*. Decontamination does not kill organisms or spores but refers to the physical removal of infected matter, e.g. cleaning the operating table. Disinfection kills most infective organisms with the exception of the most resistant such as spores. This can be achieved by pasteurization (heating to 70°C for 20 min, 80°C for 10 min), boiling (5 min), chlorhexidine and glutaraldehydethe and is useful for endoscopy equipment, etc.

5.40 A.T B.T C.T D.F E.T
Nocturia usually occurs with polyuria caused as a result of excessive intake of water, increased excretion of solute as in hyperglycaemia, or defective concentrating ability as with end-stage renal failure or vasopressin (ADH) deficiency. Chronic pyelonephritis commonly results from incompetent or absent one-way valves at the vesicoureteric junction, which allows urine to pass back up the ureters to the kidney. Although reflux usually ceases at puberty with growth of the bladder, scarring has already occurred and it frequently progresses (often without further infection) to end-stage renal failure. Acute glomerulonephritis encompasses a wide spectrum of diseases, all of which cause immune destruction of the glomeruli which may lead to end-stage renal failure and hence reduced concentrating ability and nocturia. Benign prostatic enlargement is a common cause of nocturia in men. Oliguria occurs with acute tubular necrosis, although polyuria can occur in the recovery phase.

5.41 A.T B.F C.T D.T E.T
The hydrogen ion concentration is twice normal, suggesting a metabolic acidosis. Normal cardiac index is $2.8–3.5 \, l/min/m^2$ and clinical features of cardiogenic shock are usually seen with a cardiac index below $1.8 \, l/min/m^2$. Urine volume is mainly determined by diet and fluid intake and lies between 800 and 2500 ml daily. The minimum volume needed is determined by amount of solute (urea and electrolytes) being excreted. This is about 800 mosmol daily and, as the maximum urine concentration is 1200 mosmol/l, the minimum volume needed is about 650 ml. A urine output of less than 0.5 ml/kg/h is usually the first indication of impaired renal function. The mixed venous oxygen saturation is probably the best single indicator of the adequacy of oxygen transport. It represents the amount of oxygen left after perfusion of the systemic circulation, and so can be regarded as the oxygen reserve or an indicator of the balance between oxygen delivery and consumption. 65% or less

in a critically ill patient suggests tissue hypoxia. An isolated systolic BP of 90 mmHg does not necessarily indicate hypotension or hypovolaemia. It can be regarded as being within normal limits, depending on the patient's previous BP.

5.42 A.F B.F C.F D.T E.F
Many diagnostic procedures have been described over the years. Few have stood the test of time, e.g. red cell osmotic fragility, chemiluminescence, platelet nucleotide depletion tests. Serum CPK is too insensitive. It is not reliably elevated in patients with MH susceptibility, but is frequently elevated as a result of trivial events such as minor trauma. Cholinesterase deficiency was initially thought to be linked to MH but this has been disproved. Abnormalities seen on muscle histology are non-specific but it is an important investigation to rule out the presence of other myopathies. MH susceptibility has been located to chromosome 19, the ryanodine receptor. This codes for the protein that controls calcium release in skeletal muscle. However, not all MH-susceptible families have this genetic defect, which supports the explanation that MH is a heterogeneous condition. Genetic studies alone, therefore, cannot be reliable although they are useful in conjunction with the most reliable method yet developed for diagnosis, the *in vitro* contracture test using caffeine, halothane or, more recently, ryanodine. This involves taking a piece of fresh skeletal muscle, placing it in physiological solution and measuring the tension induced by the addition of the test drug. MH susceptibility is confirmed with development of significant contracture. (See: Ording H (1988) Diagnosis of susceptibility to malignant hyperthermia in man. *British Journal of Anaesthesia* **60**, 287–302. Also: Hopkins PM, Halsall PJ, Ellis FR (1994) Editorial: Diagnosing malignant hyperthermia susceptibility. *Anaesthesia* **49**, 373–375.)

5.43 A.T B.F C.T D.T E.F
Adverse drug reactions are either dose-dependent and related to known actions of the drug, e.g. propofol decreases BP, or are unrelated to dose and not associated with predictable drug actions. The latter involve either *immune* anaphylactic reponses mediated primarily through IgE or IgG or *non-immune* (anaphylactoid) responses. Immune responses tend to require previous exposure, although there is some cross-sensitivity in patients with high levels of IgE (asthmatics, atopic individuals).

Non-immune anaphylactic responses occur without previous exposure, e.g. curare causing histamine release. Other potential immune-mediated pathways include cytotoxic (type II) reactions, e.g. blood transfusion, protamine; complement-mediated (type III) reactions caused by soluble antigen/antibody complexes, e.g. thiopentone; and delayed (type IV) reactions involving T cells combining with antigen, e.g. thiopentone again! Adverse drug reactions have been reported with most of the commonly used anaesthetic drugs. With suxamethonium the incidence is 1 in 1200, while with thiopentone it is 1 in 20 000. Penicillin has a reported incidence of 1–10% and of these 2–8% have cross-sensitivity to cephalosporins. LAs are generally very unlikely to cause an adverse drug reaction. However, if one occurs it is more likely to be with an ester LA, e.g. procaine, as these are derived from para-aminobenzoic acid (PABA). Some opiates cause sensitivity reactions by direct histamine release (e.g. morphine), but fentanyl is relatively safe.

5.44 A.T B.T C.T D.F E.T
Malignant hypertension consists of accelerated hypertension (diastolic pressure exceeding 120 mmHg) associated with raised intracranial pressure (hence papilloedema) and retinopathy. The pathophysiology includes necrotizing arteritis, proliferative endarteritis and fibrinoid necrosis with increased vascular reactivity due to vasoconstricting hormones (angiotensin II, noradrenaline, ADH). Causes include chronic essential hypertension, acute renal failure, head injuries, stroke, phaeochromocytoma, pregnancy and acute withdrawal of antihypertensive agents. It is a medical emergency requiring prompt treatment, but the decision to lower BP rapidly should not be based on arterial pressure alone as the aim is to prevent and reverse end-organ damage which can manifest as unstable angina, left ventricular failure, myocardial infarction, aortic dissection, CVA and renal failure, amongst others. A reduction in BP of 15–25% per 24 hours is considered adequate as impaired BP autoregulation can cause organ ischaemia with a more rapid fall.

5.45 A.F B.F C.F D.F E.T
Calcium channel antagonists reduce myocardial contractility, depress initiation and propagation of cardiac electrical impulses, and cause vasodilatation by interfering with slow

channel calcium entry into cells. Halothane, enflurane and isoflurane also exert significant calcium channel blocking activity and an additive effect does occur. In practice, this is rarely a problem but greater perioperative vigilance is necessary. MAOIs are antidepressant drugs which have no significant interaction with inhalational agents, adversely interacting with pethidine, sympathomimetic agents, (ephedrine, metaraminol) and tyramine-rich foods (cheese and red wine) to cause excessive central 5-HT activity which can result in agitation, hypertension and convulsions. Warfarin antagonizes the action of vitamin K, involved in the synthesis of coagulation factors II, VII, IX and X in the liver. Efficacy is reduced by hepatic enzyme-inducing drugs (e.g. phenytoin) and enhanced by drugs which displace it from protein binding sites (e.g. sulphonamides and NSAIDs). It has no significant interactions with inhalational agents. Similarly, NSAIDs and hypoglycaemic agents have several important drug interactions, but not with inhalational.

5.46 A.F B.F C.T D.F E.F
Difficult intubation in a neonate is due to several factors including a large head-to-body size ratio, short neck, a relatively big tongue in a small mouth and a floppy epiglottis. This projects posteriorly and requires lifting with the tip of a straight blade to allow visualization of the glottis. Neonates also have a more cephalad larynx (C4 as opposed to C6 in an adult). The narrowest point of the airway is at the level of the cricoid cartilage just below the vocal cords. This has no bearing on the ease or difficulty of intubation; its significance is that the epithelial lining easily becomes oedematous after minimal trauma, potentially leading to significant airway narrowing. The trachea is short (only 4–5 cm), leaving little margin of error regarding the length of the endotracheal tube, which can thus more easily fall out or pass endobronchially. In addition neonates have a flat, relatively wide face, causing difficulties in obtaining a good seal for mask ventilation, and narrow, easily blocked nasal passages. These factors can make oxygenation difficult between intubation attempts, particularly as a high metabolic rate relative to adults leads to more rapid desaturation.

5.47 A.T   B.T   C.F   D.T   E.T

A metabolic acidosis is caused either by an increase in acid or by loss of the alkaline buffer (bicarbonate) that normally maintains physiological pH/H^+ concentration within strict limits. Causes include:

1. Increased acid ingestion, e.g. salicylate overdose.
2. Increased production of acid, e.g. ketone bodies in diabetes mellitus (DM), lactic acidosis.
3. Decreased excretion of acid, e.g. renal failure, renal tubular acidosis, acetazolamide.
4. Loss of bicarbonate, e.g. chronic diarrhoea, pancreatic and gastrointestinal fistulae.

Fanconi's syndrome is a disease of childhood due to defective renal tubular reabsorption of bicarbonate, amino acids, glucose, phosphate and urate. The loss of bicarbonate results in renal tubular acidosis with a systemic hyperchloraemic acidosis. In adults, an acquired syndrome occurs secondary to renal disease or heavy metal poisoning. Zollinger–Ellison syndrome (gastrinoma) arises from G cells in the pancreas to produce large amounts of gastrin which stimulates gastric acid secretion. Hyperventilation is a compensatory mechanism for metabolic acidosis.

5.48 A.T   B.T   C.F   D.T   E.T

Gastric emptying occurs by peristaltic contraction at a rate of 3 per min. Liquids leave first, then carbohydrates, proteins and fats. Delay can be multifactorial and includes physiological (age, anxiety state), pharmacological (opioids, anticholinergics, salbutamol, dopamine, alcohol, etc.) and pathological (obstruction, diabetes, renal failure, trauma, hypothyroidism, anorexia nervosa) factors. Obesity has a variable effect but usually increases delay. Cisapride increases acetylcholine in the myenteric plexus of the gut wall to increase lower oesophageal sphincter tone, gastric emptying and intestinal motility.

5.49 A.F   B.T   C.F   D.F   E.T

Thermal injury to skin occurs at temperatures above 45°C. Three zones of burn can be delineated: a central zone of coagulation, surrounded by a zone of stasis, viable only with adequate resuscitation, and a distant zone of hyperaemia which will recover. Oedema formation occurs due to protein loss and fluid shifts caused by increased vascular permeability (due to

cytokines, vasoactive substances, e.g. oxygen radicals, histamine), low oncotic capillary pressure and increased interstitial
osmotic pressure. Oedema is maximal within the first 24 hours.
Burns over 20%, or 15% if there is an associated inhalational
injury, require urgent fluid resuscitation to avoid circulatory
collapse. There is no consensus on the ideal fluid regime but it
is probably a mixture of albumin and crystalloid. Crystalloid
alone (Hartmann's, normal saline) should be administered at
2–4 ml/kg/day per % body surface area (BSA) burnt while a
suitable combination therapy of albumin and crystalloid would
be 1 ml/kg/day each per % BSA burnt. The aim is to give at
least 50% of the daily fluid requirement in the first 8 hours
after injury and titrate the rest to maintain urine output of 1–
2 ml/kg/hour. This may require invasive haemodynamic
monitoring. Other interventions include early intubation if
there is significant inhalational injury and prompt wound
debridement and grafting to reduce infection and improve
survival. Early nutrition is required as burns cause greater
nitrogen loss than any other form of trauma. Antibiotics are
required only if infection is established. Mortality is high at
extremes of age and when more than 60% BSA is involved.

5.50 A.T **B.**T **C.**T **D.**F **E.**T
Cholelithiasis is very common. Women are three times more
likely to develop stones, as are first degree relatives of patients
with gallstones. Predisposing factors include obesity, pregnancy
(but not the OCP) and dietary factors such as a high
consumption of unrefined carbohydrate and a diet low in fibre.
Crohn's disease, terminal ileal resection and a jejuno-ileal bypass
for obesity also give rise to increased incidence of gallstones.
Diseases associated with gallstones include DM, type IV
hyperlipoproteinaemia and cirrhosis of the liver. Patients with
haemolytic anaemia, sickle cell disease and thalassaemia also
show increased prevalence of pigmented stones.

5.51 A.T **B.**F **C.**T **D.**F **E.**T
The incidence of Down's syndrome is 1 in 660 live births. Non-
dysjunction of chromosomes during germ cell formation
(trisomy 21) is the commonest cause; it is rarely due to
chromosomal translocation in parental cells. About 50% have
congenital heart disease, the most common being septal
defects or AV canal defects. Many go on to develop a floppy
mitral valve (50%) or aortic regurgitation (10%) as adults.

Potential problems as regards anaesthesia include a difficult intubation as a result of a flat face, small mouth, large tongue, mandibular hypoplasia, pharyngeal hypotonia and possibly subglottic stenosis. In addition, approximately 20% have ligamentous laxity of atlanto-axial joint which may allow C1–C2 subluxation and spinal cord injury. As most patients are asymptomatic, radiological screening is wise prior to surgery. Although susceptible to leukaemia, immune function is normal. Patients with Down's syndrome are no more susceptible to MH than the general population.

5.52 A.F B.T C.T D.F E.T
Anterior uveitis is due to inflammation of the uveal tract. It is subdivided into iritis and iridocyclitis (if the iris and anterior part of the ciliary body are both involved) and can be acute or chronic. Patients present with photophobia, pain, redness and decreased vision in the affected eye. Inflammatory cells and protein can be found in the aqueous humour. Some of the more common causes include sarcoidosis, syphilis, tuberculosis, inflammatory bowel disease and psoriatic arthropathy. Treatment is with mydriatic agents to reduce ciliary spasm and prevent development of posterior synechiae, and topical or systemic steroids to suppress the immune response. Complications of uveitis include cataracts, glaucoma and retinal detachment. Toxoplasmosis and cytomegalovirus (CMV) cause posterior uveitis or chorioretinitis (inflammation behind the posterior border of vitreous base). Uveitis occurs in 20% of patients with juvenile RA but association in adult RA is strictly coincidental; these patients are more likely to suffer from scleritis.

5.53 A.F B.T C.T D.F E.F
It is vital to recognize MH as soon as possible. Prolonged masseter spasm, an unexplained tachycardia and a raised end-tidal CO_2 with tachypnoea are usually the first abnormal signs. If adequate treatment is not initiated promptly, the maximal possible oxygen delivery will not be enough to sustain the massively elevated oxygen consumption. Thus aerobic metabolism will give way to anaerobic and a severe metabolic acidosis will prevail, together with cell death.

5.54 A.F B.T C.F D.T E.T
ACE inhibitors, e.g. captopril, enalapril and lisinopril, prevent conversion of angiotensin I (produced by the action of renin

on angiotensinogen) to angiotensin II. This prevents angio-tensin II-induced vasoconstriction, catecholamine release from the adrenal medulla and aldosterone production by the adrenal cortex. The resulting vasodilatation decreases periph-eral vascular resistance to reduce both preload and afterload, making ACE inhibitors useful as first-line treatment in both essential hypertension and heart failure. A diuretic action from increased sodium and water loss further improves heart failure. Side-effects can include profound hypotension following the first dose, tachycardia, loss of taste, gastrointestinal distur-bances, cough, proteinuria and bone marrow suppression. Renal function can deteriorate and hyperkalaemia may be a problem if pre-existing renal disease is present. Patients with renal artery stenosis require high levels of angiotensin II to generate an adequate filtration pressure at the glomerulus. Use of ACE inhibitors leads to a rapid but reversible deterioration in renal function, so much so that this can be used as a diagnostic test. Unlike beta blockers and aspirin, it has not been shown to improve survival after a myocardial infarction. ACE inhibitors are contraindicated in pregnancy as they reduce uterine blood flow. (See: Kellow NH (1994) The renin-angiotensin system and angiotensin converting enzyme inhibi-tors. *Anaesthesia* **49**, 613–622.)

5.55 A.T B.F C.F D.T E.F
Potassium is the principal intracellular cation present at 135–150 mmol/l with 3.5–5.0 mmol/l in plasma. Sodium is the principal extracellular cation with a normal plasma level of 135–145 mmol/l. Daily requirements are of the order of 2 mmol/kg/day. Men require 8 mg of iron daily, about half of the amount needed for menstruating women. Opinion is divided on the minimum calcium intake for adults: WHO recommend 500 mg/day, USA 800 mg/day (about 0.1 mmol/kg/day). Normal water intake is in the order of 20–60 ml/kg/day.

5.56 A.T B.F C.F D.T E.T
Blood is mixed with an anticoagulant, a stabilizer and other substances to preserve and prolong shelf-life. The original acid citrate dextrose (ACD) was replaced by CPD-A with added phosphate and adenine to improve red cell function and longevity. Nowadays most blood that is given has had all its components (platelets, immunoglobulins, clotting factors,

plasma, albumin) removed by centrifuge to leave red blood cells which are then resuspended in SAG-M mixture. This has the advantage of further extending shelf-life to about 42 days and decreasing viscosity to give better flow characteristics, despite the blood having a haematocrit of 55%. Although blood is stored at 4°C some metabolism continues and results in the production of lactate and degeneration of ATP and 2,3-DPG levels with time. In addition, oxidant damage to cell membranes increases fragility and membrane permeability, leading to swelling, spherocyte formation and potassium leakage. Stored blood thus becomes increasingly acidotic with pH falling to about 7.0 at 12 days. Bicarbonate will be reduced to about 10 mmol/l and potassium may rise to over 10 mmol/l. There will be virtually no platelet activity after 2 days, even in whole blood. Clotting factors (particularly V and VIII) also deteriorate, thus impairing the coagulation ability of stored blood over 1 week old. Stored blood has had its calcium chelated out by citrate to prevent it from clotting and rapid transfusion can result in a fall in ionized calcium. This, in turn, has negatively inotropic actions on cardiac output and requires treatment with intravenous calcium supplements.

5.57 A.F   B.T   C.T   D.F   E.T
Metastases from a follicular carcinoma of the thyroid are blood-borne and are most often found in bone, lungs and brain, whereas papillary thyroid carcinomas tend to be found in cervical lymph nodes. Carcinoma of the prostate accounts for 70% of all cancers in men and metastatic bone pain is a common presentation. Hypernephroma has a direct haematogenous spread to bone, liver and lung. Hepatocellular carcinomas are the commonest primary liver tumour. Most frequently associated with chronic hepatitis B, the tumour tends to invade the portal and hepatic veins and spreads to abdominal lymph nodes, lungs and bone. Bronchial carcinoid is no longer considered to be as benign as once thought. Many are locally invasive and about 30% spread to regional lymph nodes with a further 10% travelling to distant organs, especially the liver and brain but not commonly to bone.

5.58 A.T   B.T   C.T   D.F   E.F
The LM became commercially available in 1988. It consists of a connecting tube attached to an inflatable oval cuff which overlies the glottis to form a low-pressure (20–25 cm H_2O)

seal. Its size prevents intubation of the oesophagus, trachea or bronchus. It maintains normal respiratory physiology and is suitable for both spontaneous and positive pressure ventilation. It cannot protect against aspiration of gastric contents. Various sizes are available ranging from neonatal (size 1: less than 6.4 kg) through to a large adult (size 5). There are also flexible reinforced tubes which resist kinking. Obstruction can occur with both types, particularly with the floppy epiglottis of an infant. Propofol as an induction agent facilitates insertion of the LM although it can be used following thiopentone. The LM has been used successfully as an aid or an alternative to difficult intubation (and is included in the American Society of Anesthesiologists difficult airway algorithm), for bronchoscopy, and in resuscitation and emergency medicine. Current controversy centres on its use with positive pressure ventilation, prolonged anaesthesia (>2 hours) and laparoscopic and non-laparoscopic intra-abdominal surgery. Latex sensitivity is not a contraindication to its use as it is manufactured from silicone and thus contains no latex. (See: Pennant JH, White PF (1993) The laryngeal mask airway: its uses in anesthesiology. *Anesthesiology* **79**, 144–163. Also: Verghese C, Brimacombe JR (1996) Survey of laryngeal mask airway usage in 11 910 patients: safety and efficacy for conventional and nonconventional usage. *Anesthesia and Analgesia* **82**, 129–133.)

5.59 **A**.T **B**.T **C**.F **D**.T **E**.T
Raynaud's disease is ischaemia of the extremities caused by arteriolar vasospasm on exposure to cold or emotional stimuli. Sympathetic block prevents the vasospasm but is more effective in the feet than in the hands. Hyperhidrosis is excessive sweating. Eccrine glands are supplied by postganglionic sympathetic fibres and, as these are effectively blocked by sympathectomy, this is a useful treatment. CRPS type II, previously called 'causalgia', is associated with peripheral nerve injuries, and sympathetic blocks are of both diagnostic and therapeutic value. Diabetic peripheral neuropathy arises from atherosclerosis obliterans to nutrient arteries of peripheral nerves. Vasospasm is not involved and therefore sympathectomy will not improve symptoms. There is mixed opinion as to the value of sympathectomy for intermittent claudication. It may possibly be useful for ischaemic rest pain when surgery is impractical. (See: Gordon S *et al.* (1994) The role of

sympathectomy in current surgical practice. *European Journal of Vascular Surgery* **8**, 129–137.)

5.60 A.F   B.T   C.T   D.F   E.T

Ventricular tachycardia (VT) can be difficult to differentiate from supraventricular tachycardia (SVT). The heart rates likely to occur are similar and usually lie between 140 and 220 beats per minute. With SVT, P waves should be distinguishable on the ECG. Although P waves are unlikely with VT, they do occur if the atria continue to depolarize independently or through retrograde conduction (when P waves will usually be inverted). A fusion beat is characteristic of VT and occurs when a P wave is conducted through the atrioventricular node and mixes with an impulse from the VT to produce the characteristic change in the ECG. Other features distinguishing VT from SVT include broad and often bizarre complexes (greater than 140 ms), extreme left axis deviation and absence of response to carotid sinus massage or adenosine.

5.61 A.F   B.T   C.F   D.F   E.T

CPAP can be used to improve ventilatory function in spontaneously breathing patients. Appropriate clinical situations for its use include acute hypoxaemic respiratory failure, weaning ventilated patients and improving oxygenation in one-lung ventilation and in obstructive sleep apnoea. At no point in the respiratory cycle should the airway pressure become negative. As such, CPAP requires either a reservoir bag or a fresh gas flow in excess of maximal inspiratory gas flow. CPAP is usually delivered via a tracheal tube but a tight-fitting face mask can also be used. Unfortunately the mask can be uncomfortable, especially for long periods, and is only suitable for patients who are alert and able to clear secretions and protect their airway. The aim of CPAP is to improve oxygenation by reducing V/Q mismatch. This is achieved by increasing functional residual capacity (FRC) as a result of reducing airway atelectasis and recruiting alveoli in already atelectatic areas. The optimal level of CPAP is unknown but it should not adversely affect cardiac output and oxygen delivery or cause barotrauma from hyperinflation and high intrathoracic pressures. The usual range is 3–15 cm H_2O. It is also important in neonates with respiratory distress syndrome and in tracheomalacia and laryngomalacia. In any baby with a tracheal tube, at least 3–5 cm H_2O CPAP is essential to replace the 'auto-PEEP'

which it normally produces as a result of being an obligate nasal
breather – a manoeuvre designed to reduce closing capacity.

5.62 A.F B.F C.F D.T E.T

The optic nerve (II) traverses the optic canal to supply the
retina. The trochlear (IV, superior oblique) and abducens (VI,
lateral rectus) pass via the superior orbital fissure. The three
branches of the trigeminal nerve – ophthalmic, mandibular
and maxillary – exit via the superior orbital fissure, foramen
ovale and foramen rotundum, respectively. The facial nerve
(VII, motor to face muscles) exits the pons to travel with the
acoustic nerve (VIII) through the IAM. The vagus shares the
jugular foramen with the glossopharyngeal (IX) and spinal
accessory nerves (XI).

5.63 A.T B.T C.T D.T E.F

Thyroid-stimulating hormone (TSH) receptor antibodies, Ha-
shimoto's thyroiditis and post ^{131}I therapy are the commonest
causes of hypothyroidism. It is 6 times more common in females,
with incidence increasing with age. The clinical features are non-
specific, particularly in the elderly. They include:

neurological	– myopathy, cerebellar ataxia, carpal tun-nel syndrome, depression
cardiac	– angina, bradycardia, hypertension
haematological	– macrocytosis, normochromic anaemia
dermatological	– dry coarse skin, malar flush, alopecia, vitiligo, oedema
reproductive	– menorrhagia, infertility
gastrointestinal	– constipation
general	– mild obesity, hoarse voice, cold intoler-ance, tiredness, goitre

Investigations show raised TSH and low T_4; antithyroid
antibodies may or may not be present. Thyroxine replacement
is essential. Myxoedema coma is a rare medical emergency that
requires urgent intravenous triiodothyronine. Body temperature may be as low as 25°C, seizures are common and the
mortality rate is up to 50%. Oligomenorrhoea is not a common
feature – it is common in hyperthyroidism.

5.64 A.T B.T C.F D.T E.T

The hazards of lasers (light amplification by stimulated
emission of radiation) are potentially catastrophic without

strict safety procedures. Eyes need protection and both patients and operating staff should wear goggles which absorb radiation of the laser wavelength. A secondary beam of light should be used to aim the laser, and patient skin protection can be achieved by water-soaked pads. Normal tracheal tubes are unsuitable for use in shared airway procedures as lasers can ignite flammable materials such as rubber and plastic. Suitable replacements include specially manufactured metallic-coated tubes that are resistant to carbon dioxide laser beams, or an all-purpose stainless steel flexible tube. As these are very expensive (and not available in paediatric sizes) an alternative is to wrap a normal tracheal tube with aluminium foil. In addition, tube cuffs, should be filled with water (preferably coloured to be seen more easily) because air in the cuff can contribute to a fire. As both oxygen and nitrous oxide support combustion, caution should be exercised during laser treatment of the airway. Consideration should be given to using helium or nitrogen as carriers for oxygen as they do not support combustion. Jet ventilation is not contraindicated with laser treatment. Fleximetallic tubes only have a spiral of steel in silicone and are thus unsuitable for use with lasers. (See: Rampil IJ (1992) Anesthetic considerations for laser surgery. *Anesthesia and Analgesia* **74**, 424–435.)

5.65 A.T B.F C.F D.F E.T
Brainstem death tests can only be performed with profound coma, where the underlying cause is known, where drugs (e.g. alcohol, sedatives, hypnotics, muscle relaxants, poisons) have been excluded and after correction of hypothermia (core temperature >35°C) and any other endocrine or metabolic conditions which may interfere with the tests. The tests must be performed by two doctors, preferably the consultant in charge of the case and another clinically independent of the first, both registered for over 5 years. The tests must be performed twice, with a time gap agreed by all the staff involved. A minimum of 6 hours must have elapsed since onset of coma or at least 24 hours after restoration of an adequate circulation. The criteria for brainstem death in the UK are:

1. Fixed unresponsive pupils to direct and consensual light, absent corneal reflexes.
2. Absent doll's eyes movement, i.e. the eyes do not move when the head is rotated.

3. Absent eye movements on instilling cold water onto the tympanic membrane.
4. Absent motor response to painful stimulation in any cranial nerve distribution.
5. Absent gag reflex to pharyngeal, laryngeal or tracheal stimulation.
6. Absent spontaneous respiration when P_aCO_2 is more than 6.7 kPa (50 mmHg).

The auditory canals must first be checked to ensure that they are patent and both must be tested. Blood:gas tensions must be measured to ensure a PCO_2 >6.7 kPa. Spinal reflexes are often preserved since they have intact neural arcs independent of central regulation. An EEG is unnecessary as it can be misleading. (See: Pallis C (1982) Diagnosis of brain stem death I and II. *British Medical Journal* **285**, 1558–1560, 1641–1644.)

5.66 A.F B.T C.F D.F E.F
Tissue damage following surgery, severe trauma or burns causes metabolic, haematological and immunological changes mediated by the release of acute-phase substances such as interleukin-6 and cytokines. The sympathetic nervous system is stimulated, increasing release of catecholamines. The hypothalamic–pituitary–adrenal axis is activated. Stimulation of adrenocorticotrophic hormone (ACTH) release increases cortisol and this, along with catecholamines, is responsible for the catabolic response which includes lipolysis and increased muscle proteolysis and protein loss. There is an increased release of aldosterone and antidiuretic hormone, which are responsible for sodium and water retention and increased urinary potassium loss. Glucagon, arginine vasopressin, growth hormone, prolactin and endorphins also increase. Blood sugar increases through catecholamine-induced glycogenolysis and suppression of insulin. There is commonly a pyrexia and or rise in white cell count without an underlying infection. Thyroid hormone (T3>T4) falls. The magnitude of the acute-phase response is proportional to the amount of tissue damage and systemic disturbance inflicted. Attempts to minimize it by the use of high-dose opioids, non-steroidal anti-inflammatory drugs (NSAIDs) and extradural blockade have limited, if any, success.

5.67 A.F **B.**T **C.**T **D.**T **E.**T

This type of question can initially appear difficult to answer as pulmonary artery (PA) enlargement as an entity is not often discussed. The way to tackle the question is to think of possible physiological states that could lead to enlargement. These include left-to-right shunts (ASD, VSD), pulmonary hypertension and post-stenotic dilatation of pulmonary valve stenosis. Enlargement may be extreme, e.g. Eisenmenger's syndrome in association with a VSD or with a pulmonary artery aneurysm.

Fallot's	– PA ranges from normal to severely hypoplastic, pulmonary oligaemia
ASD	– PA enlargement with increased pulmonary blood flow
mitral stenosis	– chronically raised left atrial pressure causes pulmonary hypertension
pulmonary stenosis	– post-stenotic turbulence often leads to PA dilatation
cor pulmonale	– pulmonary hypertension and right ventricular enlargement

Decreased pulmonary artery diameter is seen in pulmonary atresia and in transposition of the great arteries.

5.68 A.F **B.**F **C.**F **D.**F **E.**F

Also known as Thomsen's disease, myotonia congenita can be either autosomal recessive or dominant. It presents early in childhood (6–8 years). Symptoms include myotonia (continued muscle contraction after cessation of voluntary effort), accentuated by immobility and cold but relieved with exercise. The condition is benign, does not progress and life expectancy is normal. A mildly impaired creatinine clearance is the only metabolic abnormality. EMG is characteristic but muscle biopsy is often inconclusive. Myotonic dystrophy is a more severe form of myotonia. It is an autosomal dominant condition that affects both sexes equally. Symptoms normally present in the late teens or twenties and usually affect the distal muscles first; this causes progressive muscle weakness and wasting. Other features include mental retardation, temporal balding, ptosis, cataracts, testicular atrophy and a progressive cardiomyopathy leading to conduction defects and arrhythmias. As with all myotonic conditions, suxamethonium is best avoided as it can induce prolonged contractures and precipitate fatal hyperkalaemia. Non-depolarizing muscle relaxants are not contraindicated but should be used with caution because of the associated muscle weakness: about half the normal dose is required but this should be titrated against effect. Local and regional techniques are safer, and overcome many of the problems of general anaesthesia.

5.69 A.T B.F C.F D.T E.T

Pre-eclampsia is a progressive disease with a variable mode of presentation developing any time after 20 weeks of pregnancy. The main features are hypertension (diastolic >90 mmHg), proteinuria (>300 mg/day) and oedema. The condition complicates about 6% of primigravid and 0.4% of multiparous pregnancies. Progression to eclampsia is rare (1 in 2000 but 10% of all maternal deaths). In normal pregnancy the spiral arteries supplying the placenta are invaded by trophoblast to convert the vascular supply to a low-pressure, high-flow system. Incomplete trophoblastic invasion occurs in pre-eclampsia, resulting in narrowed spiral arteries, placental ischaemia and release of factors which damage maternal vascular endothelial cells. These, in turn, produce procoagulents, vasoconstrictors, mitogens and other factors which have a further adverse effect on endothelial function. As this is important for maintaining fluid compartments, modifying smooth muscle contractility, preventing intravascular coagulation and controlling immune and inflammatory responses, the protean effects of pre-eclampsia are thus explained. Raised peripheral vascular resistance with increased permeability of the capillary membrane compounded by reduction in oncotic pressure from proteinuria results in fluid shifts from intravascular compartment into the tissues to cause laryngeal, peripheral and pulmonary oedema. CNS disturbances include headaches, hyperreflexia and seizures. Severe hypertension may cause intracranial haemorrhage. Epigastric pain and hepatic and renal dysfunction may occur when pre-eclampsia is severe, as does thrombocytopenia from increased consumption. Prevention is difficult. Aspirin, despite early hopes, has not proved helpful. Treatment focuses on reducing maternal and fetal complications. This includes controlling blood pressure, cautious rehydration to reverse intravascular hypovolaemia and administration of anticonvulsant agents. Ultimately, definitive treatment requires delivery of the baby. (See: Mushambi MC *et al.* (1996) Recent developments in the pathophysiology and management of pre-eclampsia. *British Journal of Anaesthesia* **76**, 133–148.)

5.70 **A.**F   **B.**T   **C.**T   **D.**F   **E.**F

Diathermy passes an alternating current at high frequency (300–3000 kHz) through the body. It creates heat and, by sequentially increasing current density, it can be used for coagulation, fulguration (destructive coagulation of the tissues), dissection and cutting. Monopolar diathermy includes the body in the electrical circuit by having two electrodes remote from each other. The indifferent electrode (diathermy plate) has a larger surface area to reduce current density and hence prevent the risk of burns. The active electrode (needle, forceps, etc.) concentrates the current to a small area to achieve the desired effect. Bipolar diathermy consists of two electrodes in one unit (forceps) so current only flows through the tissue being gripped to achieve greater accuracy, safety and less tissue damage, but at the expense of being less powerful. There is no need for an indifferent electrode and it is safer than monopolar diathermy in patients with cardiac pacemakers. Complications of monopolar diathermy include interference with monitoring equipment, pacemaker function, electrocution and burns from a poorly applied diathermy plate or flammable preparatory solution. Explosion from gas in obstructed bowel has also been reported. (See: Memon MA (1994) Surgical diathermy. *British Journal of Hospital Medicine* **52**, 403–407.)

5.71 **A.**T   **B.**F   **C.**T   **D.**T   **E.**T

There have been many tests devised to assess recovery of concentration, cognition, perception and motor function after anaesthesia. Steward devised a postanaesthetic recovery score that awards points for the patient's level of awareness, airway maintenance and movement. The p deletion test involves rows of random characters and assesses the speed with which the patient can find and delete the letter 'p'. The EEG is sensitive but expensive. The Maddox test assesses ocular divergence. The patient looks into an instrument in which the two eye fields are separated: the right eye sees an arrow and the left a scale; the patient states where the arrow seems to point to on the scale. The ideal test should be quick, simple, reproducible, inexpensive, without needing to be learned or requiring a skilled operator. The vast number of tests suggests that there is no singularly good one available. The Romberg test assesses dorsal column integrity. (See: Lockwood GG (1994) In: *Day Case Anaesthesia and Sedation* (Whitwam JG, ed), pp. 104–116. Blackwell Scientific, Oxford.)

5.72 **A**.F **B**.F **C**.F **D**.T **E**.T

Cyclo-oxygenase acts on arachidonic acid found in cell membranes to produce cyclic endoperoxidases. These precursor prostaglandins are converted into prostaglandins whose complex function and structure are dependent on the tissue where they are found. NSAIDs block cyclo-oxygenase production, and their action and side-effects can be inferred from this non-specific prostaglandin (PG) inhibition. Analgesia is achieved as prostaglandins sensitize nerve endings to nociceptive polypeptides produced by tissue injury. Anti-inflammatory and anti-pyretic actions result from reduction of PGE_2. Adverse features include: gastric irritation, as PGI_2 and PGE have a protective function; impairment of renal function from reduction in renal blood flow and glomerular filtration rate; increased bleeding time from inhibition of platelet thromboxane synthesis; and exacerbation of asthma from increased arachidonic acid available for lipoxygenase conversion to leukotrienes (which mediate allergic responses). They also promote sodium and fluid retention and hyperkalaemia. They have a low incidence of nausea and vomiting, do not cause respiratory depression and have significant opioid-sparing effect. Platelet numbers are not decreased although function may be impaired. (See: Souter AJ, Fredman B, White PF (1994) Controversies in the perioperative use of nonsteroidal anti-inflammatory drugs. *Anesthesia and Analgesia* **79**, 1178–1190. Also: Power I (1993) Editorial: Aspirin induced asthma. *British Journal of Anaesthesia* **71**, 619–620.)

5.73 **A**.T **B**.F **C**.T **D**.T **E**.T

Most supraventricular tachyarrhythmias require conduction through the atrioventricular (AV) node for their continuation and expression at ventricular level. An increase in vagal tone increases AV nodal conduction and recovery time and is useful in the immediate management of the condition. This can be achieved by carotid sinus massage, ocular compression, the diving reflex (immersion of the face in water) and the Valsalva manoeuvre. If physical measures have not been successful, intravenous adenosine may be tried. It is a very short-acting (half-life <10 s), naturally occurring purine nucleoside that works specifically in the atria to reduce sinoatrial node activity and conduction velocity in the AV node. Adenosine can temporarily induce complete heart block. Side-effects include negative inotropism, induction of atrial flutter and fibrillation, bronchospasm and chest pain. An alternative treatment is verapamil, although it is best not to give either of these if beta blockers have been previously given. If medical therapy fails, rapid atrial pacing or DC cardioversion can be considered. Lignocaine is used for short-term management of ventricular dysrhythmias.

5.74 A.T   B.F   C.T   D.T   E.T
A normal FEV_1/FVC ratio is in the order of 70–75%. Gas transfer factor estimates the ability of the lungs to exchange gases by measuring uptake of carbon monoxide from a single breath of a 0.3% mixture in air. This is useful in the assessment of severity of interstitial lung disease, e.g. sarcoidosis and emphysema. While simple spirometry measures FEV_1/FVC, FRC (residual volume and expiratory reserve volume) can also be measured by connecting the patient to a spirometer containing a known concentration of helium. As this is insoluble in blood, the concentration of helium present in the body will equal that present in the spirometer after several breaths. Thus, when equilibrium is reached the new concentration of helium is measured and FRC calculated. Closing capacity is the lung volume at which airway closure occurs: it is a combination of closing volume plus residual volume. Total lung capacity is the volume of gas in the lungs after maximal inspiration and is about 6 litres in a 70 kg man. Like FRC, lung capacity can be measured by helium dilution or body plethysmography.

5.75 A.T   B.F   C.T   D.T   E.T
The majority of halothane-associated hepatitis cases presents with transient jaundice and moderately deranged liver function tests. The mortality is low with only a very small number developing severe hepatic necrosis (mortality 50–70%). The incidence is difficult to state authoritatively but has been estimated at 1 in 35 000 in adults and 1 in 100 000 in children. It is twice as common in women. Significant risk factors include repeated exposures, particularly at short intervals, obesity and middle age. Length of exposure and type of surgery are immaterial. The importance of pre-existing liver disease in halothane hepatitis is debatable. The causes are not fully elucidated, but are probably multifactorial involving toxic metabolites and an immune reaction which may be compounded by hypoxia, hypotension or genetic predisposition.

Enflurane, isoflurane and desflurane have also been linked to hepatotoxicity. One proposed mechanism is from potential cross-sensitization from previous administration of halothane. All volatile agents undergo metabolism to produce TFA (trifluroacetyl) proteins, which in turn stimulate antibody production against them. As halothane is metabolized most, it effectively produces more antibodies than the others. Thus, previous exposure to it is presumed to sensitize the body to the comparatively small amount of TFA proteins produced by enflurane, etc. As sevoflurane does not produce TFA proteins, hepatotoxicity is unlikely. (See: Elliot RH, Strunin L (1993) Hepatotoxicity of volatile anaesthetics. *British Journal of Anaesthesia* **70**, 339–348. Also: Kenna JG, Neuberger J *et al.* (1989) Halothane hepatitis in children. *British Medical Journal* **294**, 1209–1211.)

5.76 A.T **B**.T **C**.F **D**.T **E**.F

Tramadol is a centrally acting synthetic analgesic for mild to moderate pain. It is an aminocyclohexanol derivative with a dual analgesic action. It has weak agonist activity at all opioid receptors including kappa, but with some selectivity for mu receptors, and a strong non-opioid action by inhibiting monoamine reuptake, thereby influencing descending inhibitory pathways. It is a racemic mixture and the two enantiomers probably confer separate opioid and non-opioid action. Its antinociceptive action is partially antagonized by naloxone. Analgesic potency is similar to that of pethidine. When given orally the peak effect is at 1 hour and duration is 4–6 hours. Hepatic metabolism produces 11 metabolites, two of which are active. The dose should be reduced with severe liver and renal disease. Tramadol has similar side-effects to opiates including nausea and vomiting, drowsiness and constipation, although the incidence of respiratory depression, tolerance and addiction is, in contrast, much less than with opiates. The dual analgesic action potentially expands its use into chronic, particularly neuropathic, pain. It can be administered by any route including spinal and epidural. The concomitant use of carbamazepine considerably reduces the plasma concentration and analgesic efficacy. It is not currently a controlled drug. (See: Eggers KA, Power I (1995) Tramadol (editorial). *British Journal of Anaesthesia* **74**, 247–249.)

5.77 A.T B.F C.F D.T E.F

Resuscitation guidelines for VF are an initial check to see whether the patient is responsive, breathing or has a pulse. If not, a precordial thump should be given in a witnessed arrest as it may cardiovert VF or VT to sinus rhythm. The following algorithm should then be followed:

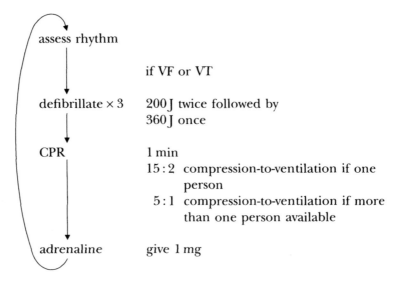

assess rhythm

if VF or VT

defibrillate × 3   200 J twice followed by
360 J once

CPR   1 min
15 : 2 compression-to-ventilation if one person
5 : 1 compression-to-ventilation if more than one person available

adrenaline   give 1 mg

Early on it is important to attempt intubation or verify the position of the tracheal tube and establish intravenous access. CPR should be in the form of 10 sequences of the appropriate compression-to-ventilation ratio. There should be no more than a 2 min delay between the two groups of shocks and adrenaline should be given every 2–3 min. This algorithm cycle should continue as long as necessary. Alkylating agents or antiarrhythmic drugs may be considered as a last resort. Sodium bicarbonate increases CO_2 production which may exacerbate any pre-existing hypercarbia, resulting in an intracellular acidosis, and antiarrhythmic agents are frequently proarrhythmogenic. Calcium chloride is only indicated in pulseless tachycardia (EMD) or if patients are taking calcium antagonists, are hypocalcaemic or hyperkalaemic. Cardiac massage should depress the lower half of the sternum by 4–5 cm and blood flow is thought to be generated either by compression of the heart between the sternum and the spine to eject blood or by raised intrathoracic pressure forcing forward flow which is maintained by venous valves. Either way it only achieves about 10–33% of pre-arrest cardiac output, most of which goes to the brain and upper trunk. (See: Advanced Life Support Working Party of the European Resuscitation Council (1992) Advanced life support working party of the European resuscitation council guidelines for advanced life support. *Resuscitation* **24**, 111–121.)

5.78 A.T **B.**T **C.**F **D.**T **E.**T

AITP results from immune destruction of platelets by IgG antibodies. It can be acute or chronic. Acute AITP is self-limiting and may occur in children following a viral illness; chronic AITP (i.e. lasting more than 6 months) is characteristically seen in women aged between 20 and 40 years. It is normally idiopathic but may occur in association with other autoimmune conditions (e.g. systemic lupus erythematosis), leukaemia and after viral infections including HIV. Common features include easy bruising, epistaxis and menorrhagia. Haemorrhage may occur spontaneously if platelets fall below 30×10^9/l. Splenomegaly is rare. The platelet count is low but they are morphologically normal. Bleeding time is prolonged and anaemia may be present, proportional to the amount of bleeding. Platelet antibodies are only detected in 70–80% of cases. Whilst 80% of all cases of AITP recover regardless of treatment, chronic ITP rarely resolves spontaneously. Steroids may improve platelet life span and suppress antibody synthesis in 20% of patients with a further 60% having a partial response. Splenectomy is reserved for those in whom steroid therapy fails. It results in 80% recovering with the platelet count rising within 24 hours. 30% of patients subsequently relapse and immunosuppressive chemotherapy (vincristine, cyclophosphamide) may then be considered as a third-line treatment. Platelet transfusion is reserved for massive haemorrhage and preoperatively for emergency surgery.

5.79 A.T **B.**T **C.**T **D.**T **E.**T

Thiazide diuretics are used for mild to moderate hypertension, oedema from congestive cardiac failure, liver cirrhosis and nephrotic syndrome. They are acidic compounds, structurally related to sulphonamides. Although actively secreted into the proximal tubule, they act primarily on the distal tubule to inhibit sodium reabsorption. They also probably cause peripheral vasodilatation by increasing vascular compliance through reduction in interstitial fluid. Hyponatraemia is a common finding with their long-term use. Although it arises mainly from natriuresis, the drop in plasma volume reduces glomerular filtration rate and stimulates release of ADH, leading to thirst and increased water intake. Hypokalaemia and hypomagnesaemia commonly occur as a result of the increase in circulating mineralocorticoids. Hyperkalaemia is also possible, more so with pre-existing renal impairment or concurrent use of angiotensin-converting enzyme inhibitors. Hypercalcaemia arises from decreased calcium excretion while volume depletion is the primary cause of hyperuricaemia. Glucose intolerance, precipitation of overt diabetes and hyperglycaemic hyperosmolar coma have all been reported. The effects are worse with age and length of use but are usually reversible on stopping therapy. Hypophosphataemia and increased serum lipids can also occur. Hypocalcaemia is uncommon due to compensatory mechanisms such as increased resorption of calcium in the loop of Henle by parathyroid hormone.

5.80 A.T B.T C.T D.F E.F
Isoflurane and enflurane are isomers. Approximately 2% of enflurane is metabolized to inorganic fluoride ions which can occasionally lead to vasopressin-resistant polyuria. Only 0.2% of isoflurane is metabolized and thus production of fluoride ions is negligible. Enflurane at more than 3% and combined with hypocarbia is associated with temporary seizure activity on EEG. Isoflurane causes cortical depression. Both cause tachycardia and hypotension, although enflurane decreases cardiac output more than isoflurane. Isoflurane is more irritant to the respiratory tract. Both decrease tidal volume but increase respiratory rate and induce mild uterine relaxation and marked potentiation of non-depolarizing neuromuscular blockade. Analgesic effects are also similar.

5.81 A.T B.T C.F D.T E.F
CVP is a reflection of right ventricular end-diastolic pressure which, in turn, is a balance between circulating blood volume, venous tone, intrathoracic pressure and right ventricular function. A tension pneumothorax, venous air embolus and a large pulmonary embolus all increase the CVP and decrease cardiac output to produce hypotension. Haemorrhage results in acute hypovolaemia decreasing central venous and systemic blood pressures. Adrenocortical insufficiency tends to cause postural hypotension from mineralocorticoid loss resulting in

hypovolaemia and sodium loss. Severe circulatory collapse is also possible.

5.82 **A.**F **B.**F **C.**T **D.**F **E.**T

Spinal shock occurs immediately after 'transection' of the spinal cord. In reality, total transection is rare but any severe injury to the cord produces a similar picture due to haemorrhage and protein extravasation which results in oedema and, eventually, necrosis of white and grey matter. The initial response is a generalized flaccid paralysis with areflexia and immediate loss of both sensation and movement at and below the level of the injury. Autonomic reflexes are variably affected, depending on the level of the injury. Hypotension occurs because of loss of sympathetic tone below the level of the injury, resulting in pooling of venous blood and disruption of the feedback regulation supplied to the baroreceptor reflexes. Temperature control is also affected, as are sacral parasympathetic nerves, resulting in loss of distal colonic and bladder reflexes. A small bowel ileus is common but usually transient. Spinal shock can last for days or weeks and may persist for longer in toxic or septic conditions. Autonomic hyperreflexia occurs with the return of reflexes, spasticity and clonus. Reflexes tend to return in a caudal to cephalad sequence. Although controversial, methylprednisolone within 8 hours of the spinal injury may reduce the incidence and severity of long-term sequelae. (See: Atkinson PP, Atkinson LD (1996) Spinal shock. *Mayo Clinic Proceedings* 71, 384–389. Also: Ducker TB, Zeidman SR (1994) Spinal cord injury: role of steroid therapy. *Spine* 19, 2281–2287.)

5.83 **A.**F **B.**F **C.**T **D.**T **E.**T

Normal values obtained during cardiac catheterization are in the region of:

	Pressures (mmHg)
RA	0–5
RV	20/5
PA	20/10
PCWP	5–10
LA	2–10
LV	120/10
AP (aortic pressure)	120/70

The principal abnormalities are raised RV and PA pressures. This implies increased resistance to pulmonary flow, and pulmonary stenosis is the most likely cause. PH, defined as a pulmonary artery systolic pressure above 30 mmHg or a mean pressure in excess of 15 mmHg, can be another cause. PH can be primary, a rare condition of unknown aetiology seen predominantly in young women, or secondary, with possible causes including:

1. Increased blood flow, e.g. left-to-right shunts with atrial or ventricular septal defect and patent ductus arteriosus (PDA).
2. Increased pulmonary capillary pressure from increased back pressure with left ventricular failure, e.g. mitral valve disease.
3. Increased pulmonary vascular resistance due to chronic lung disease, e.g. cor pulmonale, asthma, pulmonary fibrosis.

Mitral valve disease can cause pulmonary hypertension but is not the diagnosis here as PCWP is within normal limits.

5.84 A.T B.F C.T D.F E.T
Magnesium is an important regulator of intracellular function, responsible for activation of over 300 enzyme systems, including those involved in energy metabolism. It is an essential cofactor in oxidative phosphorylation and vital for manufacture of RNA, DNA and protein. It also regulates many of the actions of calcium. Serum levels of 0.75–1.0 mmol/l are mainly controlled by renal excretion and reabsorption. Magnesium deficiency can occur from decreased intake and absorption, increased requirements, e.g. pregnancy, and increased losses from acute tubular necrosis, drug therapy (particularly thiazide diuretics, digoxin, adrenaline and dopamine) or diarrhoea. Lack of magnesium is common in the critically ill but is rarely considered and often difficult to diagnose as it is mainly an intracellular ion and serum levels do not reflect the true level. In addition, hypomagnesaemia normally accompanies hypokalaemia and hypocalcaemia. The consequences of deficiency are ill-defined but are similar to hypocalcaemia as magnesium regulates calcium release from nerve endings and sarcoplasmic reticulum. The commonest symptom is therefore muscle weakness; this is often important as it can delay weaning in ventilated patients. Tetany is also possible. Myocardial contractility decreases and susceptibility to arrhythmias, both supraventricular and ventricular, increases. CNS changes include

psychosis, agitation, depression and confusion. Convulsions have been infrequently described. Magnesium is a major regulator of vascular tone as it inhibits calcium influx and acts as a direct alpha blocker in smooth muscle. Thus hypomagnesaemia is important in certain forms of hypertension. In excess it is a powerful vasodilator, particularly in the brain, kidney, coronary, splanchnic and uterine vessels.

5.85 A.T **B.**T **C.**T **D.**F **E.**F

Quality is a difficult term to define but it is probably safe to assume that in some way it refers to improved onset, duration or depth of anaesthesia. Adrenaline induces vasoconstriction, thereby reducing distribution of LA to prolong and intensify extradural blockade whilst reducing peak systemic blood levels. Adrenaline is more effective with LAs that cause vasodilatation (e.g. lignocaine compared with bupivacaine). Most opiates, particularly fentanyl, improve the quality of block. Longer-acting opiates such as morphine have a slower onset of action due to poor lipid solubility and have a higher incidence of side-effects. Extradural clonidine is an α_2 agonist and when given in combination with LAs it does improve blockade but at the expense of increasing plasma concentration of LAs and causing a significant incidence of hypotension. It has therefore not gained widespread acceptance. Both dextran and hyaluronidase have been used to improve the efficacy of intraorbital eye blocks but no effect has been seen with extradural anaesthesia. Moreover dextran is potentially immunogenic and possibly neurotoxic. Attempts have been made to improve the action of LAs by alkalization and carbonation. *In vitro* alkalization shortens latency whilst the carbonation enhances the quality and duration of anaesthesia. In clinical practice these effects have been less clear-cut and, despite certain individual enthusiasm, they are not commonly used. Current research incorporating LAs into liposomes (3–10 µm vesicles of bilayers of phospholipid surrounding an aqueous phase) to prolong duration of action and reduce toxicity may be of more value. (See: Duncan L, Wildsmith JAW (1995) Editorial: Liposomal local anaesthetics. *British Journal of Anaesthesia* **75**, 260–261.)

5.86 A.F **B.**T **C.**F **D.**T **E.**F

ATN is the commonest (75%) cause of acute renal failure and is usually due to ischaemia or toxins, either chemical or bacterial. Along with increases in serum urea, creatinine and potassium, urinary changes include:

urine volume	– reduced to 50–500 ml daily (anuria suggests obstruction, not ATN)
specific gravity	– <1.010 ⎱ due to inability to
urine osmolality	– <350 mosmol/l ⎰ concentrate urine
urine sodium	– high (>40 mmol/l)
urine chloride	– high (>40 mmol/l)
urea U:P ratio	– <5
creatinine U:P ratio	– <20

Diuretic therapy will alter the findings and the values are reversed for prerenal failure. Recovery is usually heralded by a polyuric phase after 10–20 days. Unfortunately, despite significant advances in supportive care and the potential for recovery to virtually normal renal function, ATN continues to have a 50% mortality.

5.87 A.F B.F C.F D.T E.T
Ranitidine is an H_2 blocker 4–10 times more potent than cimetidine. It reduces gastric acid secretion by 70–90% and accelerates healing of both duodenal and gastric ulcers. Advantages over cimetidine include less confusion in elderly patients (as it is poorly absorbed through the blood–brain barrier), absence of antiandrogenic activity, and it does not inhibit cytochrome P-450 to decrease metabolism of drugs such as warfarin, phenytoin and diazepam. It has no effect on acid already present in the stomach and in obstetric emergencies a non-particulate antacid is required to neutralize acid prior to anaesthesia. Omeprazole is a proton pump inhibitor, i.e. it blocks gastric parietal cell H^+/K^+ ATPase secretion of gastric acid to produce almost total inhibition of 24-hour intragastric acidity. Clinical trials have shown it to be superior to H_2 antagonists for symptomatic relief and healing of duodenal ulcers and in controlling hypersecretion of acid by gastrin-producing tumours as in the Zollinger–Ellison syndrome.

5.88 A.F B.T C.T D.F E.F
MAC is the minimum concentration of an inhalational agent needed to prevent movement to skin incision in 50% of subjects breathing 100% oxygen at atmospheric pressure. It is a measure used to compare the relative potency of individual agents. There is a direct correlation between MAC and the

oil:gas coefficient. MAC is affected by pharmacological and physiological factors. It is increased in neonates, hyperthyroidism, in the presence of catecholamines and with chronic alcohol intake. It is decreased in the elderly (10% per decade), hypothermia, pregnancy and with concomitant administration of sedatives, opiates and other inhalational agents. Length of anaesthesia, anaemia, hypertension and naloxone has no effect.

5.89 A.T B.F C.T D.T E.F
Rhesus incompatibility arises when a rhesus-negative mother has a rhesus-positive baby. Maternal sensitization can occur during pregnancy or, more commonly, at delivery when fetal blood finds its way into the maternal circulation. Some mothers develop antirhesus agglutinins which can cross the placenta in this or subsequent pregnancies. These act on a rhesus-positive fetus to cause haemolysis, anaemia and jaundice. Prevention is by post-partum administration of antirhesus antibodies to the mother at delivery.

5.90 A.T B.F C.T D.T E.T
Myasthenic syndrome (Eaton–Lambert) causes proximal muscle weakness as a result of defective release of acetylcholine from presynaptic nerve endings. It is most often due to an underlying carcinoma or thyroiditis. Symptoms can precede clinical evidence of a carcinoma by 1–2 years. Patients show improvement in muscle strength on exercise but this is usually followed by a prolonged period of fatigue. Reflexes are depressed or absent. In EMG studies, marked post-tetanic facilitation is often seen associated with a steady growth of potential on tetanic stimulation. Sensitivity to depolarizing and non-depolarizing muscle relaxants occurs. Anticholinesterase medication is of no value, although oral guanidine hydrochloride may be useful. Striking but temporary improvement has been seen with excision of the primary tumour, which has led to the theory that the tumour produces antibodies to the presynaptic membrane.

Appendix

Abbreviations used in this book

ABG	arterial blood gases
ACE	angiotensin converting enzyme
Ach	acetylcholine
ACTH	adrenocorticotrophic hormone
ADH	anti-diuretic hormone
AF	atrial fibrillation
AIP	acute intermittent porphyria
AITP	autoimmune thrombocytopenic purpura
AML	acute myeloid leukaemia
APKD	adult polycystic kidney disease
ARDS	acute respiratory distress syndrome
AS	aortic stenosis
ASD	atrial septal defect
AV	arteriovenous
AVP	arginine vasopressin
BBB	bundle branch block
BMI	body mass index
BSA	body surface area
CBF	cerebral blood flow
CF	cystic fibrosis
CML	chronic myeloid leukaemia
CMV	cytomegalovirus
CO	cardiac output
COPD	chronic obstructive pulmonary disease
CP	coeliac plexus
CPAP	continuous positive airway pressure
CPB	coeliac plexus block
CPK	creatinine phosphokinase
CRF	chronic renal failure
CRPS	chronic regional pain syndrome (eg type 1)
CSF	cerebrospinal fluid
CT	computerized tomography
CTZ	chemoreceptor trigger zone
CVA	cerebrovascular accident
CVP	central venous pressure
CVS	cardiovascular system
DC	direct current
DIC	disseminated intravascular coagulation
DKA	diabetic ketoacidosis
DM	diabetes mellitus
DPQ	Dartmouth pain questionnaire
DVT	deep vein thrombosis
ECF	extracellular fluid
EDTA	ethylenediaminetetraacetic acid

ECMO	extracorporeal membrane oxygenation	Ig	immunoglobulin
		IOP	intraocular pressure
EMLA	eutectic mixture of local anaesthetics	IPPV	intermittent positive-pressure ventilation
ENT	ear, nose and throat	IVH	intraventricular
ESR	erythrocyte sedimentation rate		haemorrhage
		IVOX	intravascular oxygenation device
FEV_1	forced expiratory volume		
FGF	fresh gas flow	JVP	jugular venous pressure
FRC	functional residual capacity		
FVC	forced vital capacity	LA	local anaesthetic
		LBBB	left bundle branch block
GABA	gamma-aminobutyric acid	LM	laryngeal mask
G6PD	glucose 6 phosphate dehydrogenase	LV	left ventricular
		LVF	left ventricular failure
GCS	Glasgow Coma Scale		
GDM	gestational diabetes mellitus	MAC	minimum alveolar concentration
GFR	glomerular filtration rate	MAOI	monoamine oxidase inhibitors
5-HIAA	5-hydroxyindoleacetic acid	MAP	mean arterial blood pressure
$5\text{-}HT_3$	5-hydroxytryptamine$_3$	MCV	mean cell volume
Hb SS	sickle cell anaemia	MH	malignant hyperthermia
HCG	human chorionic gonadotrophin	MI	myocardial infarction
		MIBG	meta-iodobenzyl guanidine
HELLP	haemolysis, elevated liver enzymes, low platelets	MPQ	Magill pain questionnaire
HFJV	high-frequency jet ventilation	MRI	magnetic resonance imaging
HME	heat and moisture exchange	MS	multiple sclerosis
HPOA	hypertrophic pulmonary osteoarthropathy	NMB	neuromuscular blockade
		NMDA	N-methyl, D-aspartate
HPV	hypoxic pulmonary vasoconstriction	NMS	neuroleptic malignant syndrome
		NO	nitric oxide
IABP	intra-aortic balloon-pump	NRS	numerical rating scale
IAM	internal auditory meatus	NSAIDs	non-steroidal anti-inflammatory drugs
ICP	intracranial pressure		
IDDM	insulin-dependent diabetes mellitus	OLV	one-lung ventilation

PA	postero-anterior
PA	pulmonary artery
	(catheter)
PAH	*para*-aminohippuric acid
PAP	pulmonary artery pressure
PBC	primary biliary cirrhois
PCA	patient controlled
	analgesia
PCP	*Pneumocystis carinii*
	pneumonia
PCOP	pulmonary artery
	occlusion pressure
PCWP	pulmonary capillary wedge
	pressure
PE	pulmonary embolus
PEEP	positive end-expiratory
	pressure
PHN	post-herpetic neuralgia
PLP	phantom limb pain
PMNLs	polymorphonuclear
	leukocytes
PONV	postoperative nausea and
	vomiting
PRI	patient rating scale
PT	prothrombin time
PTH	parathyroid hormone
PTT	partial thromboplastin
	time

RA	rheumatoid arthritis
RDS	respiratory distress
	syndrome
RIF	right iliac fossa
RSD	reflex sympathetic
	dystrophy
RSV	respiratory syncytial virus
RV	residual volume

SBE	subacute bacterial
	endocarditis
SIRS	systemic inflammatory
	response syndrome
SLE	systemic lupus
	erythematosis
SLN	superior laryngeal nerve
SVR	systemic vascular resistance

TENS	transcutaneous electrical
	nerve stimulation
TIA	transient ischaemic attack
TLC	total lung volume
TMJD	temporomandibular joint
	dysfunction
TNF	tumour necrosis factor
TOE	transoesophageal
	echocardiography
TOF	tracheo-oesophageal fistula
TOF	train of four
TPN	total parenteral nutrition
TSH	thyroid-stimulating
	hormone
TT	tracheal tube
TURP	transurethral resection of
	the prostate

| URTI | upper respiratory tract |
| | infection |

VAS	visual analogue scale
VF	ventricular fibrillation
VMA	vanillylmandelic acid
VSD	ventricular septal defect
VT	ventricular tachycardia

| WPW | Wolff–Parkinson–White |
| | (syndrome) |

Bibliography

I am always amazed at the amount of references that other 'examination' type books exhort you to read and without which any prospect of passing will seemingly be a vague and forlorn hope. This is complete nonsense. The aim of the examination is, as always, to make sure you are a safe, experienced anaesthetist with a broad base of knowledge. If you don't have the knowledge then at least you should be able to work things out from first principles. This can be obtained, by and large, from a good anaesthetic textbook, a general medical book and reading editorials and review articles in the anaesthetic journals for a few months before the examination.

The books you will use for the exam will depend on a number of factors including how much money you are prepared to spend and how many books you are able to beg, borrow or steal from your friends. My one plea is to try and avoid stealing from hospital postgraduate medical libraries as, from personal experience in writing this book, they have hardly any books left!

Listed below are a small fraction of the books I used. Please do not feel compelled to buy them. If you feel that they are vital to your revision, ask your anaesthetic department first if they will part with the money as they should have some responsibility for providing reasonably up-to-date books and there is often a slush fund somewhere for just this sort of thing.

Anaesthetics and related subjects

American Society of Anaesthesiologists (1996) 47th Annual Refresher Course Lectures.

Datta S (1995) *Common Problems in Obstetric Anaesthesia*, 2nd edn. Mosby, London.

Davis PJ, Motoyama EK (1996) *Smith's Anesthesia for Infants and Children*, 6th edn. Mosby, London.

Dolin S, Padfield N, Pateman J (1996) *Pain Clinic Manual.* Butterworth-Heinemann, Oxford.

Hinds CJ, Watson D (1996) *Intensive Care: A Concise Textbook*, 2nd edn. WB Saunders, London.

Kaufman L, Taberner P (1996) *Pharmacology in the Practice of Anaesthesia.* Edward Arnold, London.

Kenny G, David PD, Parbrook GD (1995) *Basic Physics and Measurement in Anaesthesia.* Butterworth-Heinemann, Oxford.

Moyle JTB, Davey AJ (1997) *Anaesthetic Equipment,* 4th edn. WB Saunders, London.

Oh TE (1997) *Intensive Care Manual,* 4th edn. Butterworth-Heinemann, Oxford.

Parbrook GD, Daus PD, Kenny G (1995) *Basic Physics and Measurement in Anaesthesia* 4th edn. Butterworth-Heinemann, Oxford.

Prys-Roberts C, Brown BR (1996) *International Practice of Anaesthesia,* vols 1 and 2. Butterworth-Heinemann, Oxford.

Rasch DK, Webster DE (1994) *Clinical Manual for Paediatric Anesthesia.* McGraw-Hill, Maidenhead.

Sykes MK, Vickers MD, Hull CJ *et al.* (1991) *Principles of Measurement and Monitoring in Anaesthesia and Intensive Care,* 3rd edn. Blackwell Science, Oxford.

Wall PD, Melzack R (1994) *Textbook of Pain,* vols 1 and 2. Churchill Livingstone, Edinburgh.

Williams NE, Calvey TN (1996) *Principles and Practice of Pharmacology for Anaesthetists.* Blackwell Science, Oxford.

Yentis S, Hirsch NP, Smith GB (1995) *Anaesthesia A to Z.* Butterworth-Heinemann, Oxford.

Others

Burkitt HG, Quick CRG, Gatt D (1996) *Essential Surgery.* Churchill Livingstone, Edinburgh.

Edwards CRW, Bouchier IAD, Haslett C, Chilvers ER (1995) *Davidson's Principles and Practice of Medicine,* 17th edn. Churchill Livingstone, Edinburgh.

Ganong WF (1997) *Review of Medical Physiology.* Appleton Lange, Connecticut.

Kumar P, Clark M (1994) *Clinical Medicine,* 3rd edn. WB Saunders, London.

Mann CV, Russell RCG, Williams NS (1995) *Bailey and Love's Short Practice of Surgery,* 22nd edn. Chapman and Hall, London.

Warrell DA, Ledingham JGG, Weatherall DJ (1995) *Oxford Textbook of Medicine.* Oxford University Press, Oxford.

Lightning Source UK Ltd.
Milton Keynes UK
UKOW040652160911

178715UK00001B/15/A